Cancer Treatment and Research

Volume 162

Series editor
Steven T. Rosen, Duarte, CA, USA

For further volumes:
http://www.springer.com/series/5808

Terrance D. Peabody
Samer Attar

Editors

Orthopaedic Oncology

Primary and Metastatic Tumors of the Skeletal System

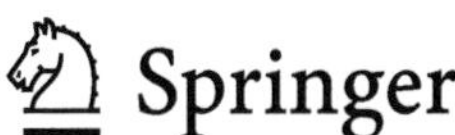 Springer

Editors
Terrance D. Peabody
Samer Attar
Department of Orthopaedic Surgery
Feinberg School of Medicine, Northwestern University
Chicago, IL
USA

ISSN 0927-3042
ISBN 978-3-319-34609-0   ISBN 978-3-319-07323-1   (eBook)
DOI 10.1007/978-3-319-07323-1
Springer Cham Heidelberg New York Dordrecht London

Contents

Principles of Musculoskeletal Biopsy 1
Raffi S. Avedian

Imaging Evaluation of Musculoskeletal Tumors 9
Nicholas Morley and Imran Omar

Benign Bone Tumors 31
Robert Steffner

Osteosarcoma 65
Drew D. Moore and Hue H. Luu

Ewing's Sarcoma of Bone 93
Drew D. Moore and Rex C. Haydon

Chondrosarcoma of Bone 117
Lee R. Leddy and Robert E. Holmes

Evaluation and Treatment of Spinal Metastatic Disease 131
Shah-Nawaz M. Dodwad, Jason Savage, Thomas J. Scharschmidt
and Alpesh Patel

Evaluation and Treatment of Extremity Metastatic Disease 151
Aaron T. Creek, Drew A. Ratner and Scott E. Porter

**Clinical Evaluation and Management of Benign Soft
Tissue Tumors of the Extremities** 171
Andrew S. Erwteman and Tessa Balach

Soft Tissue Sarcomas 203
Andre Spiguel

Principles of Musculoskeletal Biopsy

Raffi S. Avedian

Abstract

The appropriate treatment of any musculoskeletal tumor is based on a correct diagnosis. In some instances, a patient's history and imaging studies provide sufficient information to guide definitive treatment. However, in many cases, a biopsy may be necessary. A biopsy, although technically simple, must be conducted in a thoughtful manner in order to obtain an accurate tissue sample while avoiding complications. Some potential complications include inaccurate sampling, improperly placed incision that complicates future surgeries, and healthy tissue contamination that can add morbidity to the definitive surgery or preclude the chance of limb salvage. This chapter will review the considerations for planning and performing a biopsy of musculoskeletal tumors.

Keywords

Biopsy · Sarcoma · Soft tissue tumor · Limb salvage

1   Introduction

The appropriate treatment of any musculoskeletal tumor is based on the knowledge of what the tumor is and its natural history. In some instances, a patient's history and imaging studies provide sufficient information to guide definitive treatment.

R. S. Avedian (✉)
Stanford University Medical Center, Redwood City, CA, USA
e-mail: ravedian@stanford.edu

T. D. Peabody and S. Attar (eds.), *Orthopaedic Oncology*,
Cancer Treatment and Research 162, DOI: 10.1007/978-3-319-07323-1_1,
© Springer International Publishing Switzerland 2014

However, in many cases, evaluation of a patient's history, physical exam, and imaging results in a differential diagnosis that requires further elucidation. This is especially true if the leading diagnosis is an aggressive tumor that would require treatment such as chemotherapy, radiation, or ablative surgery. As such, confirming the diagnosis with a biopsy prior to subjecting the patient to therapies with potentially morbid and permanent side effects is mandatory. Similarly, missing a diagnosis of an aggressive or malignant tumor may result in unnecessary morbidity or a lost opportunity for cure.

2   Evaluation Prior to Biopsy

Prior to doing a biopsy, the clinician should perform a thorough history and physical exam and should scrutinize plain radiographs in the case of suspected bone pathology. In certain situations, the information obtained with this will be sufficient to yield a diagnosis or at least limit the differential to a benign etiology that may not need tissue sampling. This is often the case with incidentally noted bone tumors that are discovered when performing the workup for an unrelated problem (Fig. 1). When evaluating a soft-tissue mass, important aspects of the history include the duration of the mass, the rate of growth of the mass, and the presence of pain or any inciting events such as trauma. Findings that would be reassuring for a benign etiology include a several year history of a small mass without any growth. Also, tumors that are painful tend to be benign such as nerve sheath tumors or vascular malformations. Although there are no validated size criteria to indicate malignancy, most surgeons consider large masses or those greater than or equal to 3 cm to be concerning enough for malignancy to warrant further evaluation. The best radiological study for the evaluation of a soft tissue mass is an MRI with an intravenous contrast agent such as gadolinium [1]. Plain radiographs may be useful to rule out a bone tumor mimicking a soft tissue mass such as a prominent exostosis or to reveal phleboliths within a hemangioma.

3   Biopsy Principles

There are several biopsy techniques for sampling bone and soft tissue tumors. An important principle common to all techniques is that definitive treatment relies on a biopsy that is accurate and does not cause harm to a patient due to technical mistakes [2, 3]. Specifically, a poorly planned and executed biopsy may result in contamination of surrounding healthy tissue which may increase the risk of local recurrence and preclude the option of a limb-sparing surgery. The biopsy site will be contaminated with cancer cells and must be incorporated into and removed during the definitive cancer surgery. Therefore, thought must be given to where the surgical incision will be made. The biopsy ideally will be planned along this incision line (Fig. 2). In almost all cases, longitudinal incisions should be used as they can more easily be incorporated into the final surgery. Neurovascular bundles

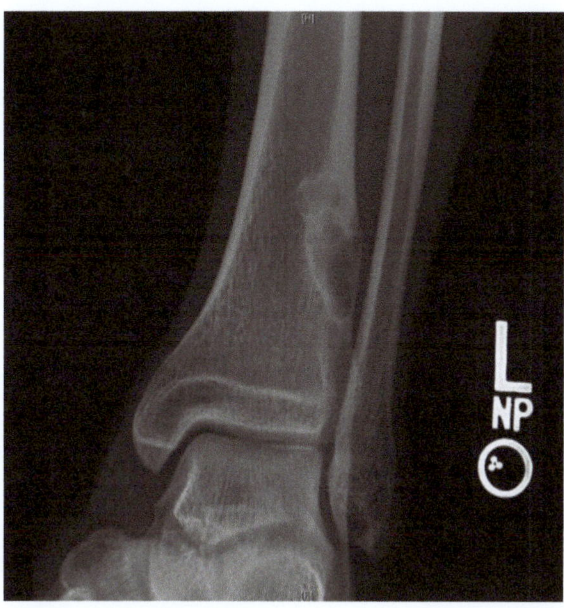

Fig. 1 Mortise oblique ankle radiograph of a 16 year old male who twisted his ankle while playing basketball and presented with anterior joint line pain. Physical exam was notable for tenderness over the anterolateral ankle but not over the lesion seen in the radiograph. Based on his history of an acute injury, exam findings suggesting an ankle sprain, and radiographs demonstrating a well-marginated lesion with a sclerotic border, a diagnosis of an ankle sprain with incidentally noted asymptomatic non-ossifying fibroma proximal to the ankle was made. A biopsy was not needed and follow-up radiographs ensured stability of the lesion

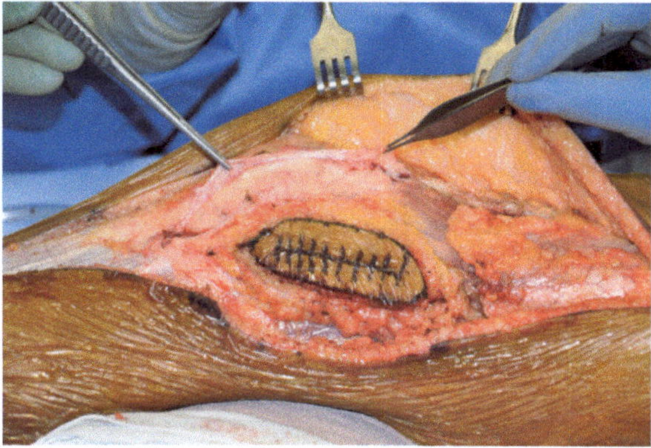

Fig. 2 Intraoperative photograph showing the surgical resection of a distal femur osteosarcoma in a 15 year old girl. Notice how the biopsy site is in line with the main incision and is being incorporated into the tumor resection. A paddle of skin and subcutaneous tissue is kept on the biopsy site as a margin of safety to ensure all potentially contaminated tissue is removed. The smaller the biopsy the easier it is to remove

Fig. 3 A 70 year old woman underwent resection of a posterior thigh mass without prior imaging. The final diagnosis was a high grade pleomorphic sarcoma. The drain was placed 6 cm lateral to the surgical incision. A local recurrence occurred along the drain path as can be seen in this T1 fat-suppressed, contrast-enhanced magnetic resonance image showing a mass between the surgical incision (*arrow*) and drain exit site (*arrowhead*)

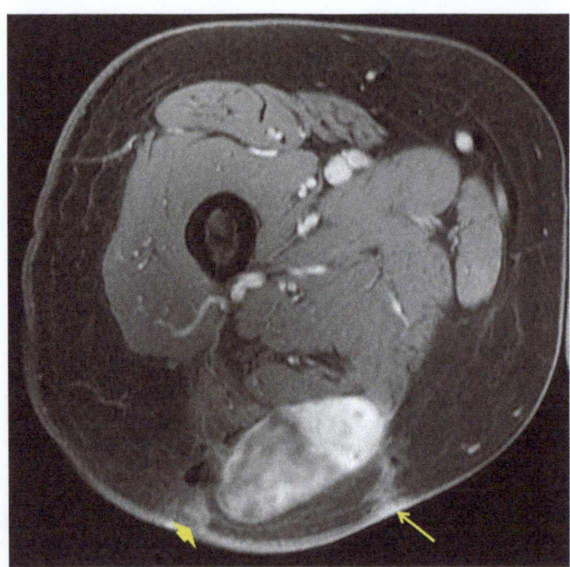

Fig. 4 Intraoperative photograph demonstrating the relationship of the principle incision (*arrow*), the drain site (*arrowhead*) and the local recurrence (*asterisk*) illustrating how an improperly placed drain site can lead to local recurrence

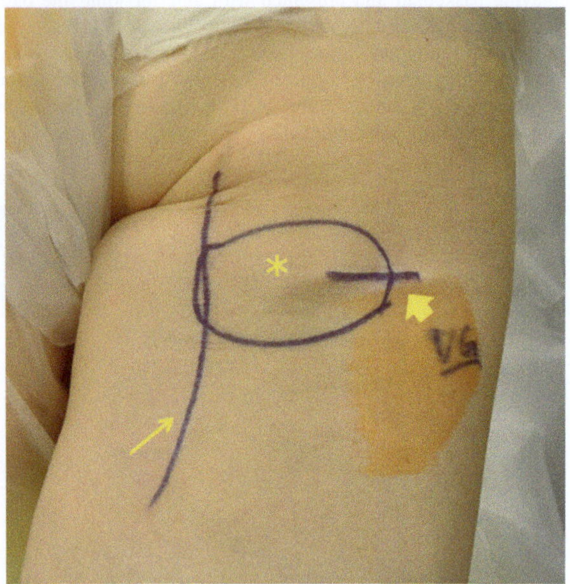

should not be dissected or manipulated, otherwise they may become contaminated and have to be resected later. The biopsy should be within a single muscle compartment rather than an intermuscular plane where multiple compartments are at risk for contamination. Skin and subcutaneous flaps should be kept to a minimum.

Meticulous hemostasis should be obtained prior to closure to avoid hematomas or bleeding that can carry tumor cells to adjacent healthy tissues. If a drain is used it should exit in line and near the incision so the drain track and exit site can be resected easily during the definitive procedure (Figs. 3 and 4).

4   Biopsy Techniques

Incisional biopsy (IB) has long been regarded as the gold standard for diagnosing musculoskeletal tumors. However, percutaneous procedures such as core needle biopsy (CNB) and fine needle aspiration (FNA) are cost-effective and reasonably accurate alternatives that have largely replaced open biopsy as the technique of choice for diagnosing soft tissue tumors in many orthopaedic oncology practices [4, 5]. The specific techniques for musculoskeletal biopsy include: FNA, CNB, IB and excisional biopsy.

The goal of an FNA is to obtain a sufficient quantity of cells to perform cytological analysis. The technique is relatively easy to perform but does not allow for evaluation of a tumor's histological characteristics such as architecture and matrix production [6].

A CNB is performed using a large diameter needle that is designed to capture a large enough piece of tissue that can be used for histological evaluation and ancillary studies such as cytogenetics [5].

Unlike FNA and CNB which are performed in the office, IB and excisional biopsy are surgical procedures that require anesthesia. An IB is performed by making a relatively small incision directly over the tumor and removing a sample of tissue. An excisional biopsy on the other hand is removal of the entire tumor by dissecting around its perimeter. The goal is to keep the tumor contained within its capsule and avoid spillage but no margin of healthy tissue is removed [7].

In a retrospective study comparing IB with CNB, Heslin et al. reported on accuracy results for 164 patients who presented to their institution with a soft tissue tumor. Sixty patients underwent CNB which had an accuracy of 95, 88 and 75 % for diagnosing malignancy, correct grade, and correct histology respectively. There was no statistical difference compared to forty-four patients who underwent IB which had an accuracy of 100, 95 and 88 % for the same variables. The authors did emphasize the significance of good technique and experience of the pathologist as important influences on the accuracy of any biopsy [8].

Yang and Damron conducted a prospective study of fifty patients comparing the accuracy of FNA with CNB. Each patient underwent a CNB that was immediately followed by a FNA. FNA achieved a diagnostic accuracy rate of 88 % for nature of lesion, 64 % for specific diagnosis, 78 % for histologic grading, and 74 % for histologic typing. CNB achieved an accuracy rate of 93 % for nature of lesions, 83 % for specific diagnosis, 83 % for histologic grading, and 90 % for histologic typing. Both biopsy methods had a higher diagnostic accuracy rate for high-grade tumors than for low-grade or benign lesions in determining the nature, specific diagnosis, and histologic grading [9].

More recently, Pohlig et al. reviewed 77 patients who had undergone either core needle or IB for a suspected bone or soft tissue malignancy [10]. Sensitivity, specificity, PPV, NPV and diagnostic accuracy were 100 % for CNB in bone tumors. Sensitivity (95.5 %), NPV (91.7 %) and diagnostic accuracy (93.3 %) for open biopsy in bone tumors showed slightly inferior results without statistical significance ($p > 0.05$). In soft tissue tumors, favorable results were obtained in open biopsies compared to CNB with differences regarding sensitivity (100 vs. 81.8 %, $p = 0.5$), NPV (100 vs. 50 %, $p = 0.09$) and diagnostic accuracy (100 vs. 84.6 %, $p = 0.19$) without statistical significance. The overall diagnostic accuracy was 92.9 % for CNB and 98.0 % for open biopsy ($p = 0.55$). A specific diagnosis could be obtained in 84.2 and 93.9 %, respectively ($p = 0.34$).

Khoja et al. compared 103 core needle biopsies with 107 incisional biopsies to determine if grade established by one technique was more accurate in predicting metastasis and disease free survival [11]. They discovered that grade predicted by CNB was not predictive of metastasis or survival, but grade determined by IB was in fact predictive of both metastasis and disease free survival. The authors concluded that CNB is a convenient tool for making a diagnosis of a soft tissue tumor. However, IB is recommended if grade is to be used to guide treatment or counseling regarding prognosis.

In summary FNA, CNB and IB are acceptable techniques for performing a biopsy of a musculoskeletal tumor. Percutaneous biopsies such as FNA and CNB obviate the potential delays due to coordinating operating room, anesthesia, and surgeon availability, are technically easy to do, and are relatively low cost. However, they do not provide as much tissue as an IB and therefore may not be as accurate [4]. An important variable that is hard to quantify in the literature is the orthopaedic oncologist's technical and cognitive skill for choosing and performing a biopsy correctly and the pathologist's experience and skill at interpreting musculoskeletal neoplasms. Ultimately, it is the treating physician's responsibility to use appropriate judgment in combining the clinical, radiological, and pathological information to determine the most appropriate care for the patient.

References

1. Demas BE, Heelan RT, Lane J, Marcove R, Hajdu S, Brennan MF (1988) Soft-tissue sarcomas of the extremities: comparison of MR and CT in determining the extent of disease. AJR Am J Roentgenol 150(3):615–620
2. Simon MA (1982) Biopsy of musculoskeletal tumors. J Bone Joint Surg Am 64(8):1253–1257
3. Mankin HJ, Mankin CJ, Simon MA (1996) The hazards of the biopsy, revisited. Members of the musculoskeletal tumor society. J Bone Joint Surg Am 78(5):656–666
4. Skrzynski MC, Biermann JS, Montag A, Simon MA (1996) Diagnostic accuracy and charge-savings of outpatient core needle biopsy compared with open biopsy of musculoskeletal tumors. J Bone Joint Surg Am 78(5):644–649
5. Welker JA, Henshaw RM, Jelinek J, Shmookler BM, Malawer MM (2000) The percutaneous needle biopsy is safe and recommended in the diagnosis of musculoskeletal masses. Cancer 89(12):2677–2686

6. Costa MJ, Campman SC, Davis RL, Howell LP (1996) Fine-needle aspiration cytology of sarcoma: retrospective review of diagnostic utility and specificity. Diagn Cytopathol 15(1):23–32
7. Simon MA, Biermann JS (1993) Biopsy of bone and soft-tissue lesions. J Bone Joint Surg Am 75(4):616–621
8. Heslin MJ, Lewis JJ, Woodruff JM, Brennan MF (1997) Core needle biopsy for diagnosis of extremity soft tissue sarcoma. Ann Surg Oncol 4(5):425–431
9. Yang YJ, Damron TA (2004) Comparison of needle core biopsy and fine-needle aspiration for diagnostic accuracy in musculoskeletal lesions. Arch Pathol Lab Med 128(7):759–764
10. Pohlig F, Kirchhoff C, Lenze U, Schauwecker J, Burgkart R, Rechl R, von Eisenhart-Rothe R (2012) Percutaneous core needle biopsy versus open biopsy in diagnostics of bone and soft tissue sarcoma: a retrospective study. Eur J Med Res 17(29):7
11. Khoja H, Griffin A, Dickson B et al (2013) Sampling modality influences the predictive value of grading in adult soft tissue extremity sarcomas. Arch Pathol Lab Med 137(12):1774–1779

Imaging Evaluation of Musculoskeletal Tumors

Nicholas Morley and Imran Omar

Abstract

In this chapter, we review different imaging modalities, including radiography, computed tomography (CT), magnetic resonance imaging (MRI), ultrasound, and nuclear medicine scintigraphy, and their application to musculoskeletal neoplasm. Advantages and limitations of each modality are reviewed, and suggestions for imaging approach are provided.

Keywords

Radiology · Medical Imaging · X–ray · Radiography · Computed Tomography (CT) · Magnetic Resonance Imaging (MRI) · Ultrasound · Nuclear Medicine

1　Introduction

Imaging evaluation of musculoskeletal tumors often involves a combination of modalities, with each modality serving a specific function in workup. Initial evaluation is typically performed with plain radiography, followed by a more advanced imaging modality, such as computed tomography (CT), magnetic resonance imaging (MRI), nuclear medicine scintigraphy, or ultrasound. Advantages and limitations of each modality are reviewed in this chapter, along with suggestions for imaging approach.

N. Morley · I. Omar (✉)
Northwestern Memorial Hospital, Chicago, IL, USA
e-mail: Imran.Omar@nmff.org

T. D. Peabody and S. Attar (eds.), *Orthopaedic Oncology,*
Cancer Treatment and Research 162, DOI: 10.1007/978-3-319-07323-1_2,
© Springer International Publishing Switzerland 2014

2 Plain Radiography

Plain radiographs form the basis for initial imaging of suspected bone tumors. Radiography provides excellent resolution, allows for assessment of lesion characteristics, and is often more specific than MRI in generating a reasonable differential diagnosis. Radiography has been the optimal modality in distinguishing nonaggressive from aggressive osseous disease [1, 2]. It should be noted that imaging studies are often able to assess how aggressive a lesion is, but the determination of whether a lesion is benign or malignant is based on pathology. Benign lesions, such as osteomyelitis, may look quite aggressive. If a lesion is pathognomonic for a specific entity, a diagnosis can be made from radiographs alone. In many situations, however, a differential diagnosis is created, and further workup is performed by a combination of advanced imaging modalities [3, 4], and if necessary, tissue sampling. In cases where tissue sampling is necessary, percutaneous biopsy using imaging guidance has been shown to be safe and effective [5]. Soft tissue differentiation is limited at radiography, and evaluation of soft tissue masses primarily involves the identification of fatty or calcified components.

Radiographic evaluation is based on the classification system described by Lodwick, which classifies lesions based on four main groups of characteristics, including destruction of bone, proliferation of bone, mineralization of tumor matrix, and location, size and shape of the tumor [6].

Patterns of bone destruction include geographic, moth-eaten, or permeative. Geographic bone destruction involves loss of bone extending to the transition between tumor and structural bone. A thin sclerotic margin (type IA) is characteristically only seen with geographic lesions, although a geographic lesion can also have a clear nonsclerotic margin (type IB, the so-called "punched out" lesion), or a poorly defined margin, typical of local infiltration (type IC). Moth-eaten bone destruction (type II) is the creation of several smaller confluent holes within the bone. Permeative bone destruction (type III) involves many punctate holes with an ill-defined transition between the involved and uninvolved bone. Moth-eaten and permeative patterns are associated with more aggressive lesions. However, some malignant lesions such as fibrosarcoma and chondrosarcoma can arise within a benign lesion, and as such radiologic-pathologic apparent discordance can arise with an aggressive histology in a benign appearing radiographic lesion [7]. Of note, the fastest margin of tumor growth would be a radiographically invisible permeative lesion, as this involves the widest of margins.

In order for a radiolucent lesion to be appreciable at radiography, there must be destruction of either cortical or cancellous bone. Since the diaphysis of long bones is comprised of primarily cortical bone that envelops a thin internal margin of cancellous bone and the marrow in the central medullary cavity, lesions arising in the medullary space may not be visible at radiography. The term "endosteal scalloping" refers to a tumor that originates in the medullary canal, and as it grows, displaces, or replaces the internal cortical margin rather than the outer surfaces of the bone. This tends to have rounded margins, hence the scalloped appearance.

Endosteal scalloping is not by itself an aggressive finding and can be seen with benign lesions, but does suggest adjacent marrow replacement.

Proliferation of bone includes both encapsulated and unencapsulated patterns, with unencapsulated growth being more aggressive. This feature is particularly characterized by different patterns of periosteal reaction. Broadly speaking, periosteal reaction can be classified as continuous, interrupted, or complex, depending on its morphology. Continuous forms include both nonaggressive and aggressive morphologies, with the terms *smooth* and *continuous* representing examples of nonaggressive periosteal reaction, and *lamellated* or *"onion-skin"* representing examples of an aggressive reaction. Interrupted patterns include the Codman's angle or triangle, which is a focal periosteal elevation, and interrupted spiculated patterns. Complex patterns include a mix of various types [8].

Tumor matrix is reflective of the type of calcification or ossification, if any, that is present within the lesion. Osteoid matrix is often described as solid, cloud-like, or ivory-like, and when in an aggressive lesion can be associated with osteosarcoma. Chondroid matrix is classically described as stippled, flocculent, or "ring and arc" configuration, and when aggressive can be seen in the setting of chondrosarcoma [9]. Fibrous matrix, as seen in fibrous dysplasia, demonstrates a "ground glass" radiographic density as a result of small, abnormally arranged trabeculae of immature woven bone [10]. Many lesions of varying cell types do not show any type of internal matrix, and this is also the case with highly dedifferentiated osteoid or chondroid malignancies.

Location, size, and shape also play a role in the evaluation of a bone tumor. Generally speaking, malignancies tend to be larger and more spherical. Differential diagnosis is aided also by location, as some tumors originate in the diaphyseal, metaphyseal, or epiphyseal location. Age of the patient also aids in formation of a differential diagnosis, as different tumors tend to favor different age groups.

Once the lesion has been assessed radiographically, if there are aggressive features, further imaging evaluation is warranted. This is particularly true in the setting of cortical destruction or suspected extension into the adjacent soft tissues. The degree of soft tissue involvement is more accurately characterized by contrast enhanced CT or MRI [11], which allow better discrimination of the extent of disease. This is often not possible at plain radiography, as both tumor and adjacent normal soft tissues are of the same density and attenuate the X-ray to the same degree (Figs. 1, 2, 3, 4, 5 and 6).

3   Computed Tomography

Computed tomography utilizes X-rays and complex computer algorithms to generate tomographic axial images, which can be reformatted in coronal and sagittal planes to aid interpretation. CT has many advantages over radiography, including allowing lesion characterization in complex regions of osseous overlap, such as the spine or pelvis, allowing determination of extent of soft tissue involvement, and in

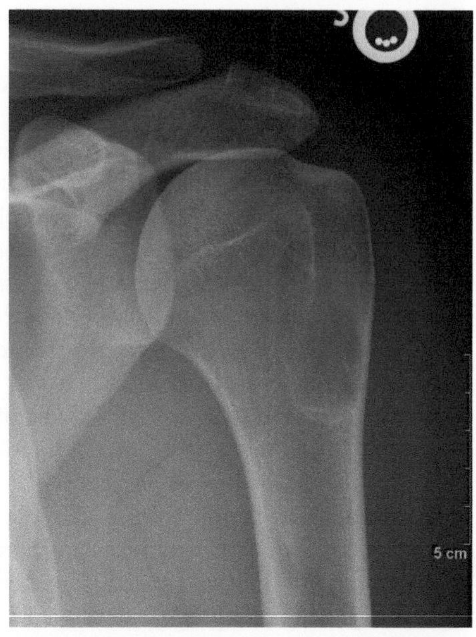

Fig. 1 Unicameral bone cyst. 18 year old man with a Lodwick type IA lesion, with a nonaggressive appearance. This does not require further evaluation

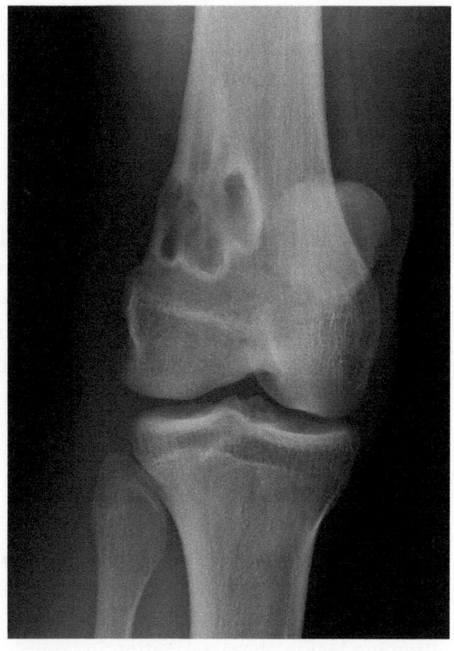

Fig. 2 Nonossifying fibroma. Another lesion typifying a type IA lesion in this 21 year old man, with a nonaggressive appearance

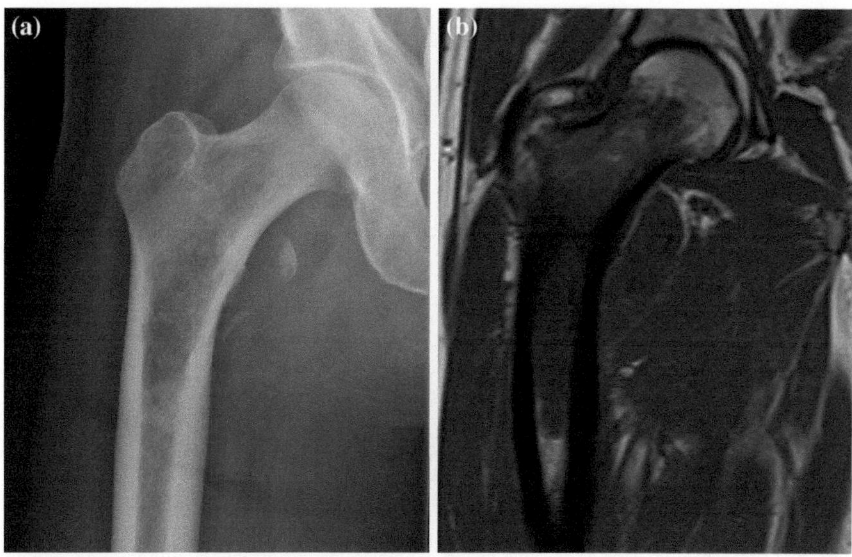

Fig. 3 a Dedifferentiated chondrosarcoma. 58 year old man with an aggressive lesion demonstrating ill-defined, permeative type III margins. Because of its dedifferentiation, no chondroid matrix is appreciable. There is a pathologic fracture of the lesser trochanter, a typical location for an underlying lesion. **b** Corresponding coronal T1-weighted MRI demonstrates replacement of the marrow by tumor

Fig. 4 Osteosarcoma, high grade. This aggressive lesion in this 30 year old woman demonstrates aggressive interrupted lamellated periosteal reaction, with permeative margins and soft tissue extension

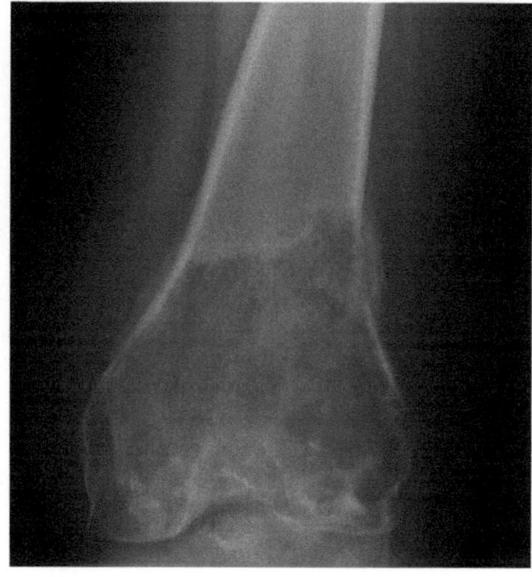

some cases, degree of intramedullary involvement. The relatively quick speed with which CT can be acquired is also of benefit in patients who are claustrophobic or unable to hold still, as motion artifact degrades all imaging. Limitations or drawbacks of CT include its inability in many cases to provide a specific histologic

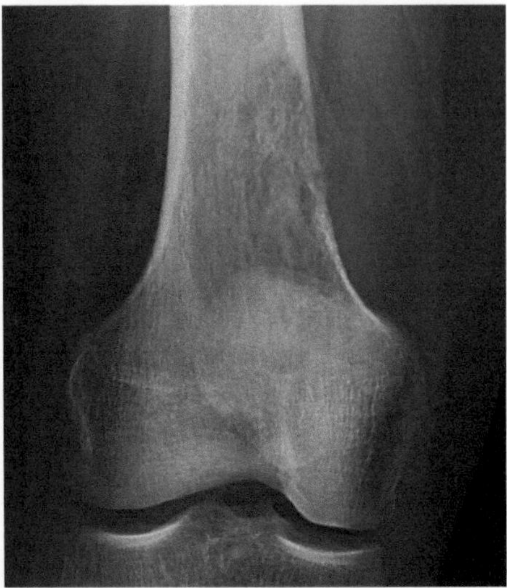

Fig. 5 Osteosarcoma. This aggressive lesion demonstrates periosteal reaction with a Codman's triangle of focal periosteal elevation in this 23 year old man. There is typical "cloud-like" osteoid matrix

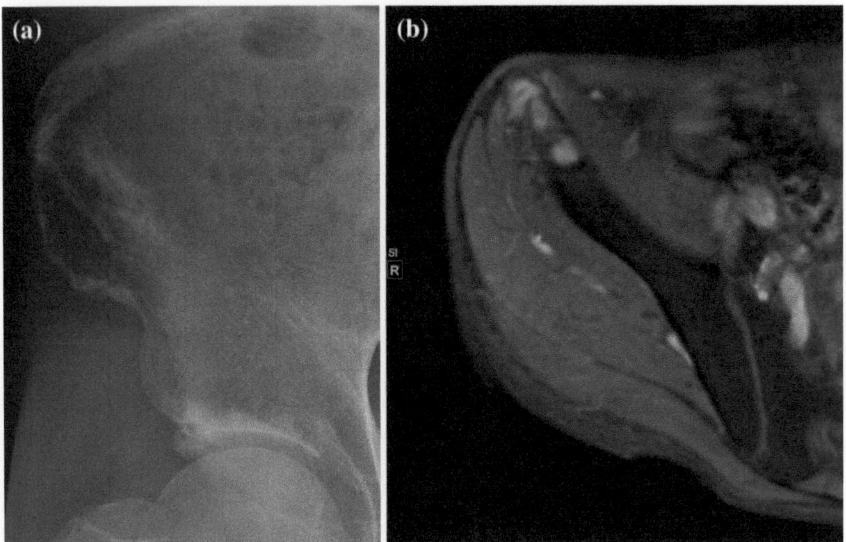

Fig. 6 **a** Multiple myeloma. 52 year old man with an ill defined right anterior iliac wing lesion, with a wide zone of transition. **b** MRI demonstrates better the extent of the lesion, showing that there is no adjacent soft tissue extension. This was subsequently biopsied and shown to be multiple myeloma

diagnosis of soft tissue tumors, and its associated radiation dose, which is particularly relevant for children and pregnant patients.

CT characterizes lesions based on their degree of attenuation of a focused X-ray beam. A specific volume of tissue is assigned a value representing this degree of attenuation, called a Hounsfield unit (HU), named for the inventor of CT, Sir Godfrey Hounsfield. Although not absolute, bone is typically +400 to +1000 HU, soft tissue +40 to +80, water 0, fat −60 to −100, and air is −1000 [12].

Although attenuation values can sometimes be helpful, such as in the setting of a lesion that contains fat or calcification, many times a lesion will be of soft tissue attenuation. This does not aid in providing a specific histologic diagnosis. Some tumors, such as osteosarcoma or chondrosarcoma, demonstrate internal matrix, which can allow for further characterization, although this information is often obtainable via radiography.

Patterns of osseous destruction seen on CT follow those seen on radiography. A slow growing process will demonstrate a narrow zone of transition and geographic margins, and more aggressive processes will have moth-eaten or permeative patterns of destruction. The endosteum is also well evaluated on CT, which can be scalloped or destroyed in the setting of tumor. The degree of marrow replacement is better evaluated on MRI, but an obvious soft tissue mass infiltrating the medullary cavity can be assessed on CT.

CT can also be helpful in identifying areas of reactive cortical destruction. CT allows direct visualization without overlying interfering attenuation from soft tissues. Cortical destruction can be assessed even in areas where several bones are in close proximity to one another or are of complex shape, such as in the spine or pelvis [13]. On X-rays, these areas of destruction can be obscured, as the three dimensional shape is flattened into two dimensions. Cortical destruction may be mistaken for overlap of other anatomic structures [14].

Extension of tumor into the adjacent soft tissues often accompanies aggressive osseous pathology, and CT can provide accurate assessment of the margins of extension. Addition of intravenous contrast can provide additional resolution between pathologic and uninvolved tissues. Despite these advantages with more well-encapsulated lesions, some tumors can be infiltrative, and the exact margin between tumor soft tissue and adjacent muscle may not be possible on CT. MRI may be advantageous in these patients as it offers superior soft tissue contrast when compared to CT, and as a result of its absence of ionizing radiation, has largely supplanted CT for the evaluation of soft tissue extent [15]. Intramedullary involvement is also better assessed on MRI [16], where subtle marrow infiltration may be detected by methods discussed below, but when grossly present may be detectable on CT by noting replacement of the marrow fat with soft tissue attenuation.

Despite the advantages of CT, in many cases, a specific histologic diagnosis of a soft tissue mass cannot be reached, and in these cases a differential diagnosis is generated. Further evaluation with MRI or tissue sampling is then performed.

Other potential limitations or drawbacks of CT include radiation dose, patient motion, and iodinated dye contrast allergy. Radiation dose associated with CT has received considerable media attention, and is particularly relevant for children and pregnant patients. Despite the attention it has received, the actual lifetime risk of developing fatal cancer from abdominopelvic CT has been the subject of a recent publication, and is by conservative estimate erring on the side of overestimation of at most 0.5 per 1,000 individuals. The risk of dying from pedestrian accident, for reference, is 1.6 per 1,000 individuals; from drowning, 0.9 per 1,000 individuals; and the risk of dying from lightning strike 0.013 per 1,000 individuals [17]. This is not to trivialize the possibility of radiation-induced cancer, but serves to provide a frame of reference of the likelihood to allow appropriate risk-benefit stratification. In general, a guiding principle with regards to medical imaging is to achieve the necessary diagnostic information using a radiation dose that is *As Low As Reasonably Achieveable* (ALARA). This can be done through both optimization of imaging protocols to include only the area of interest, and also by using techniques that do not involve ionizing radiation, such as ultrasound or MRI when appropriate. Additionally, newer generations of CT scanners have included features, such as dose modulation or iterative reconstruction, to marked reduce radiation exposures.

Patient motion degrades all imaging, regardless of modality. Although this can be a drawback on CT when a patient cannot hold still, CT is less susceptible to this limitation than is MRI, as imaging times are shorter. Sedation can be considered if the patient is a candidate when motion limits interpretation.

Iodinated contrast allergy is not uncommon. Severe anaphylaxis following contrast administration is rare, but can result in life-threatening complications that require immediate treatment [18]. Most reactions tend to be minor, and premedication regimens with steroids prior to contrast administration have been advocated. Of note, there is no specific cross-reactivity between allergy to iodinated contrast materials and allergy to gadolinium based contrast materials, so that a patient who has a history of severe allergic reaction to iodinated CT contrast material is often a candidate for contrast-enhanced MRI (Figs. 7, 8 and 9).

4   Magnetic Resonance Imaging

Magnetic resonance imaging has traditionally been utilized for staging of bone lesions and as such has been extremely valuable in planning management, but the advent of more advanced pulse sequences allows for some increased lesion characterization as well. Conventional MRI sequences do not usually allow for lesion characterization, as both benign and malignant processes show increased relaxation times on both T1 and T2 sequences. Main strengths of MRI in bone tumor imaging include the ability to assess extent of marrow involvement, to determine the presence of discontinuous, or "skip" lesions within the same bone, and to determine the extent of any soft tissue component extending beyond the

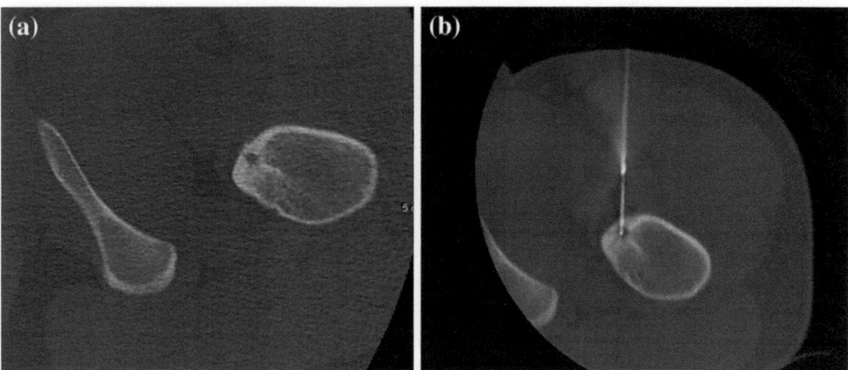

Fig. 7 **a** Osteoid osteoma. CT demonstrates focal cortical thickening with a central lucent nidus in this 19 year old man. **b** Under CT guidance, a radiofrequency ablation probe was directed to the nidus, providing relief of symptoms following ablation

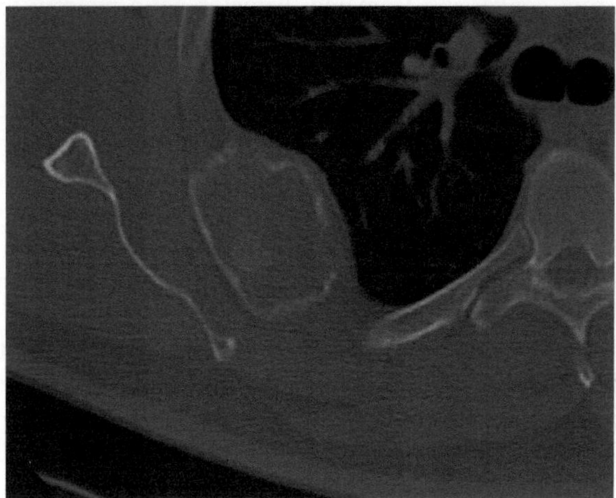

Fig. 8 Fibrous dysplasia. For complex locations such as the ribs, where there is osseous overlap with the adjacent scapula at radiography, CT is helpful in providing additional information. In this 37 year-old man, this lesion demonstrates the typical ground glass matrix of fibrous dysplasia, which was suggested at the initial CT examination. Biopsy was performed because of cortical breakthrough superiorly, and pathology confirmed fibrous dysplasia

cortex. For these reasons, continuous images extending from the joint above the lesion to the joint below are typically obtained. Additionally, MRI carries the advantage of absence of ionizing radiation. However, limitations of MRI include susceptibility artifact from metallic hardware, which is often placed in the surgical treatment of musculoskeletal tumors, and inability to safely image many patients with pacemakers or other metallic devices.

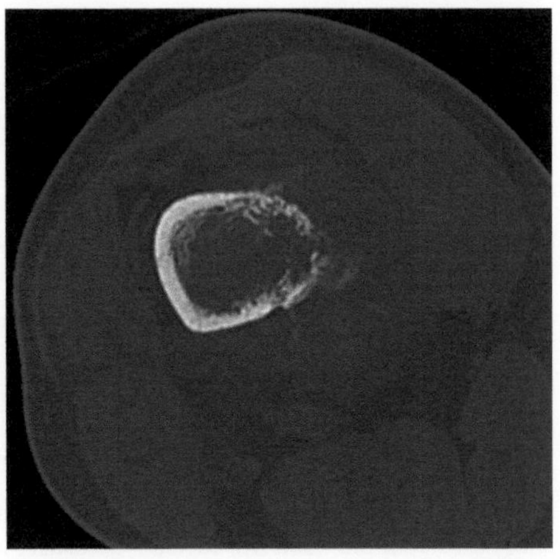

Fig. 9 Osteosarcoma. CT of the same patient as in Fig. 5. The extent of soft tissue involvement is better assessed on CT

For evaluation of marrow infiltration, T1-weighted images are the workhorse sequence. Marrow conversion from red, hematopoietic marrow to yellow, fatty marrow in a normal patient occurs in a predictable distribution with advancing age. This can be appreciated on T1-weighted images as an increase in marrow signal correlating with increased fat content. When an area that should contain yellow marrow loses its bright signal, this may represent either marrow infiltration by a pathologic process or red marrow reconversion in response to increased hematopoietic needs. On T1 images, this can many times be differentiated by assessing the signal intensity with respect to muscle. Red marrow reconversion will typically be hyperintense to skeletal muscle, whereas a pathologic process typically will be isointense to hypointense.

Extent of disease involvement is assessed as areas of T1 hypointensity. This is evaluated both for the primary lesion, which is measured and reported, as well as for the presence of any concurrent lesions within the same bone. T1-weighted images can also suggest a diffuse pattern of marrow replacement, as is often seen in the setting of metastatic disease, myeloma or lymphoma.

Local infiltration of soft tissues adjacent to bone can usually be best characterized on T2-weighted images or T1-weighted images following the administration of intravenous contrast. T1-weighted images without IV contrast may demonstrate loss of fat planes or a demarcation between tumor and normal adjacent muscle if there is a difference in signal intensity, but these findings are often subtle, and small areas of involvement can be easily overlooked.

Pathological conditions are usually more conspicuous on fluid-sensitive sequences, such as T2-weighted imaging or with *short tau inversion recovery* (STIR), since the signal intensities of these areas are brighter than skeletal muscle. Additionally, fluid sensitive sequences are commonly performed with fat saturation. Decreasing the signal from fat further increases the conspicuity of abnormal fluid content within tissues. Thus, T2-weighted images increase the conspicuity of tumor infiltration. Chemically selective fat saturation sequences tend to have higher spatial resolution but may suffer from areas of inhomogeneous fat suppression or may be more prone to other artifacts. On the other hand, STIR images demonstrate uniform fat suppression over larger fields of view but have poorer spatial resolution and may take longer to perform. T2-weighted images also increase the conspicuity of fluid-fluid levels. Although fluid–fluid levels are not specific, a lesion comprised of a higher percentage of fluid-fluid levels has a higher likelihood of being benign [19].

While the mainstay of MRI has been in assessing the extent of disease, the advent of advanced pulse sequences has allowed for some lesion characterization as well [20]. Chemical shift imaging, diffusion weighted imaging, and post-contrast imaging provide additional information for problem solving.

Chemical shift imaging is also called in and opposed phase imaging. The basic principle behind chemical shift imaging is that when water and fat molecules are located within the same sampled space and imaged while in phase, their signals will be additive, producing bright signal on the image. When imaged during the opposed phase, their signals will cancel one another out, resulting in a signal drop. Yellow marrow contains predominantly fat, and as such, will remain bright in signal on opposed phase imaging. Red marrow contains more hematopoietic elements, and as such is more cellular. With increased cellularity comes increased water content, although there is also usually some fatty marrow in these areas as well [21]. On opposed phase imaging, these signals then cancel, resulting in a signal drop.

Both marrow replacing processes and hematopoietic red marrow may be lower in signal intensity than fatty marrow on a T1-weighted image, and sometimes it can be difficult to distinguish between them simply by using comparison to internal references, such as muscle. This principle of chemical shift imaging can be applied to allow differentiation of an aggressive marrow replacing process from hematopoietic marrow. Marrow replacing processes are unlikely to spare the normal fatty marrow, and as a result, only cellular, water-heavy components are likely to remain. Thus, unlike with red marrow, there will be no signal drop on opposed phase imaging.

The role of diffusion-weighted imaging in the musculoskeletal system is less well defined. Diffusion-weighted sequences have been used extensively in the evaluation of stroke and many other intracranial processes, but have been less extensively studied with regard to bone tumors. Diffusion weighted sequences are created based on Brownian motion at the microscopic level, and in tumor imaging, increased cellularity results in restricted diffusion. This is displayed on two sets of sequences. One of these is referred to by their *b value*, which is a representation of the diffusion weighting used to generate the image, and the other is called the *apparent diffusion coefficient*, or *ADC map*. Some authors have attempted to classify neoplastic versus normal marrow signal based on absolute ADC values [22]. However, the application of this technique for this usage is early, and absolute cutoffs may vary based on vendor and institution specific techniques used to generate the ADC map.

Although contrast-enhanced imaging is often unnecessary in the setting of a primary osseous tumor [23], contrast-enhanced MRI may provide additional information for the assessment of a suspected soft tissue mass. Additionally, contrast-enhanced imaging may provide additional valuable information when staging for local extent, biopsy planning, tissue characterization, monitoring preoperative chemotherapy, and detection of recurrence [24]. Musculoskeletal malignancies often demonstrate high T2 signal, which can mimic a ganglion cyst, meniscal cyst, or synovial cyst on unenhanced images. If the lesion demonstrates any internal T1 heterogeneity or septations, further evaluation with contrast-enhanced images are requisite to exclude a solid malignancy mimicking a benign process [25]. Contrast can also be useful for allowing identification of any cystic regions within the mass. When biopsy is performed of a mixed solid and cystic mass, it should be directed toward the solid components.

Recent studies have focused on the utilization of dynamic contrast-enhanced MRI in evaluation of the prognosis of patients with osteosarcoma. Dynamic contrast-enhanced MRI utilizes a bolus of IV gadolinium contrast, with serial images of the tumor after administration allowing assessment of parameters related to tumor vascularity, which may serve as a marker for treatment response. Early results are promising although further studies are needed [26].

MR spectroscopy is an emerging technology for the characterization of musculoskeletal neoplasms. Spectroscopy is a technique that uses MRI to determine the chemical composition of a volume of tissue. A tissue containing a discrete choline peak has been shown to have a sensitivity of 88 % and specificity of 68 % in the detection of malignancy [27]. Limitations include inaccuracy as a result of magnetic field inhomogeneity and difficulties arising from the varying shapes of the musculoskeletal system. Because people are of varied body habitus, different coils need to be used to optimally image different sized extremities, which further complicates analysis.

Ultimately, evaluation of many lesions solely on MRI yields nonspecific results, and studies have shown less than 50 % accuracy in determination of malignancy from benign processes. Correlation with plain radiographs can aid in assessing whether a process is likely to be aggressive, and the need for further evaluation with tissue sampling (Figs. 10, 11, 12, 13, 14 and 15).

5   Nuclear Medicine Scintigraphy

Nuclear medicine scintigraphy is used to look for areas of increased bone turnover, and its power in the diagnosis of musculoskeletal tumors lies in its sensitivity to detect lesions. Bone scintigraphy is typically performed with technetium 99 m methylene diphosphonate (MDP), although a variety of other isotopes are also available for medical imaging. Bone scintigraphy for tumor imaging is best

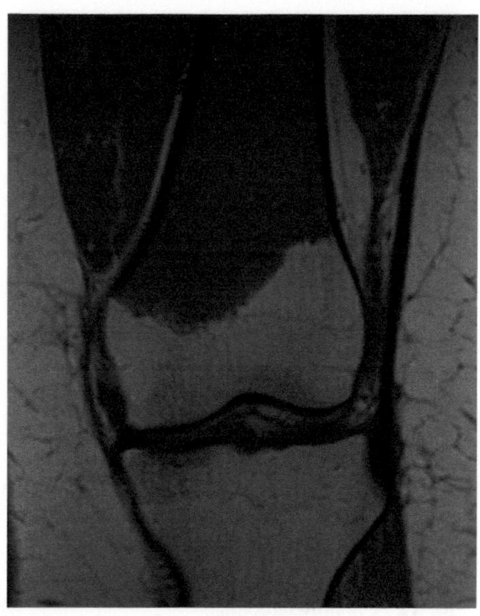

Fig. 10 Lymphoma. T1 coronal MRI demonstrates confluent marrow replacement in the femoral diaphysis in this 30 year-old woman with lymphoma

performed in patients with a known primary tumor, particularly to assess for the presence and extent of metastatic disease [28]. Bone scan is more sensitive than radiography in depicting a reactive process, as approximately 50 % of bone must be lost before a lytic lesion will become radiographically visible.

Multifocal disease will be seen as several discontiguous areas of increased uptake. This will allow detection of both local and remote disease spread, as bone scintigraphy is most commonly acquired as whole body imaging, with spot views of areas of concern for higher magnification. Primary bone lesions uncommonly present with metastatic disease, and bone scan is not initially indicated in the setting of a known primary osseous tumor [29].

Following detection of a lesion with bone scan, radiographic correlation is the appropriate next step to ensure that the lesion does not represent a non-tumor area of osseous pathology, such as an infectious or arthritic process. Particularly in the setting of a solitary lesion in a patient with low grade primary disease, specificity for tumor on bone scan alone is low. Biopsy may be necessary, as even in the setting of known primary malignancy, biopsy may reveal no malignancy or a second malignancy as frequently as 12 % of the time [30].

Positron emission tomography, or PET, is typically performed with a fluorine-18 fluorodeoxyglucose (FDG) tracer. This radiolabeled analog of glucose is injected intravenously and trapped in cells that are metabolically active. As a result, it has a predilection for some tumor cells, which tend to have higher metabolic needs. PET is often performed in combination with CT, with hybrid fused images allowing precise anatomic localization.

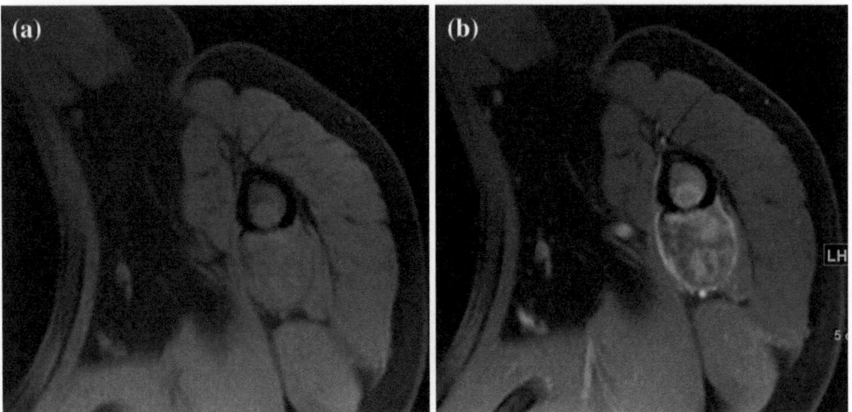

Fig. 11 **a** and b Osteosarcoma. Axial T1 pre and post contrast images demonstrate the added value of contrast in the evaluation of soft tissue extension of tumor in this 48 year old man

Fig. 12 Chondrosarcoma. Coronal STIR demonstrates diffuse marrow replacement with tumor in this 60 year old woman

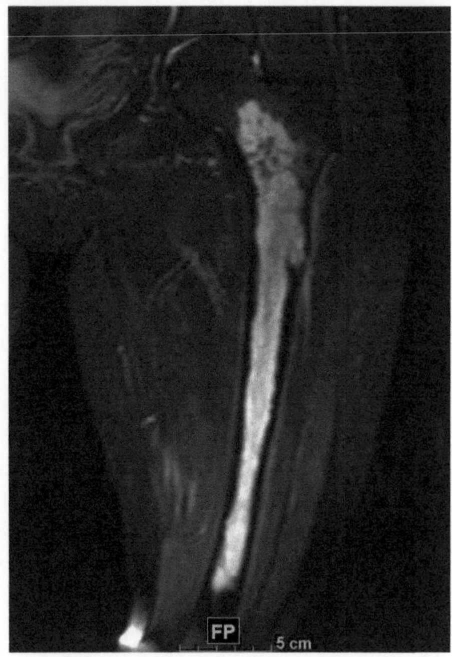

FDG PET has shown particular benefit in imaging of patients with sarcomas. Many types of childhood sarcoma, including Ewing's sarcoma, rhabdomyosarcoma, osteosarcoma, and leiomyosarcoma, can be detected both at their primary site and at sites of metastasis as areas of increased metabolism [31]. This has also been shown of value in adult sarcoma as well [32].

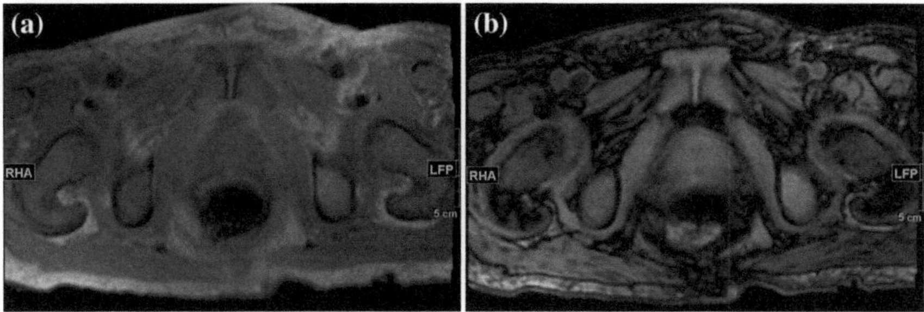

Fig. 13 **a** and **b** Hematopoetic red marrow. In and opposed phase images demonstrate loss of signal on opposed phase images in the intertrochanteric regions, consistent with the presence of both water and fat. This is compatible with hematopoetic red marrow in this 60 year old man with mantle cell lymphoma

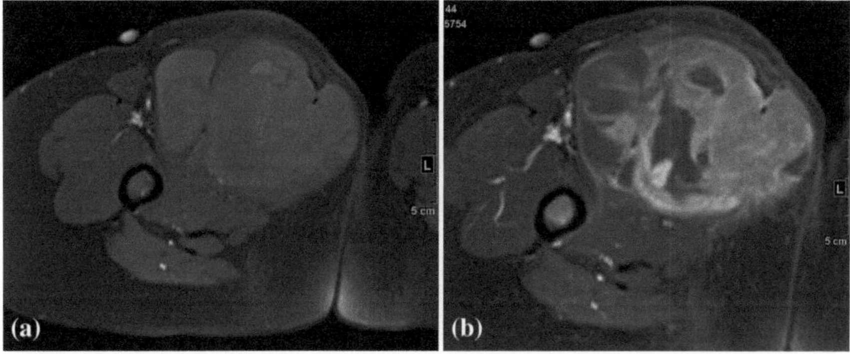

Fig. 14 **a** and **b** Synovial sarcoma. Pre- and post-contrast axial T1 images (**a** and **b** respectively) illustrating the value of postcontrast imaging for a soft tissue mass in this 23 year old woman. There are lobulated areas of enhancing residual tumor interspersed with areas of necrosis following treatment. Although the lesion increased in overall size compared with the prior exam, there was also an increase in the necrotic component, suggestive of treatment response

Although other nuclear medicine techniques provide specific information regarding secondary osseous metastatic disease, they are not discussed here as they are beyond the scope of this chapter (Figs. 16 and 17).

6 Ultrasound

Although there is little indication for its use in characterizing bone lesions, ultrasound can also be helpful in the characterization of extraosseous musculo-skeletal soft tissue tumors. Although ultrasound is not specific enough to allow histologic diagnosis, it can provide information regarding the cystic versus solid nature of a lesion, and in some settings may allow differentiation of a tumor from a

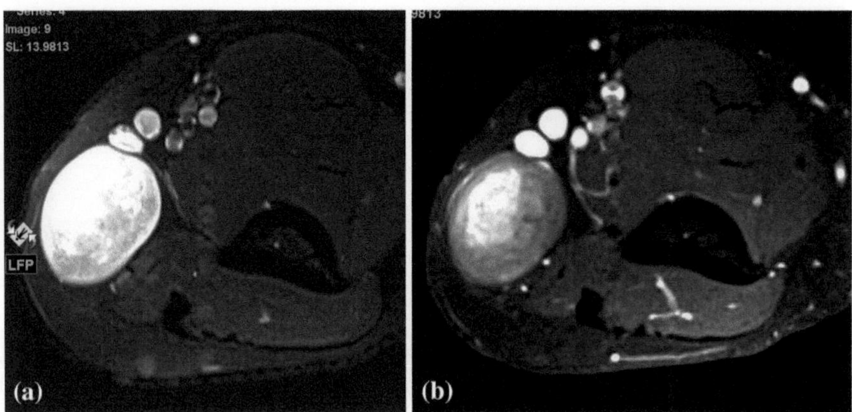

Fig. 15 **a** and **b** Schwannoma. T2 axial fat saturated image (**a**) of the left distal humerus demonstrates a fluid-bright lesion in the medial soft tissues in this 39 year old woman. Post contrast T1 image (**b**) demonstrates that this lesion is a solid enhancing mass, and not a cyst

simple fluid collection [33]. Color Doppler flow imaging can also aid in distinguishing solid from cystic lesions (Figs. 18 and 19).

Patients may present with a palpable subcutaneous lesion, in which case an ultrasound is often the first line of imaging. Ultrasound allows for further characterization without ionizing radiation, and is not as expensive as MRI. Benign fluid collections, such as typical ganglion cysts or Baker's cysts, may be differentiated from solid lesions, which have malignant potential. Although specific histologic diagnosis is not possible on ultrasound, aggressive sonographic features such as invasion of adjacent structures or a lack of well defined margins can prompt further workup with MRI. Ultrasound also offers excellent resolution of very small superficial structures when a high frequency linear transducer is employed, and may also be useful in distinguishing foreign body reaction from a true tumor.

Grayscale imaging may allow suggestion of specific lesions if there is a classic morphology, such as in the setting of plantar fibromatosis, abscess, or ganglion cyst. However, any lesions that appear suddenly, are painful, or that exceed 5 cm in diameter need further evaluation, often with biopsy. Also, if a lesion is deep seated and as such not well evaluated with a superficial transducer, or if all margins of the tumor cannot be well delineated, further evaluation with MRI, and if necessary, biopsy, is warranted [34]. Although a lipoma may be suggested if a solitary lesion has typical sonographic features, sonography has been shown not to be specific for diagnosis [35], as lipomas may have variable echogenicity, ranging from hypoechoic to hyperechoic depending on the adjacent soft tissues. Other lesions with classic features include hemangiomas, which may include phleboliths, and peripheral nerve sheath tumors, which follow the course of a specific nerve. Peripheral nerve sheath tumors may produce symptoms in the distribution of the

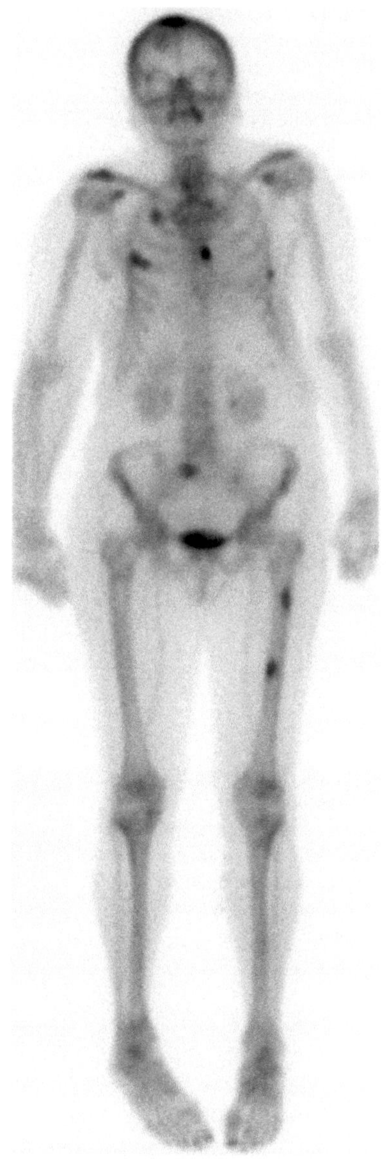

Fig. 16 Metastatic breast cancer. Whole body MDP bone scan in a patient with breast cancer demonstrates several scattered sites of increased uptake, compatible with metastatic disease in this 79 year old woman

nerve, and as such, dynamic sonography is of value as the sonographer is able to elicit typical signs and symptoms in real time during the examination [36].

Following grayscale evaluation, color Doppler flow evaluation of all lesions is necessary, as some solid tumors, most commonly fibrous lesions, may appear hypoechoic to anechoic at grayscale imaging. These may even have smooth margins, further mimicking a cyst [37].

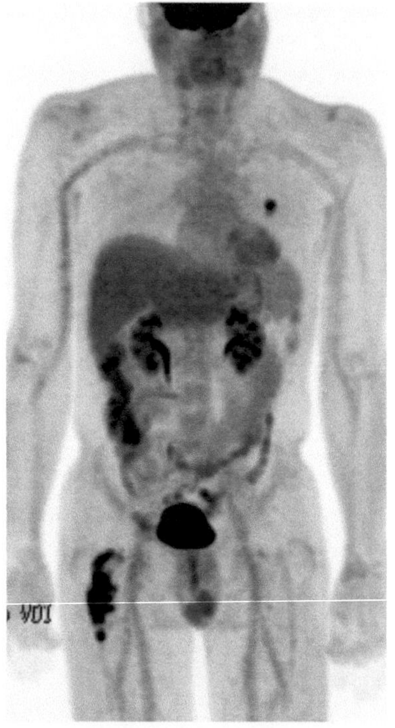

Fig. 17 Metastatic chondrosarcoma. Whole body PET demonstrates a primary chondrosarcoma of the right femur with a metastasis to the left lung in this 58 year old man

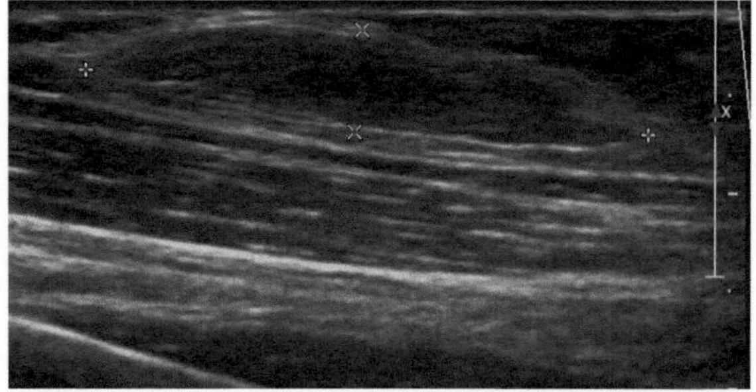

Fig. 18 Soft tissue lipoma. Ultrasound image demonstrates an encapsulated mass that is isoechoic to the adjacent fat, compatible with a lipoma in this 67 year-old woman

Color Doppler flow imaging also aids in distinguishing cystic from solid masses. Cystic lesions will not demonstrate internal pulsatile color Doppler flow; therefore, if a lesion contains flow, it is at least in part solid and not a simple cyst. The absence of flow does not exclude malignancy, as a tumor may have slow flow that is not detectable by Doppler, but the presence of flow excludes a simple cyst. Arrangement of color Doppler flow in morphology suggestive of neoangiogenesis includes disorganized blood vessels, occlusions, stenoses, or trifurcations [38]. Power Doppler flow is a similar technique to color Doppler. Instead of directional information being displayed as alternating colors, power Doppler displays only an absolute value, but may be more sensitive to small amounts of flow.

Fig. 19 Soft tissue
malignancy. Transverse
ultrasound image
demonstrates a lobulated
hypoechoic mass deep to the
gastrocnemius muscle in the
popliteal fossa in this 44 year
old man

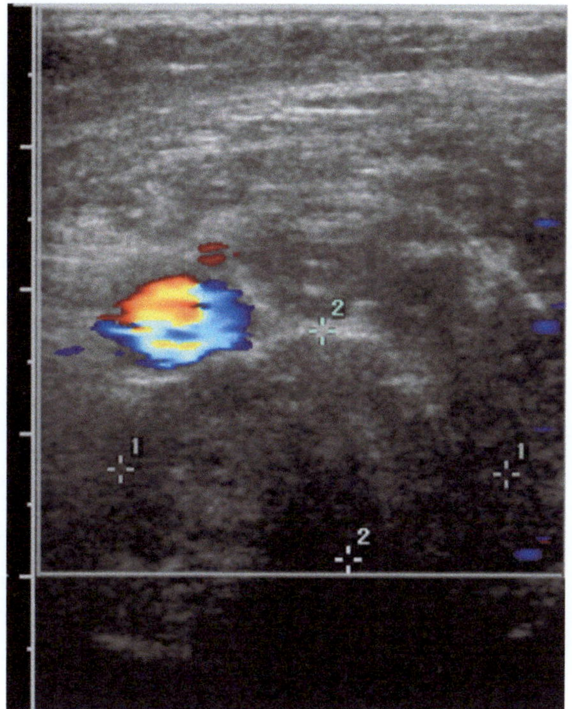

7   Suggestions for Imaging Approach

Initial evaluation of a primary bone tumor should be performed using radiography. If initial radiography is negative but the patient has persistent symptoms, the next study of choice is MRI. However, if the patient is not a candidate for MRI, Tc99 m MDP bone scan or CT may be performed instead.

If the initial radiographic evaluation is positive, and shows suspicious characteristics for malignancy, MRI is the next evaluation of choice. CT and PET/CT may also be helpful to evaluate the cortex and for additional lesions as detailed above. In the setting of a positive radiographic evaluation with benign characteristics, such as in the setting of osteoid osteoma, further characterization with CT can be performed to aid in treatment planning.

Soft tissue lesions, which are often radiographically negative, are ideally further evaluated with MRI. However, patients with abnormal renal function are at increased risk for nephrogenic systemic fibrosis, and as a result may be ineligible to receive gadolinium contrast. Ultrasound may be of value in this setting.

For further details, please refer the ACR appropriateness criteria for primary bone tumors [39].

References

1. Sundaram M, McLeod RA (1990) MR imaging of tumor and tumorlike lesions of bone and soft tissue. AJR Am J Roentgenol 155(4):817–824
2. Colleran G, Madewell J, Foran P et al (2011) Imaging of soft tissue and osseous sarcomas of the extremities. Semin Ultrasound CT MR 32(5):442–455
3. Hwang S, Panicek DM (2009) The evolution of musculoskeletal tumor imaging. Radiol Clin North Am 47(3):435–453
4. Rajiah P, Ilaslan H, Sundaram M (2011) Imaging of primary malignant bone tumors (nonhematological). Radiol Clin North Am 49(6):1135–1161
5. Jelinek JS, Murphey MD, Welker JA et al (2002) Diagnosis of primary bone tumors with image-guided percutaneous biopsy: experience with 110 tumors. Radiology 223(3):731–737
6. Lodwick GS (1965) A probabilistic approach to the diagnosis of bone tumors. Radiol Clin North Am 3(3):487–497
7. Madewell JE, Ragsdale BD, Sweet DE (1981) Radiologic and pathologic analysis of solitary bone lesions. Part I: internal margins. Radiol Clin North Am 19(4):715–748
8. Ragsdale BD, Madewell JE, Sweet DE (1981) Radiologic and pathologic analysis of solitary bone lesions. Part II: periosteal reactions. Radiol Clin North Am 19(4):749–783
9. Sweet DE, Madewell JE, Ragsdale BD (1981) Radiologic and pathologic analysis of solitary bone lesions. Part III: matrix patterns. Radiol Clin North Am 19(4):785–814
10. Greenspan A (2011) In orthopedic imaging: a practical approach. Chapter 19. In: 5th edn Benign tumors and tumor-like Lesions III: Fibrous, Fibroosseous and Fibrohistiocytic Lesions
11. Oudenhoven LF, Dhondt E, Kahn S et al (2006) Accuracy of radiography in grading and tissue-specific diagnosis–a study of 200 consecutive bone tumors of the hand. Skeletal Radiol 35(2):78–87 Epub 2005 Oct 25
12. Brant WE, Helms CA (2012) In fundamentals of diagnostic radiology. Chapter 1. Diagnostic imaging methods, Fourth Edn
13. deSantos LA, Bernardino ME, Murray JA (1979) Computed tomography in the evaluation of osteosarcoma: experience with 25 cases. AJR Am J Roentgenol 132(4):535–540
14. Egund N, Ekelund L, Sako M et al (1981) CT of soft-tissue tumors. AJR Am J Roentgenol 137(4):725–729
15. Aisen AM, Martel W, Braunstein EM et al (1986) MRI and CT evaluation of primary bone and soft-tissue tumors. AJR Am J Roentgenol 146(4):749–756
16. Ilaslan H, Sundaram M (2006) Advances in musculoskeletal tumor imaging. Orthop Clin North Am 37(3):375–391
17. McCollough CH, Guimarães L, Fletcher JG (2009) In defense of body CT. AJR Am J Roentgenol 193(1):28–39
18. ACR manual on contrast media (2013)
19. O'Donnell P, Saifuddin A (2004) The prevalence and diagnostic significance of fluid-fluid levels in focal lesions of bone. Skeletal Radiol 33(6):330–336
20. Fayad LM, Jacobs MA, Wang X et al (2012) Musculoskeletal tumors: how to use anatomic, functional, and metabolic MR techniques. Radiology 265(2):340–356
21. Vogler JB 3rd, Murphy WA (1988) Bone marrow imaging. Radiology 168(3):679–693
22. Padhani AR, van Ree K, Collins DJ et al (2013) Assessing the relation between bone marrow signal intensity and apparent diffusion coefficient in diffusion-weighted MRI. AJR Am J Roentgenol 200(1):163–170
23. Stacy GS, Mahal RS, Peabody TD (2006) Staging of bone tumors: a review with illustrative examples. AJR Am J Roentgenol 186(4):967–976
24. Verstraete KL, Lang P (2000) Bone and soft tissue tumors: the role of contrast agents for MR imaging. Eur J Radiol 34(3):229–246

25. Ma LD, McCarthy EF, Bluemke DA et al (1998) Differentiation of benign from malignant musculoskeletal lesions using MR imaging: pitfalls in MR evaluation of lesions with a cystic appearance. AJR Am J Roentgenol 170(5):1251–1258
26. Guo J, Reddick WE, Glass JO et al (2012) Dynamic contrast-enhanced magnetic resonance imaging as a prognostic factor in predicting event-free and overall survival in pediatric patients with osteosarcoma. Cancer 118(15):3776–3785
27. Subhawong TK, Wang X, Durand DJ et al (2012) Proton MR spectroscopy in metabolic assessment of musculoskeletal lesions. AJR Am J Roentgenol 198(1):162–172
28. Sanders TG, Parsons TW 3rd (2001) Radiographic imaging of musculoskeletal neoplasia. Cancer Control 8(3):221–231
29. Roberts CC, Daffner RH, Weissman BN et al (2010) ACR appropriateness criteria on metastatic bone disease. J Am Coll Radiol 7(6):400–409
30. Toomayan GA, Major NM (2011) Utility of CT-guided biopsy of suspicious skeletal lesions in patients with known primary malignancies. AJR Am J Roentgenol 196(2):416–423
31. McCarville MB, Christie R, Daw NC et al (2005) PET/CT in the evaluation of childhood sarcomas. AJR Am J Roentgenol 184(4):1293–1304
32. Treglia G, Salsano M, Stefanelli A et al (2012) Diagnostic accuracy of ^{18}F-FDG-PET and PET/CT in patients with Ewing sarcoma family tumours: a systematic review and a meta-analysis. Skeletal Radiol 41(3):249–256
33. Van der Woude HJ, Vanderschueren G (1999) Ultrasound in musculoskeletal tumors with emphasis on its role in tumor follow-up. Radiol Clin North Am 37(4):753–766
34. Widmann G, Riedl A, Schoepf D et al (2009) State-of-the-art HR-US imaging findings of the most frequent musculoskeletal soft-tissue tumors. Skeletal Radiol 38(7):637–649
35. Inampudi P, Jacobson JA, Fessell DP et al (2004) Soft-tissue lipomas: accuracy of sonography in diagnosis with pathologic correlation. Radiology 233(3):763–767
36. Lin J, Jacobson JA, Fessell DP et al (2000) An illustrated tutorial of musculoskeletal sonography: part 4, musculoskeletal masses, sonographically guided interventions, and miscellaneous topics. AJR Am J Roentgenol 175(6):1711–1719
37. Lee MH, Kim NR, Ryu JA (2010) Cyst-like solid tumors of the musculoskeletal system: an analysis of ultrasound findings. Skeletal Radiol 39(10):981–986
38. Bodner G, Schocke MF, Rachbauer F et al (2002) Differentiation of malignant and benign musculoskeletal tumors: combined color and power Doppler US and spectral wave analysis. Radiology 223(2):410–416
39. Morrison WB, Zoga AC, Daffner RH, et al (2009) Expert panel on musculoskeletal imaging. ACR appropriateness Criteria® primary bone tumors [online publication]. American College of Radiology (ACR), Reston

Benign Bone Tumors

Robert Steffner

Abstract

Benign bone lesions are a broad category that demonstrates a spectrum of activities from latent to aggressive. Differentiating the various tumors is important in order to properly determine necessary intervention. This chapter focuses on the presentation, imaging, diagnostic features, and treatment of the most common benign bone tumors in order to help guide diagnosis and management.

Keywords

Incidental · Latent · Observation · Aggressive · Curettage · Adjuvant

1 Introduction

The true incidence of primary bone lesions is unknown as many are asymptomatic and go undetected unless incidentally discovered. Such lesions can arise due to developmental aberrancies, reactive changes, or localized neoplastic processes. Activity lies on a spectrum from latent to aggressive. All, however, are categorized as benign because their action for the most part is local.

R. Steffner (✉)
Orthopaedic Oncology, UC Davis Comprehensive Cancer Center,
Sacramento, CA, USA
e-mail: robert.steffner@ucdmc.ucdavis.edu

T. D. Peabody and S. Attar (eds.), *Orthopaedic Oncology*,
Cancer Treatment and Research 162, DOI: 10.1007/978-3-319-07323-1_3,
© Springer International Publishing Switzerland 2014

More common in younger individuals, benign bone lesions have varied presentations and varied treatments, ranging from mere observation to en bloc resection. While many benign bone lesions exist, this chapter will focus on the most common. Characteristic features will be described to assist diagnosis and guide appropriate treatment. On a whole, bone tumors are not common. Any uncertainty with diagnosis or management should prompt the consideration to refer to an orthopedic oncologist.

2   Clinical Presentation

Review of demographic information and a detailed history can help to form a working differential diagnosis. It is important to have the patient characterize the location of symptoms and detail events leading up to the evaluation. A clear understanding of symptom onset, duration, intensity, change over time, alleviating/exacerbating factors, attempted interventions, associated constitutional symptoms, and any significant past history such as infection or metabolic problem, is imperative. Surgical and family history is also quite valuable. Specific inquiry should ask about related trauma, pain at rest or at night, and patient's perception of symptom progression. Physical exam localizes the symptomatic area, which is inspected for visible swelling and overlying skin changes. Palpation assesses tenderness, presence of a mass, and pulsations. Nearby joints should be ranged and the neurovascular status of the involved area cataloged. A broader inspection should look for associated deformity, leg-length discrepancy, skin café-au-lait spots, and lymph node swelling.

The physician has a clinical sense after taking a history. If symptoms seem more indicative of another process such as tendon inflammation, if symptoms developed acutely after trauma, or if symptoms are resolving, a latent lesion, perhaps found incidentally, is suspected. Increasing pain localized to a bone or joint, a palpable mass growing in size, pain at rest or at night, or associated weight loss or night sweats—these signs and symptoms raise concern that an active or malignant process may be taking place.

3   Imaging

Radiographs are the next step in management. They are economical, accessible, and provide a wealth of information (Fig. 1). Orthogonal views should be obtained. Additional views are helpful in complex areas such as the ribs, scapula, spine, pelvis, and foot. In addition to location and size, radiographs give an impression of the host bone response to the tumor. The zone of transition from tumor to normal bone characterizes the margin, which reflects the growth rate. A narrow transition is often radio-dense and well-defined—features of a slow process. Surrounding bone has had a chance to react. In a wide transition, it is difficult to delineate the end of tumor and the beginning of normal bone. It reflects a more

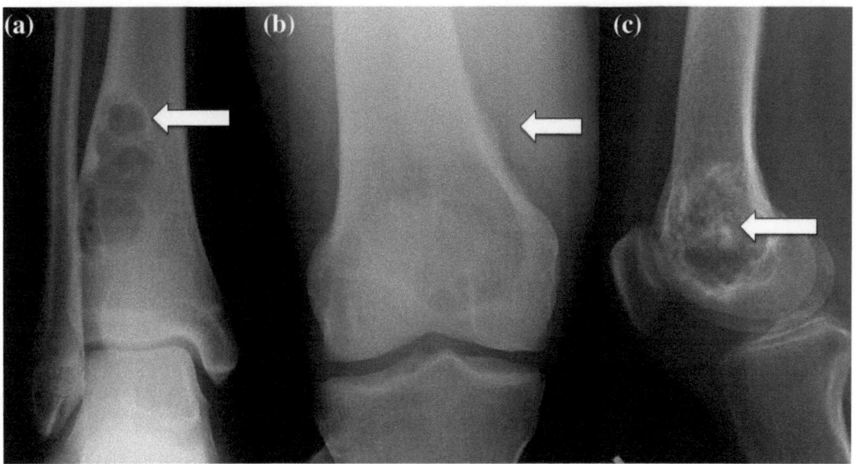

Fig. 1 Host bone response to tumor: zone of transition (**a**) and periosteal reaction (**b**). Intralesional matrix mineralization of a benign bone tumor (**c**)

aggressive process that is overwhelming native bone. Bone destruction is seen on radiographs, which represents at least 30–50 % loss of mineral [1]. Periosteal reaction depicts biologic behavior of the tumor. Benign reaction is often unilaminar while more aggressive lesions have a multilaminar appearance with triangular interfaces where the periosteum is lifted away at the edges from host bone, a phenomenon known as Codman's Triangle [2]. Intralesional mineralization is another feature assessed on radiographs. Its presence offers a clue to the histologic composition of the tumor. Osteoid appears as a fluffy radiodensity; cartilage as stippled or arc calcifications; fibrous as a hazy radiodensity described as "ground glass" [2]. Patients should be asked about any prior imaging of the same region. Comparison gives some perspective on lesion occurrence and progression. Enneking has described features of benign lesions on radiographs. They are characterized as latent, active, or aggressive [3]. Latent appearing lesions do not need further imaging studies. Active or aggressive lesions do.

A computed tomography (CT) scan is indicated in tumors with aggressive features, lesions with suspected matrix mineralization (Fig. 2), and in areas of heavy anatomic overlap such as the sternum, pelvis, acetabulum, and spine. CT provides the best assessment of bony anatomy and excels at qualifying erosion, perforation, and occult fracture. It is the choice study for cortically based lesions and for the risk assessment of impending fractures.

Magnetic resonance imaging (MRI) with intravenous gadolinium adds information about soft tissue, bone marrow, and intra-articular involvement. Signal characteristics on different sequences can be used to gauge lesion composition as well as presence of hemorrhage and/or necrosis (Fig. 3). Comparison of pre and postcontrast fat-suppressed T1 images determines the enhancement of the lesion, which is an indication of its blood supply and an indirect measure of biologic

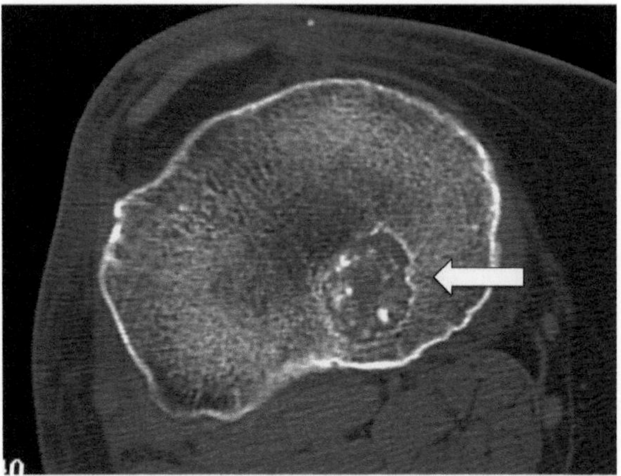

Fig. 2 Matrix mineralization on CT scan

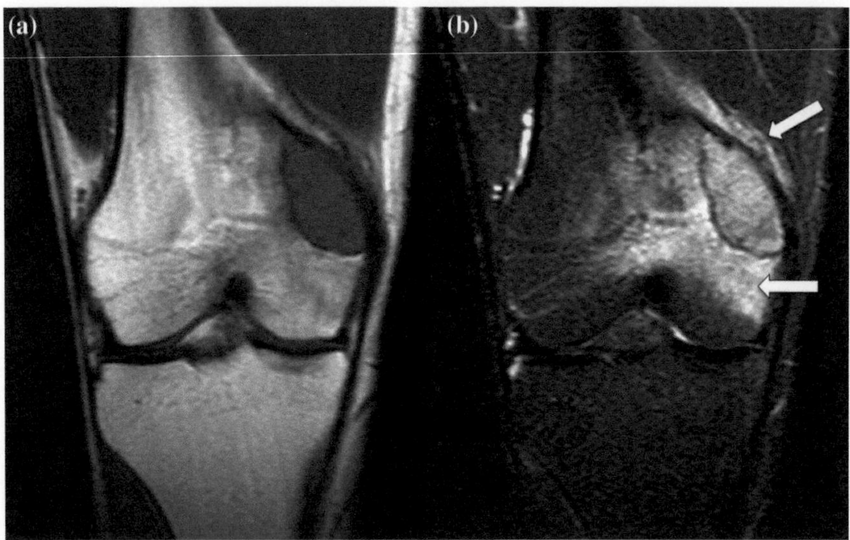

Fig. 3 MRI of a benign bone tumor of the medial femoral condyle: low T1 signal with well-defined anatomy (**a**), High T2 signal with sensitivity to soft tissue and bony edema (*arrows*) (**b**)

activity. Additional MRI sequences further characterize tumor aspects that improve diagnostic accuracy. Dynamic Enhanced MRI differentiates reactive bony edema from tumor extension into bone [4]. Quantitative Dynamic MRI best qualifies the degree of tumor necrosis, an indication of tumor growth [5, 6]. Diffusion Weighted MRI helps in the spine by distinguishing osteoporotic from pathologic vertebral compression fractures [7]. MRI Spectroscopy measures the quantity of certain metabolites in tumors, which helps with diagnosis [8].

Bone scanning with Technetium-99 m assesses osteoblast activity in the primary lesion as well as uncovers additional sites of disease in the skeleton (Fig. 4) [9]. In benign disease this represents multifocal or polyostotic disease, which can be seen with Fibrous Dysplasia, Enchondroma, and Nonossifying Fibroma.

Positron emission tomography (PET) imaging alone or combined with CT or MRI is a diagnostic measure of metabolic activity (Fig. 5). Its role in bone tumors is undetermined. The tracer Fluorodeoxyglucose (^{18}F) is preferentially taken up by cells utilizing cellular glycolysis [8] The degree of uptake, measured in Standard Uptake Values (SUV), can help distinguish benign from malignant tumors. Moreover, SUV can be used to determine lymph node involvement, guide biopsy placement, gauge treatment response, and monitor for recurrence after treatment. The average SUV uptake for benign lesions is 2.18 compared to 4.34 for malignant [10]. The addition of CT and MRI to PET is being investigated as an all-encompassing staging tool but is hampered by an unacceptable rate of false negatives [11].

Most benign bone tumors are evident after clinical evaluation and imaging. There are times, however, when the diagnosis is still unclear and the possibility of malignancy cannot be excluded. Biopsy is then necessary to guide treatment. For bone lesions, CT-guided biopsy is preferred as it allows accurate localization, identifies mineralized areas for sampling, and can be done under anesthetic titrated to patient comfort. The radiologist and orthopedic surgeon should collaborate to plan the biopsy. This avoids unnecessary contamination of normal tissues and maintains a tract that could be excised if needed. In addition, cultures should be taken at the same time as the biopsy.

4   Diagnosis

While pathognomonic findings are rare, a constellation of findings can often be used to sufficiently narrow a differential diagnosis to make treatment decisions. This section will review the characteristic findings for the most common benign tumors of bone as well as elaborate on a few of the common reactive and residual bony changes that mimic bone tumors.

5   Nonossifying Fibroma

Also called fibroxanthoma or, when smaller, fibrous cortical defect (FCD), these lesions are thought to be an abnormal development extending from the growth plate (Fig. 6). They are common, found in, approximately, 30 % of people, and most present as asymptomatic, incidental findings in the first two decades of life [12]. Pain from pathologic fracture can occur and most lesions are found in the lower extremities [13]. On radiographs, lesions are typically radiolucent, eccentric, and cortically based in the metaphysis. They often elongate with skeletal growth and eventually extend into the diaphysis. Bony trabeculae are maintained and the

Fig. 4 Bone scan showing
activity in the distal femur

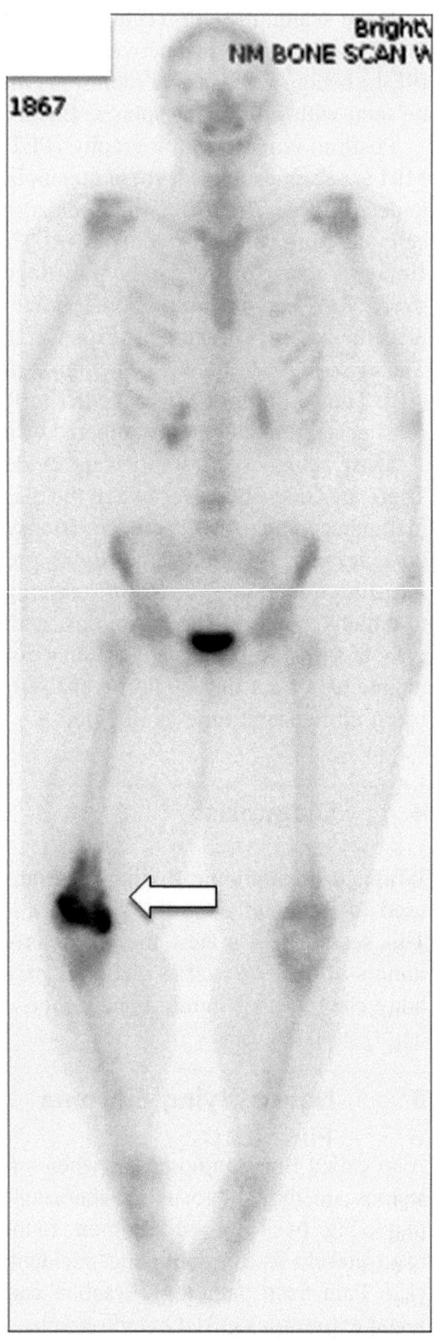

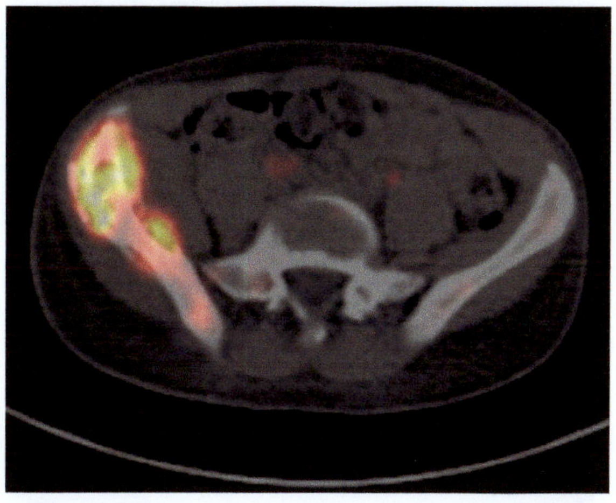

Fig. 5 PET scan with increased metabolic activity in the right ilium

zone of transition is narrow but thin. MRI demonstrates a characteristic low signal on both T1 and T2 sequences without enhancement. High signal on T2 can be seen with an associated stress fracture. Histologically, there is an appearance of fibrous bundles with a mixture of giant cells, lipid-laden macrophages, and hemosiderin with cholesterol clefts. Osteoid can be seen if there has been a recent fracture. The natural history is spontaneous resolution with skeletal maturity. An expanded sclerotic region is typically all that remains in adults [14]. Observation with serial radiographs is adequate for most lesions. The majority of pathologic fractures are treated with weight bearing or activity restrictions with or without immobilization. Twisting is often the mechanism leading to fracture and should be avoided during recovery. Treatment with curettage, grafting, and possibly internal fixation should be considered with displaced fractures, multiple fractures, large lesions at high-risk of fracture, and those that develop a secondary aneurysmal bone cyst (ABC). Recurrence is uncommon and malignant transformation is very rare. Multiple NOFs, café-au-lait skin lesions, and mental retardation characterize Jaffe-Campanacci Syndrome. These patients need to be monitored for symptomatic lesions. There is no increased risk of malignant transformation [15, 16].

6 Fibrous Dysplasia

FD is a spontaneous developmental anomaly leading to an area of fibrous tissue and nonossified bone (Fig. 7), usually diagnosed in the first three decades of life, it is commonly located in the femur, tibia, ilium, skull, and rib. Most cases present as incidental findings or as pain secondary to pathologic fracture. Eighty percent of lesions are monostotic with the remainder polyostotic [17]. Radiographs demonstrate a centered, medullary based radiolucent lesion in the metaphysis and/or diaphysis with bony expansion and loculations. Sclerotic rims are seen in the

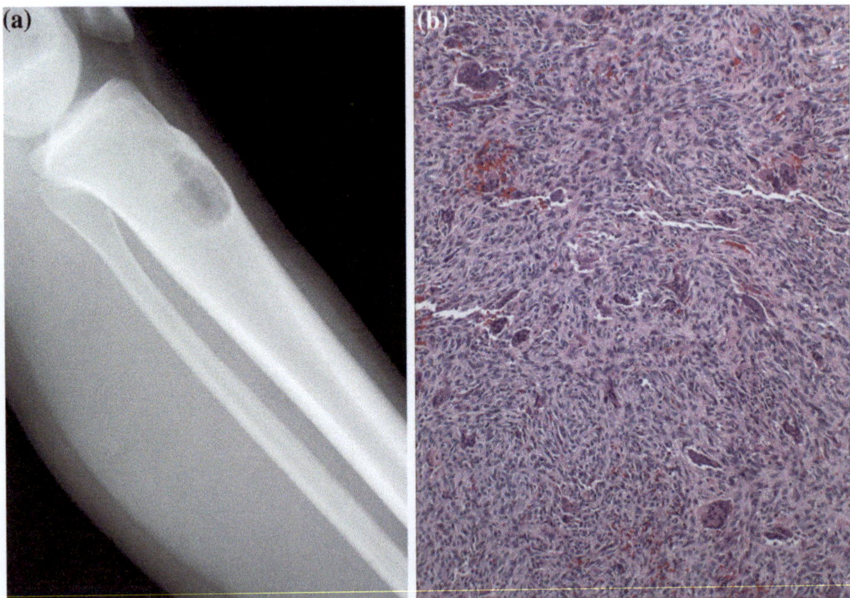

Fig. 6 Radiograph (**a**) and histology (**b**) of a Nonossifying Fibroma

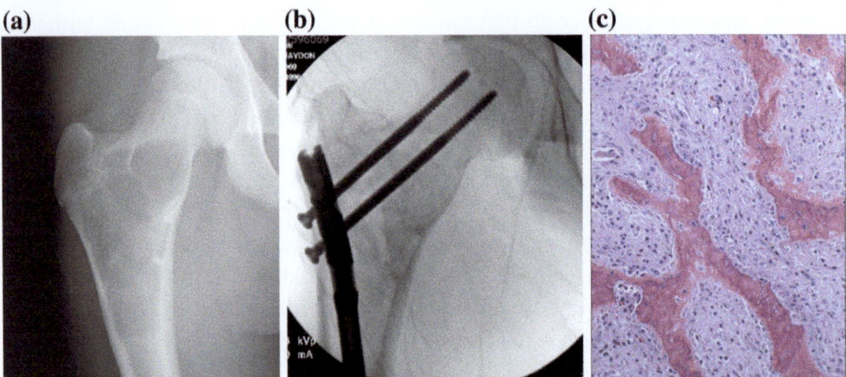

Fig. 7 Fibrous dysplasia of the right femur on radiograph (**a**), after internal fixation for impending fracture and developing varus deformity (**b**), and on histology (**c**)

proximal and distal aspects of the lesion within the medullary canal. The zone of transition is narrow and often sclerotic. Internal matrix on radiographs has a hazy central appearance described as "ground glass" with a radiolucent rim [14]. Deformity can occur through repeated stress fractures with varus alignment of the proximal femur (Shepherd Crook's Deformity) being common [18]. MRI is low on T1 and variable on T2. T2 high signal may represent bony edema secondary to fracture. Enhancement is serpiginous. Bone scan demonstrates activity. These lesions get larger with skeletal growth and rarely resolve spontaneously. They are usually present throughout life. Histology shows fibrous tissue with islands of woven bone absent of osteoblastic rimming. Pathologists describe spicules of woven bone as having an "alphabet soup" appearance. Most are observed with serial radiographs. Nondisplaced fractures or stress responses can be treated with weight bearing or activity modification with or without immobilization. Curettage, grafting, and possible internal fixation is indicated with displaced fractures, multiple fractures, worsening deformity, impending fractures, and secondary ABC (arising out of FD). Due to the metabolic origin most lesions recur after curettage, and therefore any internal fixation should be placed with long-term intention for structural support. Any resolved areas will show patchy sclerosis on radiographs. Transformation into malignancy is rare. It is foreshadowed by increasing pain, swelling, cortical destruction, and an associated soft tissue mass [13]. Polyostotic FD usually affects one side of the body and can be associated with precocious puberty and café-au-lait spots in McCune-Albright and with soft tissue intramuscular myxomas in Mazabraud Syndrome [8, 19]. Polyostotic forms are best detected on bone scan and benefit from evaluation by an endocrinologist. Bisphosphonate or RANK ligand inhibitor therapy may be considered in adults.

7   Osteofibrous Dysplasia

OFD is a fibrous defect of unknown origin in bone (Fig. 8). It presents as painless, progressive swelling or as local tenderness when associated with pathological fracture. Most cases occur in the first decade of life and are localized to the anterior tibial cortex, rarely the fibula [13]. Radiographs demonstrate a cortically based radiolucent area with multiloculated cysts and expansile features. Internal matrix is generally mixed lytic and sclerotic. Anterior or anterolateral bowing of the tibia can be seen. MRI shows intermediate T1 and high T2 signal as well as enhancement with contrast. Bone scan is active. Histology shows a vascularized fibrous stroma with spicules of woven bone rimmed by osteoblasts. Mitoses and giant cells can be present [20, 21]. Treatment is observation. Most lesions remain static and regress with advancing age [22]. Deformity can be braced and rarely requires osteotomy. There is a low threshold to biopsy of these lesions because of the similar appearance to the low-grade epithelial malignancy adamantinoma. Adequate sample should be sent during biopsy to avoid sampling error. Curettage, grafting, and possible internal fixation can be considered for persistent pain, risk of pathologic fracture, and worsening deformity. Follow-up is life-long to assure OFD is not an indolent adamantinoma. Sudden growth, invasion of the medullary canal, and development of a soft tissue mass are indications to pursue biopsy.

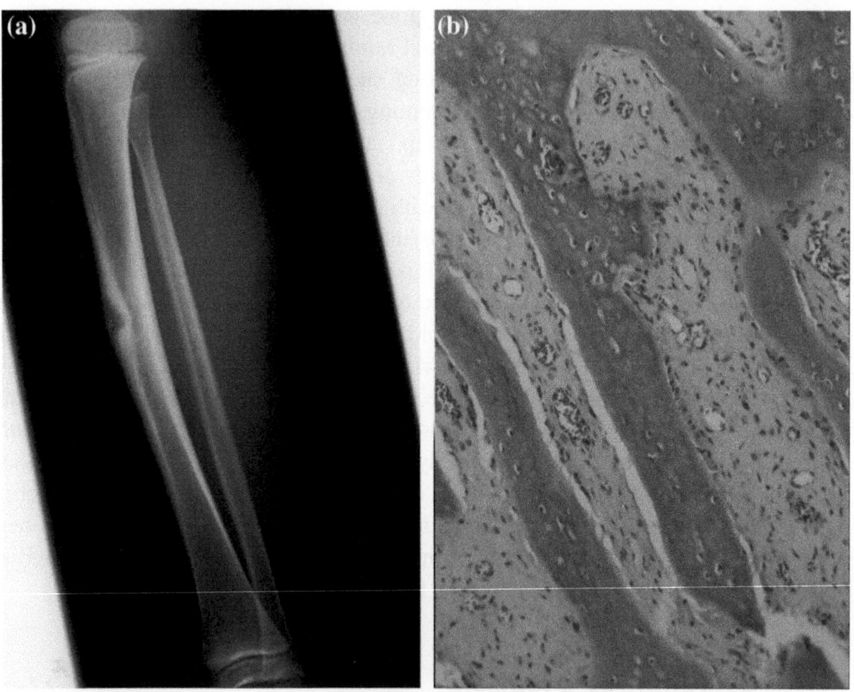

Fig. 8 Radiograph (**a**) and histology (**b**) of osteofibrous dysplasia

8   Enchondroma

EC is a rest of hyaline cartilage within the medullary canal of long bones and tubular bones of the hands and feet (Fig. 9) comprising 12–24 % of benign bone tumors, they are often painless and incidentally found [23]. EC can present with pain due to pathologic fracture. Peak incidence is in the third decade of life. Radiographs generally show a central radiolucent lesion in the metaphysis with lobular margins and a narrow zone of transition [24]. Matrix mineralization can be variable, but characteristically occurs as "rings and arcs" and is best identified on CT scan [13]. Mineralization is usually absent in the hands and feet. MRI shows uniform low signal on T1 sequence. T2 sequence has a high signal secondary to the water content of hyaline cartilage with small areas of low signal representing mineralization. There should not be MRI enhancement or bone scan activity. Histology demonstrates hyaline cartilage with sparse chondrocytes with no nuclear atypia or mitotic figures. Hand ECs look more aggressive under the microscope. Treatment consists of observation with serial radiographs. Curettage and grafting with optional internal fixation may be considered for multiple fractures, impending fracture, or painful lesions. EC should not progress or recur. Any clinical indication of increasing pain or imaging showing progressive growth, endosteal scalloping,

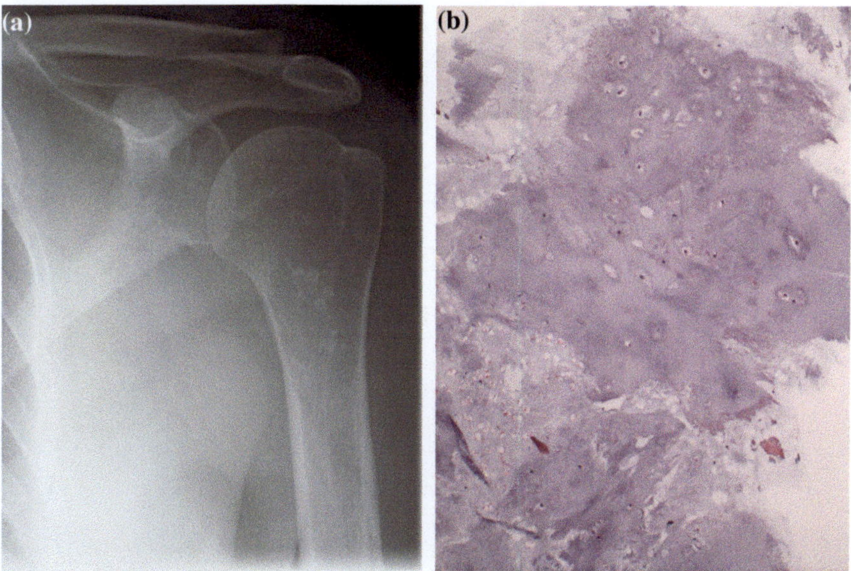

Fig. 9 Radiograph (**a**) and histology (**b**) of an enchondroma

cortical destruction, or a soft tissue mass should warrant a biopsy to assess for secondary chondrosarcoma [24]. Isolated lesions rarely transform. Larger and more proximal lesions are at greatest risk [14]. Hand ECs are exceedingly rare to transform despite their histologic appearance [13]. Noninherited conditions with multiple ECs exist. They often affect one side of the body and are at greater risk of secondary transformation, which occurs in adulthood. Ollier's Disease consists of multiple EC whereas Maffucci Syndrome is multiple EC with soft tissue hemangiomas and/or lymphangiomas. With either, there is a 20–30 % chance of malignant transformation [25]. In adulthood, these patients should be monitored with periodic chest CT and whole body bone scan. Areas with activity on bone scan are investigated further with MRI. There is a fine line between the diagnosis of EC and grade 1 chondrosarcoma. The latter is treated with intralesional curettage and grafting. More aggressive chondrosarcomas are widely excised.

9 Osteochondroma

OC or exostosis is a surface lesion of bone (Fig. 10). It is thought to be physeal cartilage displaced onto the longitudinal surface of bone. A common benign bone tumor, it is noticed as a painless mass near joints in the first two decades of life. Symptoms may be present from traumatic fracture or mass effect, as OCs grow with the patient. Affected extremities should be inspected for associated deformity and leg-length discrepancy. Lesions can occur in any bone undergoing endochondral

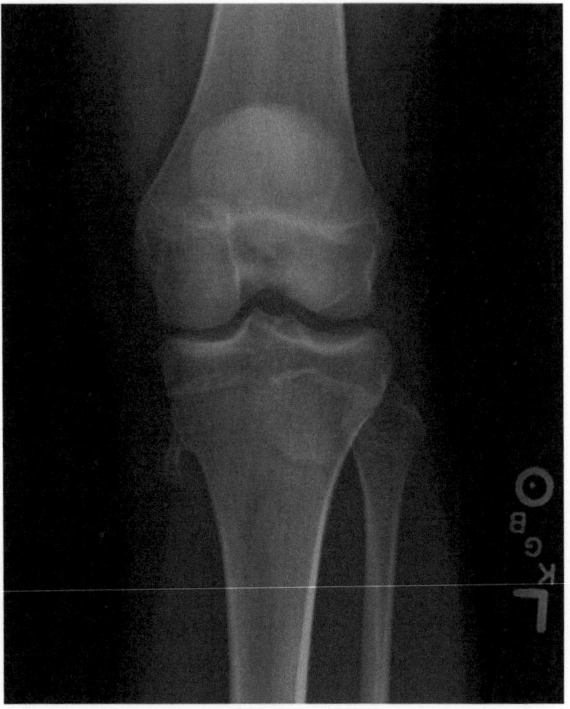

Fig. 10 Radiograph of an osteochondroma

ossification. The knee, ilium, and scapula are common locations. On radiographs, a bony growth is seen at the metaphysis aiming away from the joint. CT scan demonstrates cortical and medullary continuity between the OC and host bone. MRI shows nonspecific low T1 and high T2 signal of the surface. The top of the OC is composed of a cartilage cap connected to native bone with a pedunculated or sessile stalk. Histology shows lamellar bone connected to a hyaline cartilage cap covered by a perichondrium of dense collagen [26, 27]. Endochondral ossification is seen in the cap until skeletal maturity. Treatment consists of observation and symptom control. If symptoms persist or worsen despite medical intervention, marginal excision is considered. It is best to wait until OCs move away from the physis to avoid growth arrest after surgery. OCs stop growing at skeletal maturity. Malignant transformation of isolated OC is rare and occurs in adulthood. It is preceded by sudden growth and increasing pain. Radiographs show cortical erosion of the osseous protuberance [18, 19]. MRI is indicated to assess the cartilage cap. An irregular cap with incomplete calcification and thickness 2 cm or more is highly suspicious for secondary chondrosarcoma [28, 29]. At times, it can be difficult to distinguish adventitial bursae from a cartilage cap. Use of ultrasound or contrast MRI can help differentiate. Patients with the familial autosomal dominant condition known as multiple hereditary exostosis (MHE) have polyostotic OCs and a 5 % risk of malignant transformation. Transformation is more likely in the pelvis, scapula, and proximal femur [30]; areas the lesion can grow undetected for some time. MHE patients need to be routinely followed with clinical exams throughout life. Symptomatic areas should be X-rayed and surveillance pelvis radiographs should be obtained every 5 years. A developmental disorder known as Trevor's Disease or Dysplasia Epiphysealis Hemimelica (DEH) is characterized by OC of the epiphysis in a single extremity [13]. These point toward the joint and are treated the same way as isolated OC with the same risk of malignant transformation.

10   Chondromyxoid Fibroma

CMF is a rare bone lesion of unknown origin that frequently presents as a palpable mass or localized swelling (Fig. 11). Pain is variable and pathologic fracture is uncommon. The majority of patients are male in the second to third decades of life [13]. Prevalent locations are the foot, pelvis, and knee. Radiographs show a well-defined radiolucent lesion that is eccentric in the metaphysis. The zone of transition is narrow with variable thickness. CT scan demonstrates lobules and a paucity of matrix mineralization. MRI signal is low on T1 and high on T2. Nodules of dense cartilage between fibromyxoid areas characterize the histology. The zonal architecture shows well-defined areas of mixed cellularity with occasional giant cells. These lesions expand and become symptomatic. Intralesional curettage and grafting with or without internal fixation is the preferred treatment. Recurrence is approximately 25 % after curettage alone [31]. En bloc excision is considered after multiple recurrences.

11   Chondroblastoma

CB is an uncommon bone tumor of unknown origin (Fig. 12). Occurrence is more frequent in males in the first two decades of life [13]. Most patients present with joint pain and restricted motion. The knee, shoulder, hip, and heel bones are typical locations. Radiographs show an epiphyseal or apophyseal radiolucent lesion with a narrow zone of transition. The thin surrounding rim may be expansile. Marked cortical destruction is associated with secondary ABC formation, which occurs in 15 % of CBs [13]. Lacelike matrix mineralization can be seen on CT, along with scalloped borders and periosteal reaction. Notable inflammation produces high signal marrow edema on T2, which surrounds the low to intermediate signal of the tumor. T1 signal is low. Bone scan is active [8]. Plump chondroblasts with giant cells are seen among calcifications spread out in a pattern described as "chickenwire" on histologic review. These lesions are progressive and increasingly painful. Treatment is intralesional with curettage and grafting with or without internal fixation. Some success has been demonstrated with radiofrequency ablation (RFA) [32]. Care must be taken with any treatment to avoid damage to nearby growth plates and articular cartilage. Recurrence depends on the type and adequacy of treatment and ranges from 5 to 20 % [33].

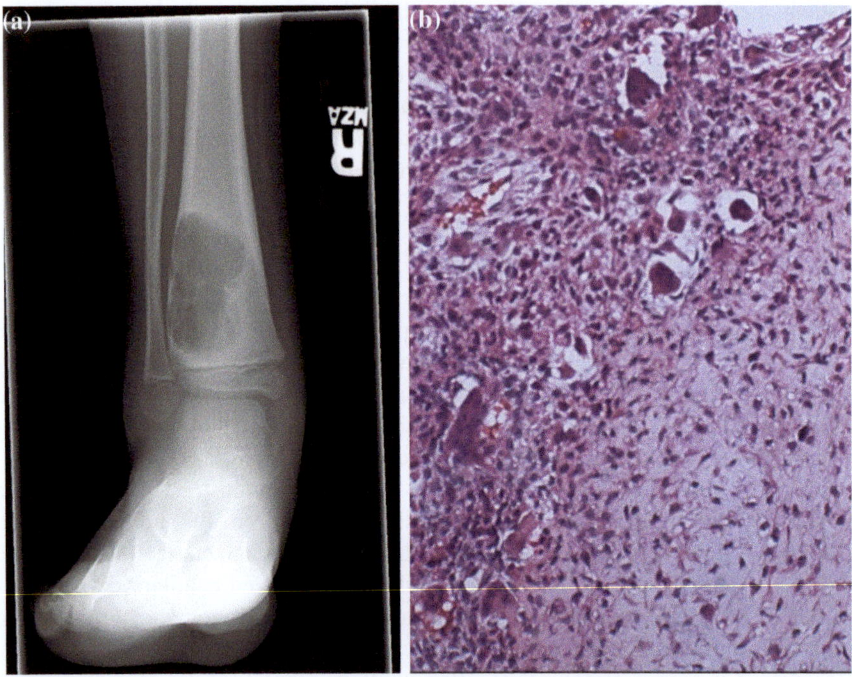

Fig. 11 Radiograph (**a**) and histology (**b**) of chondromyxoid fibroma

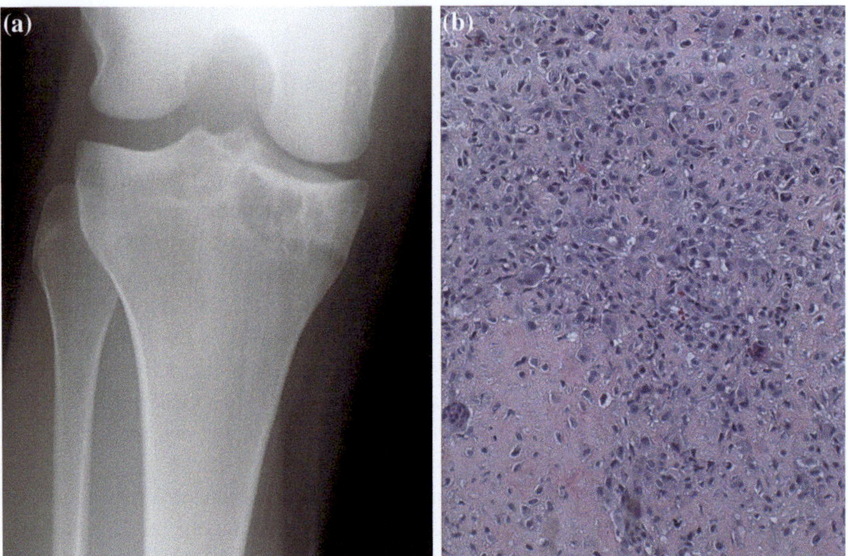

Fig. 12 Radiograph (**a**) and histology (**b**) of Chondroblastoma

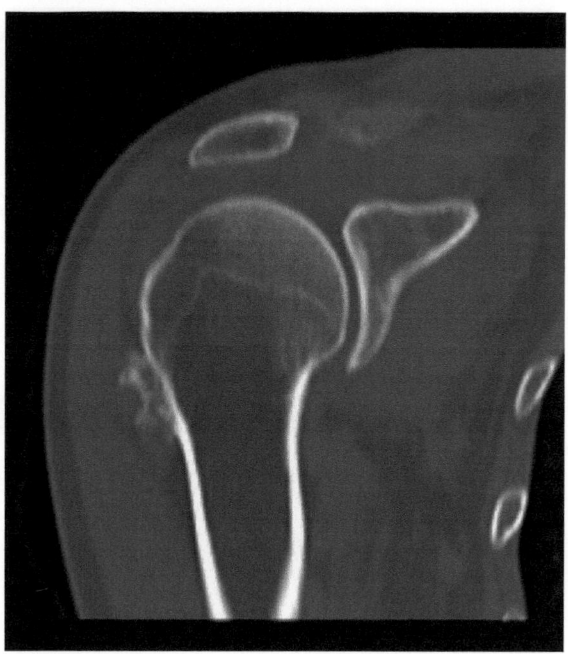

Fig. 13 CT scan of a proximal humeral periosteal chondroma

12 Periosteal Chondroma

Periosteal or juxtacortical chondroma is rare and the origin unknown (Fig. 13). Focal swelling is the most common presentation and men in the second and third decades of life are the most affected [13]. Frequent locations include the distal femur, proximal femur, proximal humerus, hands and feet. Radiographs show a lesion extending from the metaphyseal cortex pushing into soft tissue, appearing as a "soap bubble." Sclerosis is prominent between the lesion and the medullary canal and the outer metaphyseal cortex is frequently saucerized from pressure. The periosteum is lifted up and some reaction may be visible. CT scan best demonstrates the thin cortical shell and variable mineralized matrix. Signals are low T1 and high T2 on MRI [13]. The lesion does not enhance but overlying bursae may. Bone scan is cold. Bland chondrocytes in lacunae with surrounding endochondral ossification is seen on histology. Lesions may be observed, but their behavior is typically progressive. When symptomatic, intralesional curettage and grafting with or without internal fixation is performed. Recurrence is unlikely.

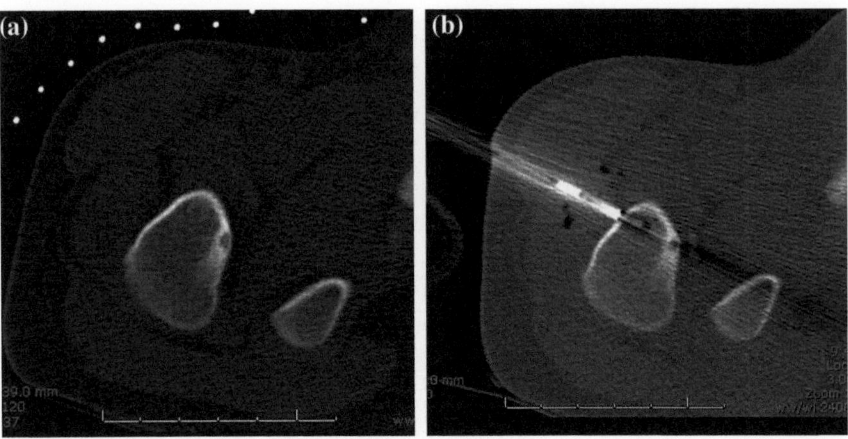

Fig. 14 Axial CT scan of an osteoid osteoma (**a**). Treatment with CT guided radiofrequency ablation (**b**)

13   Osteoid Osteoma

Osteoid osteomas comprise around 12 % of benign bone tumors [34, 35] (Fig. 14). Their cause is unknown. They characteristically present in the first three decades and occur more often in males [36]. Most patients have localized pain that worsens at night. Additional symptoms vary by location. Long bone OOs, most common in the metadiaphysis of the femur and tibia, have tenderness, swelling, and muscle atrophy [37–39]. Intra-articular lesions close to growth plates may have a joint effusion, limb overgrowth, limb deformity, abnormal gait, joint contracture, and limited range of motion [38, 40]. Twenty percent of OOs occur in the posterior elements of the spine, they present with back pain and scoliotic deformity. The curve is secondary to muscle spasm and the lesion can be found on the concave side of the curve [13]. Tumors are usually less than 1 cm and are most often cortically based, although they can be subperiosteal, intraarticular, or in cancellous bone. OOs can be hard to see on radiographs. An isolated area of reactive cortical thickening from periosteal bone formation can be seen. Close scrutiny of X-rays and a high-index of suspicion lead to further imaging with thin slice CT or bone scan. Axial CT shows a mineralized osseous nidus with a lucent halo and surrounding thick spherical or ovoid sclerosis. Bone scan shows increased activity. MRI can be misleading as intense soft tissue and bone marrow edema obscures the lesion and appears as a large mass. This can lead to a futile work-up for malignancy or infection [32, 41]. Osteoid and woven bone lined with osteoblasts and richly innervated with surrounding hypervascular connective tissue with osteoclasts is seen on histology [42]. OOs do not malignantly transform [37, 43]. Debilitating symptoms justify treatment. Pain has been linked to elevated cyclooxygenase expression and subsequent increased prostaglandin (PG) synthesis

[44, 45]. Nonsteroidal Antiinflammatory Drugs (NSAIDs) or salicylates inhibit PG synthesis and are the first-line of treatment. Patients must be screened for renal insufficiency, gastrointestinal bleeding, and stomach ulcerations before initiating treatment. Concomitant use of a medication to reduce stomach acid as well as periodic lab draws to assess anemia and renal function is recommended. It takes an average of 33 months on therapy for symptoms to resolve [46]. When NSAIDs are contraindicated or the patient/family does not want to pursue medical therapy because of progressive deformity, growth disturbance, arthritis, rigid scoliosis, or pain, percutaneous, or open techniques are employed. CT-guided excision and RFA are both effective percutaneous techniques. Excision obtains sufficient pathologic tissue for a more reliable histologic diagnosis, but creates a larger bone defect raising the risk of postoperative fracture [47]. RFA has become very popular and eliminates 80 % of lesions with one treatment, 96 % with two [48]. Pathologic diagnosis can be obtained, but it is not as reliable. RFA is cost-effective and allows early weight bearing with only activity modification for 3 months [49, 50]. Subcutaneous and intra-articular lesions as well as OOs close to critical structures are best treated with open curettage or en bloc resection with or without internal fixation. The risk to adjacent structures is too great to use RFA. Recurrence is most common in the 6 months following a procedure [51]. Risk is around 10 % with an indirect correlation with age [32]. Recurrence is treated in the same manner as the sentinel lesion.

14 Osteoblastoma

A rare osteoid producing tumor that is histologically indistinguishable from OO (Fig. 15). OB has a larger nidus ($\geq$2 cm) and clinical behavior that is more aggressive. It comprises 3 % of benign bone tumors, presents in the second and third decades, and is two times more common in men [34]. Long bone location is common. Symptoms are progressive swelling and achy pain. One-third of patients have lesions in the posterior elements of the spine, most often the lumbar and sacral regions [52]. Symptoms are neurologic compression and scoliosis. Pain is not worse at night and is not relieved by NSAIDs [13]. On average, patients have 2 years of symptoms before presenting for evaluation [53]. A geographic eccentric lesion with a narrow zone of transition, expansion, and variable ossified matrix is typically seen. Four to fourteen percent have a multifocal central nidus [53, 54]. Aggressive features such as cortical disruption, periosteal reaction, and soft tissue mass are possible. Matrix mineralization, cortical margin, and spinopelvic location are best visualized on CT. MRI detects bone marrow and soft tissue inflammation, but it does not obscure the lesion as in OO. Signal is low to intermediate on T1 and intermediate to high on T2 [55]. MRI shows lesion proximity to neural foramina and spinal cord [56]. Bone scan is active due to increased osteoblast activity. Secondary ABC occurs in approximately 15 % of lesions. Imaging shows aggressive changes when this occurs [57]. An osteoid nidus with rimming osteoblasts surrounded by a fibrovascular stroma with osteoclasts is the histologic

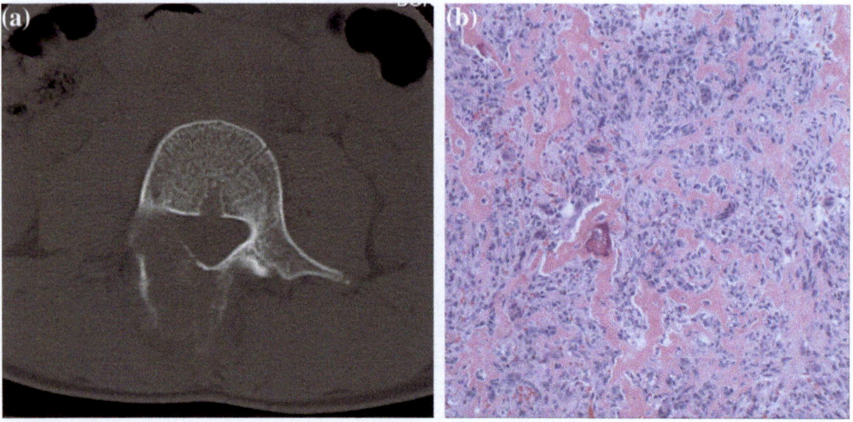

Fig. 15 Axial CT scan of the spine (**a**) and histology (**b**) of an Osteoblastoma of the posterior elements of the L4 lumbar vertebrae

appearance [36]. More aggressive lesions tend to have large epitheloid-like osteoblasts that are mitotically active [54, 55]. OBs do not have malignant or metastatic potential, but they are progressive and lead to pain, bone destruction, spine instability, and neural compression if untreated. Intralesional curettage and grafting with or without internal fixation for stability is the preferred treatment. Recurrent, refractory, or particularly aggressive lesions should be considered for en bloc resection. Recurrence risk is related to the adequacy of resection and is higher than OO at 10–24 % [52]. It is important to distinguish OB from low-grade osteosarcoma as both form osteoid and bone.

15 Unicameral Bone Cyst

UBCs are true cysts with unknown origins (Fig. 16). They occur more frequently in males and are diagnosed in the first two decades. Pathologic fracture and incidental finding are the most common presentations. Frequent locations include the proximal humerus and proximal femur in children [14]. Adults may have lesions in the calcaneus and ilium, which usually appear adjacent to the sacroiliac joint. Radiolucent central metaphyseal lesions with mild expansion and a narrow zone of transition characterize radiographs. UBCs often abut growth plates and move away with skeletal growth. A "fallen leaf" sign, where a fracture fragment falls to the dependent portion of the lesion, is seen in approximately 5 % of lesions [18, 19]. Loculations and pathologic fracture can best be seen on CT. MRI shows low T1 and high T2 signal with rim enhancement typical of a cyst [14]. A single layer of mesothelial cells comprises the cyst wall and is seen in conjunction with pressurized serous fluid on histology [13]. Osteoid may be seen when there is a pathologic fracture. UBCs tend to elongate with skeletal growth and then spontaneously fill-in at maturity. Most can be observed with pathologic fractures

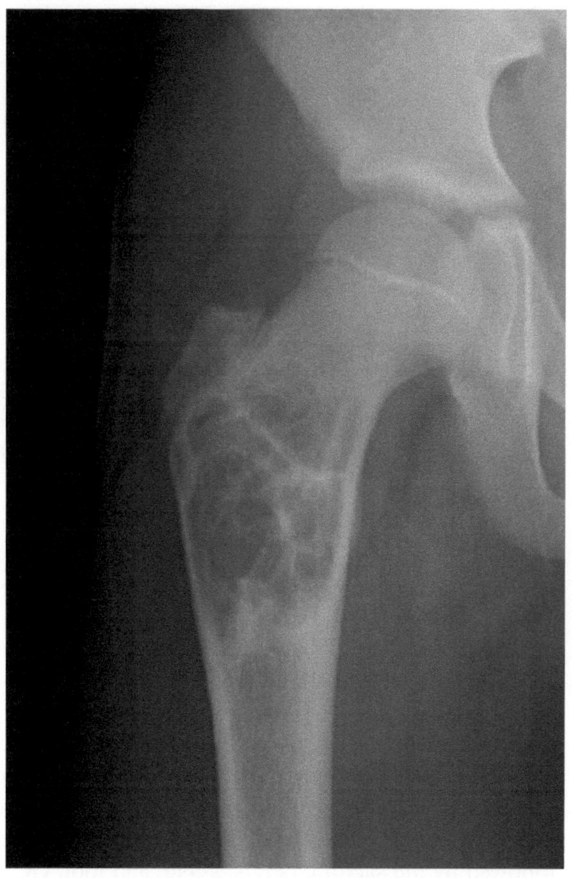

Fig. 16 Radiograph of a right proximal femur unicameral bone cyst

treated conservatively. Patients with large lesions at a young age or multiple fractures can be considered for treatment. Aspiration of the brown fluid for cytologic diagnosis, followed by injection of various substances can be done to try and stimulate healing and spontaneous filling. Common injected substances include steroids, bone marrow aspirate, and demineralized bone matrix (DBM). Multiple injections are usually needed. Venting is done during injection to prevent pressurization and embolization. Injections close to the physis can risk growth arrest and should be done with caution. Curettage and grafting with or without internal fixation is performed in older children and adolescents. These lesions are safe for an open procedure because they are further away from the physis and articular cartilage. Recurrence risk is 25–50 % with a greater likelihood associated with younger age [58]. UBCs in high-risk locations such as the femoral neck are treated with weight bearing and/or activity restrictions, aspiration and injection, or rarely, curettage with either placement of allograft cortical strut (younger patients) or internal fixation (postpubertal or >13 years old).

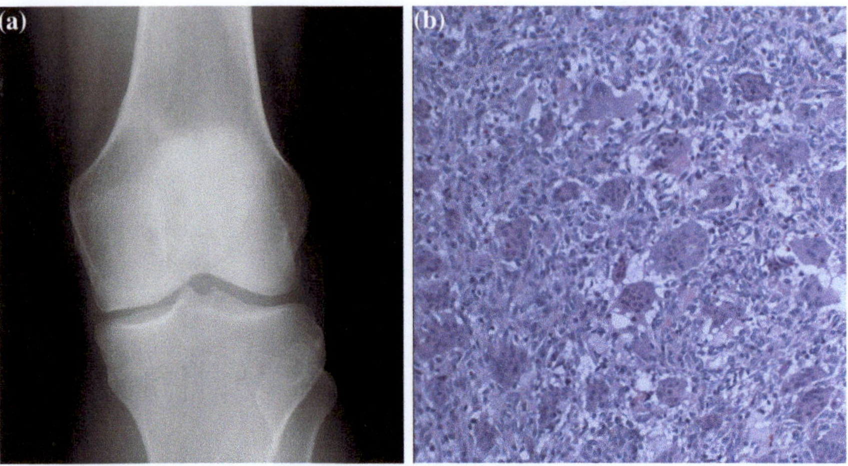

Fig. 17 Radiograph (**a**) and histology (**b**) of a lateral femoral condyle giant cell tumor

16   Giant Cell Tumor

GCTs are neoplasms of unknown origin (Fig. 17). They comprise 15–20 % of benign bone tumors [59]. Occurrence is usually in the third to fourth decades with a slight prevalence in females. Clustering has been identified with Paget's Disease, Chinese ancestry, and some families [13, 60–63]. Progressive pain and swelling are presenting symptoms. Pathologic fracture is associated in 30 % of patients [64, 65]. The distal femur, proximal tibia, and distal radius are the most common locations, followed by the sacrum, pelvis, ankle, and foot. GCT may be hormone responsive and worsen during pregnancy or with oral contraceptives [13]. Demonstrated as an eccentric radiolucent expansile mass in the epiphysis on X-ray, there is a narrow zone of transition that may be faint. Aggressive features such as cortical destruction, periosteal reaction, and bone loss are not uncommon. The cortical rim, remaining subchondral bone, and lack of internal matrix are best appreciated on CT. MRI may show a soft tissue component along with low to intermediate T1 and low T2 signal, which is secondary to high cellularity and hemosiderin [66, 67]. Lesions are vascular and show MRI enhancement [8]. PET activity is enhanced due to an elevated level of ATP-dependent proton pumps in the giant cells [68, 69]. Numerous multinucleated giant cells are seen among a bland mononuclear background with similar appearing nuclei on microscopic review [70]. GCT is a progressive, destructive tumor. Secondary ABC is common and can be responsible for sudden aggressive behavior. Treatment is intralesional with curettage and grafting/cementing with or without internal fixation. Around 3 % of GCTs metastasize to the lung [71]. All newly diagnosed patients should obtain chest imaging. Any metastatic foci are often indolent and are either observed or marginally excised via thoracotomy [72]. Progressive or numerous metastases warrant Imatinib (Novartis, East Hanover, NJ) or

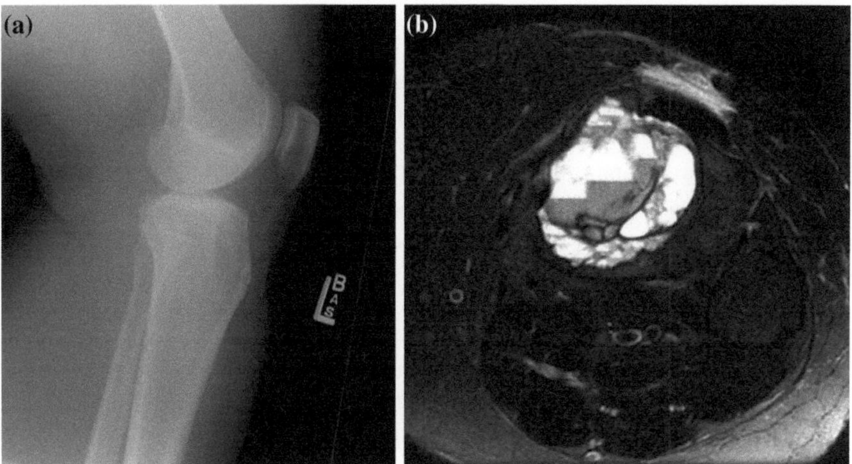

Fig. 18 Lateral radiograph (**a**) and T2 axial MRI (**b**) of a left proximal tibia aneurysmal bone cyst with characteristic fluid-fluid levels

chemotherapy, often with Adriamycin and Cisplatin [73]. Refractory, multiply recurrent, and particularly aggressive lesions may undergo en bloc excision. Inaccessible and difficult to treat areas such as the spine, skull base, pelvis, and sacrum in adults and adolescents have few options. Recently approved by the FDA, systemic treatment with monoclonal antibody to RANK ligand appears effective. Immature osteoblast-like cells in the GCT stroma lead to high expression of RANK ligand by the tumor. Blocking RANK ligand binding to the RANK receptor on monocytes prevents osteoclast-like giant cell activation and bone destruction [74]. Uncoupling osteoblast activation of osteoclasts removes bone as a source of calcium, putting patients on RANK ligand inhibitors at risk of hypocalcemia [75]. The safety of these medications, especially in the developing skeleton and with long-term use, is relatively unknown. Bisphosphonates can also be used. Zoledronic Acid (Novartis, East Hanover, NJ) is the most effective and works through the direct inhibition of osteoclasts [76]. Radiation, embolization, and RFA are other considerations infrequently used. Local recurrence rates are approximately 20 % after curettage. Most receive a second curettage, which works as well as primary curettage [77]. Patients need to be monitored with radiographs for lesion recurrence and pulmonary metastases, which develop an average of 3.8 years after initial diagnosis [73].

17   Aneurysmal Bone Cyst

ABCs have a controversial etiology (Fig. 18). Currently, they are thought to result from a translocation where a ubiquitin-specific protease becomes over-expressed and leads to activation of matrix metalloproteinases that remodel bone matrix and increase vascular endothelial growth factor (VEGF) [78]. Primary ABCs occur in the first two decades and present with localized pain and swelling. On average, patients endure 6 months of pain before presenting to a physician [27]. In the spine, patients can present with nerve root or spinal cord impingement. Long bones are the most common site, followed by the pelvis and posterior elements of the spine [13]. The thoracolumbar region is most affected and 30–40 % of lesions extend multiple levels [27]. A radiolucent eccentric expansile lesion in the metaphysis is the typical radiographic appearance. The zone of transition is narrow. ABCs actively enlarge and a thin outer rim develops that can show signs of destruction and periosteal reaction, which is best seen on CT scan. No mineralized matrix is present. MRI demonstrates variable T1 and T2 signal due to internal blood products of different age and surrounding bone edema [79]. Reactive edema can be an indicator of aggression. The most characteristic finding is fluid-fluid levels, best seen on axial MRI. Internal septa enhance with contrast [8]. Secondary ABCs develop out of preexisting benign bone tumors, most commonly GCT, OB, and CB [14]. Spindle cell fibrous septae with numerous lining osteoclast-like giant cells around woven bone trabeculae and cavernous blood-filled spaces is the histologic appearance [80]. There is no endothelial lining and vessels are thin-walled [27]. Given the progressive nature of ABCs, their treatment is surgical. Accessible lesions receive intralesional treatment with curettage and grafting with or without internal fixation. Preoperative embolization is considered to minimize intraoperative blood loss. Aggressive and recurrent lesions as well as lesions in expendable bones should be considered for en bloc resection. Inaccessible lesions are treated with embolization or alcohol-based sclerotherapy. Recurrence is best detected with MRI and the risk is approximately 10–20 % with curettage. Repeating prior treatment is acceptable and effectiveness is equivalent. Most recurrences are in the 2 years following treatment [27]. It is important to differentiate these lesions from telangiectatic osteosarcomas.

18 Eosinophilic Granuloma

EOG is an inflammatory bone lesion from Langerhan Cell Histiocytosis (LCH), which is considered a disease of the reticuloendothelial system (Fig. 19). It presents in the first decade, more often in males, and usually as a solitary lesion, although it can be multifocal [81, 82]. Multifocal involvement occurs in one-third of spine lesions and is typically seen in younger patients [27]. Pain, restricted motion, and spine deformity are frequent presenting symptoms. Flat bones, long bones, and anterior elements of the spine are common locations. The thoracic region is often affected in the spine. An aggressive mixed density lesion with variable zone of transition and associated periosteal reaction with a central location in the vertebral body or long bone diaphysis is the classic radiographic appearance. Vertebral bodies can show asymmetric wedge collapse or symmetric flattening known as "vertebrae plane." This can lead to a kyphotic deformity [81, 83]. Disk spaces are maintained and soft tissue mass is absent. CT defines cortical anatomy and MRI is

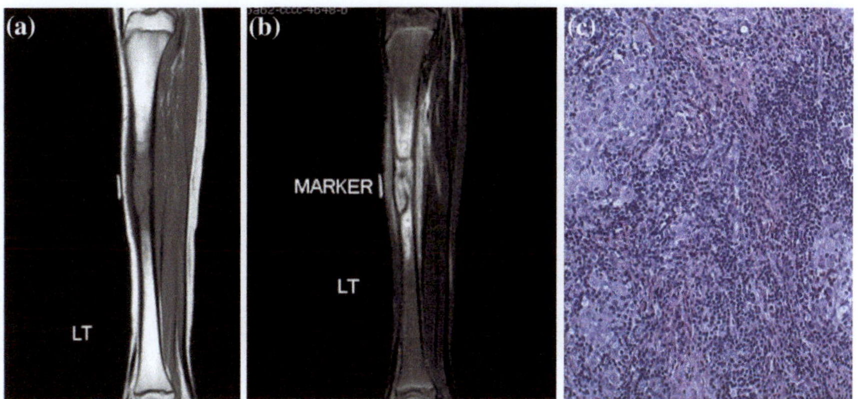

Fig. 19 T1 MRI (**a**), T2 MRI (**b**), and histology of Eosinophilic Granuloma

nonspecific low T1 and high T2 signal with contrast enhancement. A ring of new lamellar bone can often be seen on axial CT and MRI, giving a target sign. Bone scan demonstrates variable activity with EOG and therefore a skeletal survey is preferred to look for multifocal involvement. Punched out radiolucent lesions are often seen in the skull in systemic disease. Histology shows a mix of histiocytes, lymphocytes, eosinophils, and polymorphonuclear cells (PMNs). Histiocytes stain S100, CD1a, and CD68 positive and have a grooved nucleus with tennis racquet shaped organelles in the cytoplasm called "Birbeck granules," which are best seen under Electron Microscopy [27]. Cells are generally uniform and lack atypia. On imaging, EOG looks very similar to marrow cell tumors and infection. Blood work may show an elevated ESR and Ferritin, which can help with diagnosis. Biopsy, however, is usually performed. It is important to take cultures at the same time as biopsy. Isolated EOG lesions resolve spontaneously and only require symptom management, activity restriction, and observation with serial radiographs in limbs and MRI in the spine. With spinal deformity, bracing helps prevent progression. Some reconstitution of vertebral body height occurs with lesion resolution [27]. When refractory to bracing, surgery may be necessary to halt progression of deformity. Intralesional curettage is recommended for aggressive and impending fracture lesions. Internal fixation may be used to support bone as the disease runs its course. Multifocal EOG exists on its own or as part of a disease constellation. Multifocal EOG warrants a CT scan to look for visceral involvement and a referral to see a medical oncologist to consider low-dose chemotherapy and/or steroids to control disease until resolution. There are two disease constellations. Letterer-Siwe is associated with hepatosplenomegaly and anemia. It is seen in children less than 3 years old and universally fatal. Hand-Schuller-Christian Disease has dissemnated visceral involvement with exopthalmos and Diabetes Insipidus [27]. Medical management is indicated. Recurrence of EOG is rare in skeletally immature patients and more likely in adults [82, 83].

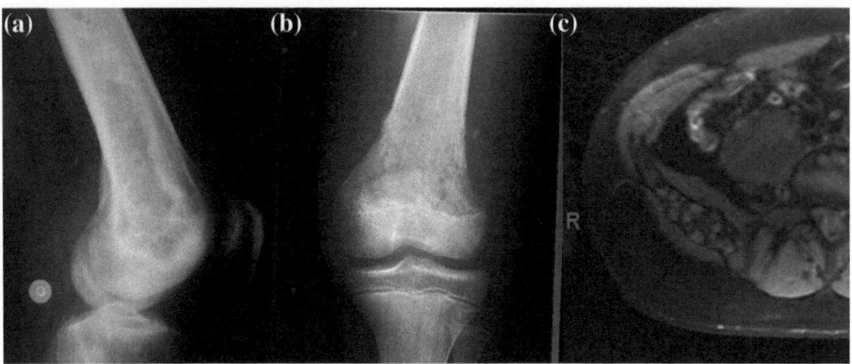

Fig. 20 Radiographs of a Bone Infarct (**a**) and osteomyelitis (**b**) in the distal femur. Axial T1 Fat-suppressed MRI of an osseous hemangioma (**c**) of the right ilium

19   Other Bone Lesions

Many processes create abnormality in bone and it is important to keep these in consideration when making a diagnosis (Fig. 20). An enostosis or bone island is a focus of dense lamellar bone with normal haversian canals [13]. It is often incidentally found on imaging. X-ray and CT show spiculated margins. MRI is low T1 and T2 signal with normal narrow and no surrounding edema [84]. Bone scan is cold. Observation is appropriate. Multiple lesions on both sides of a joint can be a benign autosomal dominant dysplasia called osteopoikilosis [13]. TUG lesion is a cortical irregularity at the medial posterior distal femur. This is an overuse injury in adolescents and only requires activity modification and observation. Intraosseous lipoma is mature fat in a cystic area of bone. The most common presentation is an incidental finding in a long bone metaphysis or calcaneus in a thirty to 50-year old [85]. MRI confirms the diagnosis by demonstrating signal consistent with fat on all sequences. Intraosseous ganglion cysts and subchondral cysts are subchondral radiolucent lesions with sclerotic margins with or without associated arthritis. Bone Infarct results from disrupted blood supply to an area of bone. There are many potential causes including fracture, dislocation, radiation, sickle cell disease, alcoholism, steroid use, and hyperlipidemia [86]. Radiographs show a serpiginous area that appears as "smoke rising from a chimney." MRI shows a characteristic mixed signal with infiltrative fat. Treatment of the lesion is observation. There is a very small chance of malignant transformation. Osseous hemangioma is usually an incidental finding in the metaphysis of long bones and in vertebral bodies of adults [13]. A striated radiographic appearance is seen in vertebral bodies. CT and MRI can show phleboliths and fat signal between vascular channels [56, 87]. Treatment is observation. Embolization is considered with refractory pain. Glomus tumors are rare focal hemangioma-like lesions that occur in the subungual region of the hand terminal phalanx. The distal phalanx frequently shows erosions [88]. Lesions are very painful and sensitive to cold. Treatment is marginal excision. Osteomyelitis is bone infection. It presents with swelling, warmth, erythema, and fever. Children are more susceptible to acute infection due to metaphyseal venous pooling [85]. ESR, CRP, and blood cultures should be obtained and aspiration considered for culture. MRI shows dark marrow signal on T1 and bright marrow on T2. Enhancement can be seen on MRI and bone scan in areas of increased blood flow [85]. Localized chronic infection is known as a Brodie's abscess. A central area of necrotic infected bone known as the sequestrum is surrounded by sclerotic host bone known as an involucrum. Acute osteomyelitis can be treated with antibiotics. Chronic osteo-myelitis or infection with necrosis, purulence, or sequestrum needs debridement and irrigation in addition to antibiotics.

19.1 Treatment

section will discuss treatment in greater detail. Lesions that appear latent are observed. Serial imaging helps to document any tumor progression. This is typi-cally done with radiographs. Areas of complex anatomy such as the acetabulum, pelvis, sacrum, spine, hands, and feet may require advanced imaging with CT or MRI. After initial patient evaluation, imaging is generally repeated at 3, 6 months, and then every 12 months. Children and adolescents should be followed until shortly after skeletal maturity. Adults need to be followed for a minimum of one to 2 years. Any concern in lesion progression in either population should prompt earlier follow-up, advanced imaging, or biopsy.

Active and aggressive lesions are progressive and treatment is necessary to limit morbidity. When pathologic fracture is present, it is best to wait 6-8 weeks to allow fracture healing. This establishes a continuous bone cavity and helps reduce the likelihood of recurrence [89]. In most cases, an open biopsy is performed first through a limited incision. Staying within one anatomic compartment is important because tumor contaminates the dissection area. Specimen should be sent for intraoperative frozen section. If a benign diagnosis is confirmed, treatment con-tinues under the same anesthetic. Any uncertainty of the diagnosis should end the procedure at biopsy and any further surgical action waits until the final diagnosis is confirmed. Diagnostic yield is better with open biopsy compared to percutaneous techniques for benign bone lesions. Frozen section can determine adequacy of tissue sampling even if a diagnosis cannot be made [8]. Definitive treatment of active and aggressive lesions is usually intralesional with open curettage. The goal is removal of all neoplastic tissue. Full exposure of the cavity with a large cortical window facilitates visualization of the tumor and allows access to all areas with a curette. High-speed burr (HSB) is used as a mechanical curette in order to extend the resection margin and remove residual microscopic tumor. Use of fluoroscopy with the burr helps prevent excessive bone removal and minimizes postoperative fracture risk. A probe is beneficial to assure that all septae and trabeculae have been violated in multicystic lesions.

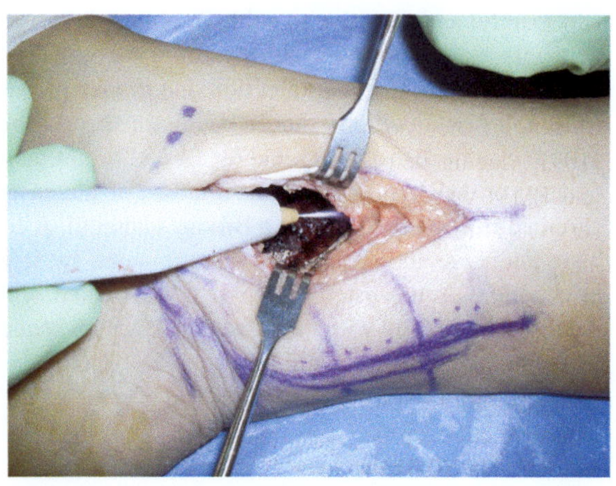

Fig. 21 Adjuvant use of the argon beam coagulator on the wall of a benign bone lesion in the distal tibia

Recurrence risk is associated with the extent of lesion resection and the technical quality of the surgery. Curettage alone is associated with a high recurrence rate of 30–50 % [90–93]. This can be diminished with use of an adjuvant treatment to 10–20 % [94–96]. Many adjuvants are available and preference is institutional. They have all demonstrated effectiveness and the ability to reduce recurrence rates with similar functional outcomes and complications [92, 94–98]. Liquid nitrogen or cryosurgery requires an intact bone cavity and works through repetitive fast freeze/spontaneous thaw cycles. Each cycle decreases tissue vascularity and increases thermal conductivity leading to the production of intracellular ice crystals, which produce mechanical cell damage [94, 99–101]. Osteonecrosis results and creeping substitution begins at 7 days. A 7–12 mm rim of necrosis is achieved [102]. Fracture risk is high and requires protected weight bearing for 3 months postoperatively. Phenol is a weak acid that directly denatures proteins and damages DNA. It is often applied to the walls of intact bone cavities with a cotton tip applicator. Dissolved in alcohol and typically used in an 85 % concentration, phenol is applied for one minute and then neutralized with sodium bicarbonate [100, 103]. It achieves a 0.5 mm rim of necrosis and is ineffective against cartilage [104]. Spill is the main risk with resultant necrosis of normal tissue [105]. Argon beam coagulation is a spray of inert argon gas that coagulates proteins and desiccates tissue [97, 106] (Fig. 21). It can be applied to incomplete bone cavities. Depth of necrosis depends upon the power of the beam and length of time it is applied. Application of 100 Watts for 5 s gives an average necrotic rim of 5.5 mm [107, 108]. Primary risk is fracture and warrants restriction of postoperative weight bearing and/or activities [89].

Created bone defects are generally large and require some filling substance to offer temporary structural support. Polymethylmethacrylate (PMMA) offers immediate long-term support. It is best used in adults and in areas adjacent to subchondral bone. There may be a secondary adjuvant effect from the heat of polymerization and the cement monomers themselves that have a direct cytotoxic effect on tumor cells. This creates a 1–2 mm fibroblastic reaction around the bony rim [102]. Further, PMMA creates a characteristic radiographic appearance that makes it easy to detect recurrence [100] and also has elution qualities that allow incorporation of antibiotics or bisphosphonates into the filler. Drawbacks are lack of biologic incorporation and damage to surrounding structures from heat necrosis [109]. Placing demineralized bone putty or gel foam between subchondral bone and PMMA may protect articular cartilage. Other fillers are more biologic; they serve as a mixture of temporary support and scaffold for host bone to incorporate. This type of filler is preferred in children and younger patients. Cancellous bone graft is frequently used although its structural support is minimal. Autograft is osteoinductive, osteoconductive, and safe, but harvest contributes donor site morbidity and supply is limited. Allograft is osteoconductive but does not have bone promoting biologic factors, although mixture with DBM may add some osteoinductive properties. There is no donor site morbidity with allograft. However, this is exchanged for the risk of disease transmission from cadaver to recipient. Synthetic fillers are additional options for osteoconduction. Current preference is use of a composite containing calcium sulfate, calcium phosphate, and β-tricalcium phosphate. The different resorption properties balance structural support with porosity to allow host vascular ingrowth and osteoblast recruitment [110]. Use in lower extremity lesions has demonstrated enough bony consolidation after an average of 7.3 weeks to allow full weight bearing and unrestricted activities [111]. Identification of lesion recurrence can be challenging with composite grafts and they need to be removed during infection [111].

En bloc resection is excessive for the majority of benign bone tumors. These tumors do not metastasize and the main concern is local recurrence and local morbidity. While GCT of bone carries a low risk of metastatic disease, the clinical behavior of these metastases does not warrant more aggressive primary treatment. Contemporary intralesional management adequately minimizes recurrence in benign bone tumors and serves as first-line treatment in accessible lesions. Resection is a consideration in a few circumstances. Aggressive lesions in expendable bones, multiply recurrent, and recalcitrant lesions producing substantial local morbidity may justify the risk of a more substantial surgery.

Percutaneous treatment for benign bone tumors, with one exception, is considered for inaccessible lesions or patients medically unfit for surgery. RFA for osteoid osteoma is considered equivalent to open curettage and used first-line in appropriate locations. The technique is safe and also serves as a secondary option in other benign bone lesions. RFA is performed under anesthesia because bone drilling and placement of a biopsy needle into the lesion is necessary [32]. Further, minimal movement aids the accuracy and limits radiation exposure with CT guidance. A monopolar electrode is centrally placed into the tumor and a temperature of around 90 °C is maintained for 5–6 min [112]. Complications are low, recovery is quick, and clinical success with one treatment is approximately 91 % [49]. Care must be exercised in subcutaneous areas and around neurovascular structures. Sclerosing therapy is another percutaneous option and has demonstrated clinical success, most notably in ABCs. The procedure is outpatient and done under anesthesia with fluoroscopic guidance [113]. Several injections are usually needed to successfully thrombose the tumor blood supply. Complications are not uncommon and include cutaneous fistula, local inflammation, hypopigmentation, abscess, and fracture [114]. External beam radiotherapy (EBRT) can also be effective against inaccessible aggressive lesions. The photon energy induces DNA damage. Multiple cycles are given over several weeks. Effectiveness is 84 % with >50 Gy of radiation [115]. Risks include local inflammation, growth arrest, tissue scarring and necrosis, fracture, and secondary sarcoma formation.

After treatment, lesions need to be monitored for local recurrence. Length of surveillance can vary but should take place for at least 5 years. One approach is to monitor with clinical exam and imaging every 3 months for the first postoperative year, every 4 months for the second postoperative year, every 6 months for the third postoperative year, and then annually for the duration of follow-up. Any clinical or radiographic concern should warrant earlier follow-up, advanced imaging, or biopsy. GCT also needs chest monitoring during follow-up.

References

1. Ardran GM (1951) Bone destruction not demonstrable by radiography. Br J Radiol 278(24):107–109
2. Costelloe CM, Madewell JE (2013) Radiography in the initial diagnosis of primary bone tumors. AJR 200:3–7
3. Enneking WF (1986) A system of staging musculoskeletal neoplasms. Clin Orthop Relat Res 204:9–24
4. Shapeero LG, Vanel D (2000) Imaging evaluation of the response of high-grade osteosarcoma and ewing sarcoma to chemotherapy with emphasis on dynamic contrast-enhanced magnetic resonance imaging. Semin Musculoskelet Radiol 4(1):137–146
5. Hwang S, Panicek DM (2009) The evolution of musculoskeletal tumor imaging. Radiol Clin North Am 47(3):435–453
6. Dyke JP, Panicek DM, Healey JH et al (2003) Osteogenic and ewing sarcomas: estimation of necrotic fraction during induction chemotherapy with dynamic contrast enhanced MR imaging. Radiology 228(1):271–278
7. Karchevsky M, Babb JS, Schweitzer ME (2008) Can diffusion-weighted imaging be used to differentiate benign from pathologic fractures? A meta-analysis. Skeletal Radiol 37(9):791–795
8. Girish G, Finlay K, Morag Y, et al (2012) Imaging review of skeletal tumors of the pelvis—part I: benign tumors of the pelvis. Sci World J. Epub May 15 PMID: 22666102
9. Roberts CC, Daffner RH, Weissman BN et al (2006) ACR appropriateness criteria on metastatic bond disease. J Am Coll Radiol 7(6):400–409
10. Aoki J, Watanabe H, Shinozaki T et al (2001) FDG PET of primary benign and malignant bone tumors: standardized uptake value in 52 lesions. Radiology 219(3):774–777
11. Buchbender C, Heusner TA, Lauenstein TC et al (2012) Oncologic PET/MRI, part 2: bone Tumors, soft-tissue tumors, melanoma, and lymphoma. J Nucl Med 53:1244–1252
12. Betsy M, Kupersmith LM, Springfield DS (2004) Metaphyseal fibrous defects. J Am Acad Orthop Surg 12(2):89–95
13. Motamedi K, Seeger LL (2011) Benign bone tumors. Radiol Clin N Am 49:1115–1134
14. Cronin MV, Hughes TH (2012) Bone tumors and tumor-like conditions of bone. Appl Radiol 41(10):6–15

15. Mankin HJ, Trahan CA, Fondren G et al (2009) Non-ossifying fibroma, fibrous cortical defect and Jaffe-Campanacci syndrome: a biologic and clinical review. Musculoskelet Surg 93:1–7
16. Jee WH, Choe BY, Kang HS et al (1998) Non-ossifying fibroma: characteristics at MR imaging with pathologic correlation. Radiology 209(1):197–202
17. Fitzpatrick KA, Taljanovic MS, Speer DP et al (2004) Imaging findings of fibrous dysplasia with histopathologic and intraoperative correlation. AJR 182(6):1389–1398
18. Brant WE, Helms CA (2007) Fundamentals of diagnostic radiology, 3rd edn. LWW, Philadelphia
19. Manaster BJ, Disler DG, May DA et al (2002) Musculoskeletal imaging: the requisites, 2nd edn. Mosby, St Louis
20. Gleason BC, Liegl-Atzwanger B, Kozakewich HP et al (2008) Osteofibrous dysplasia and adamantinoma in children and adolescents: a clinicopathologic reappraisal. Am J Surg Pathol 32(3):363–376
21. Ishida T, Iijima T, Kikuchi F et al (1992) A clinicopathological and immunohistochemical study of osteofibrous dysplasia, differentiated adamantinoma, and adamantinoma of long bones. Skeletal Radiol 21(8):493–502
22. Most MJ, Sims FH, Inwards CY (2010) Osteofibrous dysplasia and adamantinoma. J Am Acad Orthop Surg 18:358–366
23. Dorfman HC, Czerniak B (1988) Bone tumors, 1st edn. CV Mosby, St Louis
24. Murphey MD, Flemming DJ, Boyea SR et al (1998) Enchondroma versus chondrosarcoma in the appendicular skeleton: differentiating features. Radiographics 18(5):1213–1237
25. Simon MA, Peabody TD, Haydon RC, et al (2009) Musculoskeletal clinicopathologic course. In: Lecture notes, University of Chicago, Chicago, 26–28 October 2009
26. Jaffe HL (1943) Hereditary multiple exostosis. Arch Pathol 36:335–357
27. Thakur NA, Daniels AH, Schiller J et al (2012) Benign tumors of the spine. J Am Acad Orthop Surg 20:715–724
28. Brien EW, Mirra JM, Luck JV (1999) Benign and malignant cartilage tumors of bone and joint: their anatomic and theoretical basis with an emphasis on radiology, pathology and clinical biology. II: juxtacortical cartilage tumors. Skeletal Radiol 28(1):1–20
29. Edeiken J (1990) Roentgen diagnosis of diseases of bone, 3rd edn. Williams and Wilkins, Baltimore
30. Pedrini E, DeLuca A, Valente EM et al (2005) Novel EXT1 and EXT2 mutations identified by DHPLC in Italian patients with multiple osteochondromas. Hum Mutat 26(3):280
31. American Academy of Orthopaedic Surgeons (AAOS) (2012) Chondromyxoid fibroma. OrthoInfo. http://orthoinfo.aaos.org/topic.cfm?topic=A00624
32. Rosenthal D, Callstrom MR (2012) Critical review and state of the art in interventional oncology: Benign and metastatic disease involving bone. Radiology 262(3):765–780
33. Petsas T, Megas P, Papathanassiou Z (2007) Radio-frequency ablation of two femoral head chondroblastomas. Eur J Radiol 63(1):63–67
34. Greenspan A (1993) Benign bone-forming lesions: osteoma, osteoid osteoma, and osteoblastoma. Clinical, imaging, pathologic, and differential considerations. Skeletal Radiol 22(7):485–500
35. Eggel Y, Theumann N, Lüthi F (2007) Intra-articular osteoid osteoma of the knee: clinical and therapeutical particularities. Joint Bone Spine 74(4):379–381
36. Jackson RP, Reckling FW, Mants FA (1977) Osteoid osteoma and osteoblastoma: similar histologic lesions with different natural histories. Clin Orthop Relat Res 128:303–313
37. Cerase A, Priolo F (1998) Skeletal benign bone-forming lesions. Eur J Radiol 27(suppl 1):S91–S97
38. Peyser A, Applbaum Y, Simanovsky N et al (2009) CT-guided radiofrequency ablation of pediatric osteoid osteoma utilizing a water-cooled tip. Ann Surg Oncol 16(10):2856–2861
39. Kiers L, Shield LK, Cole WG (1990) Neurological manifestations of osteoid osteoma. Arch Dis Child 65(8):851–855

40. Lindner NJ, Ozaki T, Roedl R et al (2001) Percutaneous radiofrequency ablation in osteoid osteoma. J Bone Joint Surg Br 83(3):391–396
41. Davies M, Cassar-Pullicino VN, Davies AM et al (2002) The diagnostic accuracy of MR imaging in osteoid osteoma. Skeletal Radiol 31(10):559–569
42. Schulman L, Dorfman HD (1970) Nerve fibers in osteoid osteoma. J Bone Joint Surg Am 52(7):1351–1356
43. Mankin HJ (2009) Osteoid osteoma and osteoblastoma: two related bone tumors, in great educator series: pathophysiology of orthopaedic diseases, vol 2. American Academy of Orthopaedic Surgeons, Rosemont, pp 79–85
44. Makley JT, Dunn MJ (1982) Prostaglandin synthesis by osteoid osteoma. Lancet 2(8288):42
45. Greco F, Tamburrelli F, Ciabattoni G (1991) Prostaglandins in osteoid osteoma. Int Orthop 15(1):35–37
46. Kneisl JS, Simon MA (1992) Medical management compared with operative treatment for osteoid osteoma. J Bone Joint Surg Am 74(2):179–185
47. Roqueplan F, Porcher R, Hamzé B et al (2010) Long-term results of percutaneous resection and interstitial laser ablation of osteoid osteomas. Eur Radiol 20(1):209–217
48. Vanderschueren GM, Obermann WR, Dijkstra SP et al (2009) Radiofrequency ablation of spinal osteoid osteoma: clinical outcome. Spine 34(9):901–904
49. Rosenthal DI, Hornicek FJ, Torriani M et al (2003) Osteoid osteoma: percutaneous treatment with radiofrequency energy. Radiology 229(1):171–175
50. Rosenthal DI, Hornicek FJ, Wolfe MW, Jennings LC, Gebhardt MC, Mankin HJ (1999) Decreasing length of hospital stay in treatment of osteoid osteoma. Clin Orthop Relat Res 361:186–191
51. Rimondi E, Mavrogenis AF, Rossi G et al (2012) Radiofrequency ablation for non-spinal osteoid osteomas in 557 patients. Eur Radiol 22(1):181–188
52. Berry M, Mankin H, Gebhardt M, Rosenberg A, Hornicek F (2008) Osteoblastoma: A 30-year study of 99 cases. J Surg Oncol 98(3):179–183
53. Lucas DR, Unni KK, McLeod RA et al (1994) Osteoblastoma: clinicopathologic study of 306 cases. Hum Pathol 25(2):117–134
54. Frassica FJ, Waltrip RL, Sponseller PD et al (1996) Clinicopathologic features and treatment of osteoid osteoma and osteoblastoma in children and adolescents. Orthop Clin North Am 27(3):559–574
55. Arkader A, Dormans JP (2008) Osteoblastoma in the skeletally immature. J Pediatr Orthop 28(5):555–560
56. Motamedi K, Ilaslan H, Seeger LL (2004) Imaging of the lumbar spine neoplasms. Semin Ultrasound CT MR 25:474–489
57. Crim JR, Mirra JM, Eckardt JJ et al (1990) Widespread inflammatory response to osteoblastoma; the flare phenomenon. Radiology 177(3):835–836
58. American Academy of Orthopaedic Surgeons (AAOS) (2013) Unicameral bone cyst. OrthoInfo. http://orthoinfo.aaos.org/topic.cfm?topic=A00081
59. Azevedo CP, Casanova JM, Guerra MG et al (2013) Tumors of the foot and ankle: a single-institution experience. J Foot Ankle Surg 52:147–152
60. Guo W, Xu W, Huvos AG et al (1999) Comparative frequency of bone sarcomas among different racial groups. Chin Med J (Engl) 112:1101–1104
61. Sung HW, Kuo DP, Shu WP et al (1982) Giant-cell tumor of bone: analysis of two hundred and eight cases in Chinese patients. J Bone Joint Surg Am 64:755–761
62. Rendina D, Mossetti G, Soscia E et al (2004) Giant cell tumor and Paget's disease of bone in one family: geographic clustering. Clin Orthop Relat Res 421:218–224
63. Jacobs TP, Michelsen J, Polay JS et al (1979) Giant cell tumor in Paget's disease of bone: familial and geographic clustering. Cancer 44:742–747
64. Campanacci M, Baldini N, Boriani S, Sudanese A (1987) Giant-cell tumor of bone. J Bone Joint Surg Am 69:106–114

65. Enneking WF, Spanier SS, Goodman MA (1980) A system for the surgical staging of musculoskeletal sarcoma. Clin Orthop Relat Res 153:106–120
66. Murphey MD, Nomikos DJ, Flemming FH et al (2001) From the archives of the AFIP. Imaging of giant cell tumor and giant cell reparative granuloma of bone: radiologie-pathologic correlation. Radiographics 21(5):1283–1309
67. Parman LM, Murphey MD (2000) Alphabet soup: cystic lesions of bone. Semin Musculoskelet Radiol 4(1):89–101
68. Skubitz KM, Cheng EY, Clohisy DR et al (2004) Gene expression in giant-cell tumors. J Lab Clin Med 144:193–200
69. Morgan T, Atkins GJ, Trivett MK et al (2005) Molecular profiling of giant cell tumor of bone and the osteoclastic localization of ligand for receptor activator of nuclear factor kappaB. Am J Pathol 167:117–128
70. WHO (2002) Pathology and genetics of tumours of soft tissue and bone. IARC Press, Lyon
71. Klenke FM, Wenger DE, Inwards CY et al (2011) Giant cell tumor of bone: risk factors for recurrence. Clin Orthop Relat Res 469(2):591–599
72. Ng ES, Saw A, Sengupta S, et al (2002) Giant cell tumour of bone with late presentation: review of treatment and outcome. J Orthop Surg (Hong Kong) 10:120–28
73. Makis W, Alabed YZ, Nahal A et al (2012) Giant cell tumor pulmonary metastases mimic primary malignant pulmonary nodules on 18F-FDG PET/CT. Nucl Med Mol Imaging 46:134–137
74. Thomas D, Henshaw R, Skubitz K et al (2010) Denosumab in patients with giant-cell tumour of bone: an open-label, phase 2 study. Lancet Oncol 11(3):275–280
75. Smith MR, Saad F, Coleman R et al (2012) Denosumab and bone-metastasis-free and survival in men with castration-resistant prostate cancer: results of a phase 3, randomised, placebo-controlled trial. Lancet 379:39–46
76. Zwolak P, Manivel JC, Jasinski P et al (2010) Cytotoxic effect of zoledronic acid-loaded bone cement on giant cell tumor, multiple myeloma, and renal cell carcinoma cell lines. J Bone Joint Surg Am 92(1):162–168
77. Klenke FM, Wenger DE, Inwards CY et al (2011) Recurrent giant cell tumor of long bones: analysis of surgical management. Clin Orthop Relat Res 469(4):1181–1187
78. Ye Y, Pringle LM, Lau AW et al (2010) TRE17/USP6 oncogene translocated in aneurysmal bone cyst induces matrix metalloproteinase production via activation of NF-kappaB. Oncogene 29(25):3619–3629
79. Kransdorf MJ, Sweet DE (1995) Aneurysmal bone cyst: concept, controversy, clinical presentation, and imaging. AJR 164(3):573–580
80. Schajowicz F (1993) Histological typing of bone tumors (international histological classification of tumors). Springer, New York
81. Garg S, Mehta S, Dormans JP (2004) Langerhans cell histiocytosis of the spine in children: long-term follow-up. J Bone Joint Surg Am 86(8):1740–1750
82. Yeom JS, Lee CK, Shin HY, Lee CS, Han CS, Chang H (1999) Langerhans' cell histiocytosis of the spine: Analysis of twenty-three cases. Spine 24(16):1740–1749
83. Huang W, Yang X, Cao D et al (2010) Eosinophilic granuloma of spine in adults: a report of 30 cases and outcome. Acta Neurochir 152(7):1129–1137
84. Cerase A, Priolo F (1998) Skeletal benign bone forming lesions. Eur J Radiol 27:91–97
85. Campbell RS, Grainger AJ, Mangham DC et al (2003) Intraosseous lipoma: report of 35 new cases and a review of the literature. Skeletal Radiol 32:209–222
86. Hermann G, Singson R, Bromley M et al (2004) Cystic degeneration of medullary bone infarction evaluated with magnetic resonance imaging correlated with pathologic examination. Can Assoc Radiol J 55(5):321–325
87. Baudrez V, Galant C, Van de Berg BC (2001) Benign vertebral hemangiomas: MR-histological correlation. Skeletal Radiol 30:442–446
88. Baek HJ, Lee SJ, Cho KH et al (2010) Subungual tumors: clinicopathologic correlation with US and MR imaging findings. Radiographics 30:1621–1636

89. Steffner RJ, Liao C, Stacy G et al (2011) Factors associated with recurrence of primary aneurysmal bone cysts: is argon beam coagulation an effective adjuvant treatment? J Bone Joint Surg Am 93(21):e1221–e1229

90. Campanacci M, Baldini N, Boriani S, Sudanese A (1987) Giant-cell tumor of bone. J Bone Joint Surg Am 69(1):106–114

91. Becker WT, Dohle J et al (2008) Local recurrence of giant cell tumor of bone after intralesional treatment with and without adjuvant therapy. J Bone Joint Surg Am 90(5):1060–1067

92. Blackley HR, Wunder JS, Davis AM, White LM, Kandel R, Bell RS (1999) Treatment of giant-cell tumors of long bones with curettage and bone-grafting. J Bone Joint Surg Am 81(6):811–820

93. Turcotte RE, Wunder JS, Isler MH et al (2002) Giant cell tumor of long bone: a Canadian Sarcoma Group study. Clin Orthop Relat Res 397:248–258

94. Malawer MM, Bickels J, Meller I et al (1999) Cryosurgery in the treatment of giant cell tumor. A long-term followup study. Clin Orthop Relat Res 359:176–188

95. Dürr HR, Maier M, Jansson V, Baur A, Refior HJ (1999) Phenol as an adjuvant for local control in the treatment of giant cell tumour of the bone. Eur J Surg Oncol 25(6):610–618

96. Gibbs CP, Hefele MC, Peabody TD et al (1999) Aneurysmal bone cyst of the extremities. Factors related to local recurrence after curettage with a high-speed burr. J Bone Joint Surg Am 81(12):1671–1678

97. O'Donnell RJ, Springfield DS, Motwani HK et al (1994) Recurrence of giant-cell tumors of the long bones after curettage and packing with cement. J Bone Joint Surg Am 76(12):1827–1833

98. Lewis VO, Wei A, Mendoza T et al (2007) Argon beam coagulation as an adjuvant for local control of giant cell tumor. Clin Orthop Relat Res 454:192–197

99. Marcove RC, Sheth DS, Takemoto S et al (1995) The treatment of aneurysmal bone cyst. Clin Orthop Relat Res 311:157–163

100. Schreuder HW, Veth RP (1997) Simple bone cysts treated by injection of autologous bone marrow. J Bone Joint Surg Br 79(5):877

101. Marcove RC (1982) A 17-year review of cryosurgery in the treatment of bone tumors. Clin Orthop Relat Res 163:231–234

102. Malawer MM, Marks MR, McChesney D et al (1988) The effect of cryosurgery and polymethylmethacrylate in dogs with experimental bone defects comparable to tumor defects. Clin Orthop Relat Res 226:299–310

103. Quint U, Vanhöfer U, Harstrick A et al (1996) Cytotoxicity of phenol to musculoskeletal tumours. J Bone Joint Surg Br 78(6):984–985

104. Lack W, Lang S, Brand G (1994) Necrotizing effect of phenol on normal tissues and on tumors. A study on postoperative and cadaver specimens. Acta Orthop Scand 65(3):351–354

105. Quint U, Müller RT, Müller G (1998) Characteristics of phenol. Instillation in intralesional tumor excision of chondroblastoma, osteoblastoma and enchondroma. Arch Orthop Trauma Surg 117(1–2):43–46

106. Rock M (1990) Adjuvant management of benign tumors; basic concepts of phenol and cement use. Chir Organi Mov 75(1 suppl):195–197

107. Bristow RE, Smith Sehdev AE, Kaufman HS, et al (2001) Ablation of metastatic ovarian carcinoma with the argon beam coagulator: pathologic analysis of tumor destruction. Gynecol Oncol 83(1):49–55

108. Heck RK, Pope WE, Ahn JI et al (2009) Histologic evaluation of the depth of necrosis produced by argon beam coagulation: implications for use as adjuvant treatment of bone tumors. J Surg Orthop Adv 18(2):69–73

109. Ozaki T, Hillmann A, Lindner N et al (1996) Aneurysmal bone cysts in children. J Cancer Res Clin Oncol 122(12):767–769

110. Fillingham YA, Lenart BA, Gitelis S (2012) Function after injection of benign bone lesions with a bioceramic. Clin Orthop Relat Res 470(7):2014–2020
111. Evaniew N, Tan V, Parasu N et al (2013) Use of a calcium sulfate-calcium phosphate synthetic bone graft composite in the surgical management of primary bone tumors. Orthopedics 36(2):e216–e222
112. Peyser A, Applbaum Y (2009) Radiofrequency ablation of bone tumors. Curr Orthop Pract 20(6):616–621
113. Rastogi S, Varshney MK, Trikha V et al (2006) Treatment of aneurysmal bone cysts with percutaneous sclerotherapy using polidocanol. A review of 72 cases with long-term follow-up. J Bone Joint Surg Br 88(9):1212–1216
114. Varshney MK, Rastogi S, Khan SA et al (2010) Is sclerotherapy better than intralesional excision for treating aneurysmal bone cysts? Clin Orthop Relat Res 468(6):1649–1659
115. Feigenberg SJ, Marcus RB Jr, Zlotecki RA et al (2003) Radiation therapy for giant cell tumors of bone. Clin Orthop Relat Res 411:207–216

Osteosarcoma

Drew D. Moore and Hue H. Luu

Abstract

Osteosarcoma is a malignant tumor that primarily affects the long bones but can also involve other bones in the body. It has a bimodal distribution with peaks in the second decade of life and late adulthood. This chapter will highlight the clinical presentation, diagnosis, and treatment of osteosarcoma.

Keywords

Osteosarcoma · Bone tumor · Limb salvage · Chemotherapy

1 Introduction

Like all sarcomas, osteosarcoma is a tumor of mesenchymal origin. However the tumor cells are unique in that they produce immature osteoid, thus providing its namesake. It is the most common primary sarcoma of bone in children and young adults and typically has a bimodal age distribution, being found predominantly in the second decade of life and in elderly individuals. There are a variety of different types of osteosarcoma which are associated with varying degrees of aggressiveness. In general, the treatment strategies are similar among them. Since 80 % of osteosarcoma patients have metastatic or micro-metastatic disease at diagnosis, nearly all patients are treated with multiagent chemotherapy in addition to surgical

D. D. Moore · H. H. Luu (✉)
Department of Orthopedic Surgery and Rehabilitation Medicine,
The University of Chicago, 5841 South Maryland, MC 3079, Chicago, IL 60637, USA
e-mail: hluu@bsd.uchicago.edu

T. D. Peabody and S. Attar (eds.), *Orthopaedic Oncology*,
Cancer Treatment and Research 162, DOI: 10.1007/978-3-319-07323-1_4,
© Springer International Publishing Switzerland 2014

resection. Advances in surgical treatment have significantly decreased the number of amputations performed as limb preservation has become the preferred surgical method when possible. Over time, the prognosis for patients has improved from less than 30 % survival to more than 70 % as the result of an evolution in treatment principles and chemotherapy. Despite these advances, there remains much room for improvement as new chemotherapeutic agents are investigated and surgical methods continue to be refined.

2 History

William Enneking in the *History of Orthopedic Oncology in the United States*, provides a detailed account of the history of osteosarcoma [1]. The term osteosarcoma was first described by the French surgeon Alexis Boyer in 1805, who also served as an army surgeon for Napoleon Bonaparte [2]. It was almost half a century later before a true description and natural history of the process was provided by Guillaume Dupuytren in 1847 [3]. Soon after in 1854, Hermann Lebert provided the first histologic description of bone tumors, which would become the basis for the work of Rudolf Virchow in creating a classification of bone tumors based on histology [4, 5]. These principals continue to this day, as osteosarcoma is defined according to the histological findings of a sarcoma which produces osteoid.

In terms of surgical management of osteosarcoma, some of the first recommendations were made by Samuel Gross in 1879, who advocated radical removal and amputation, since he found more conservative limb sparing procedures had an unacceptably high mortality rate [6]. However, as Enneking mentions, these aggressive procedures did little to increase survivability [1].

In the early 1900s as roentgenograms became more available, so did radiographic descriptions of bone tumors. Ernest Codman in 1909 described many of the features that osteosarcomas demonstrate on X-rays, including the periosteal elevation which continues to be known as Codman's Triangle [7]. Figure 1 demonstrates an example of an osteosarcoma with robust periosteal reaction and associated Codman's Triangle.

In those early days, there were not many alternatives to amputation, as reconstructive procedures were limited as a result of poor instrumentation. A major breakthrough in limb preservation surgery was the use of allografts and bone graft to reconstruct bony defects. Dallas Phemister pioneered this work in the 1920–1940s at the University of Chicago [8]. In the years after World War II, advances in orthopedic techniques in general and surgical implants made it possible to perform increasingly complex reconstructions following tumor removal. Despite this, the survival rates associated with osteosarcomas remained low.

The modern age of osteosarcoma treatment really began with the discovery of chemotherapeutic regimens in the 1970s. There was a major jump in the survival rates from about 30 % to almost 70 % during this time period, as is described in more detail in the section on chemotherapy. Unfortunately, despite major technological

Fig. 1 An anteroposterior view of a distal femur osteosarcoma showing sclerosis of the metaphysis and ossification of a soft tissue mass with a wide zone of transition and periosteal elevation suggesting aggressive behavior. The arrow demonstrates Codman's Triangle

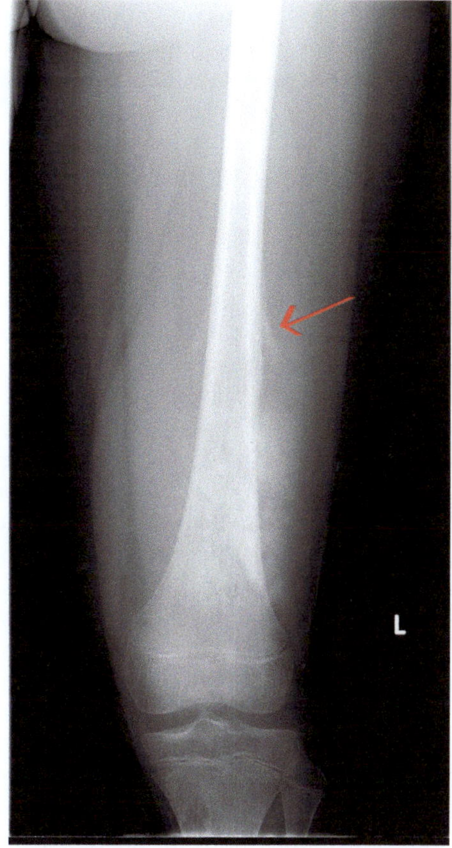

advances in systemic chemotherapy and surgical techniques in the past 40 years, the survival rates for osteosarcoma have reached a plateau over that time period. As a result, this continues to be an area of intense research.

3   Epidemiology

The most comprehensive data regarding the epidemiology of osteosarcoma in the United States comes from the Surveillance, Epidemiology, and End Results (SEER) Program from the National Institute of Health. This is a collection of cancer statistics drawn from a variety of cancer centers throughout the United States, which serves as an accurate cross-section of the population. Most recently, Mirabello et al. specifically examined the SEER data from 1973 to 2004 for osteosarcoma, which included 3,482 patients [9]. Their data confirmed that osteosarcoma does indeed have a bimodal age distribution with an adolescent and an elderly peak in incidence. The adolescent peak was centered at about age 15 and consisted predominately of primary osteosarcoma. The incidence of osteosarcoma in the 0–24 year-old group was 4.4 per million. The second peak was centered at age 75 and consisted predominately of secondary osteosarcomas associated with Paget's disease or other bony lesions. While there are occasional temporary increases or decreases in the incidence for an age group, the overall incidence of osteosarcoma does not appear to be trending in a specific direction over the past 35 years. When examining for race and gender, males have a slightly higher incidence compared to females at a ratio of 1.22:1 [9].

In terms of the most common anatomic locations for osteosarcoma, it seems to have a predilection for the metaphyseal portions of long bones. According to the work of Dahlin et al. the most common bones of involvement include the femur at about 40 %, three quarters of which are in the distal femur, the tibia at about 20 %, the humerus at 10 % and the pelvis at 8 %. Therefore, these sites comprise almost 80 % of the reported cases. The remaining cases are scattered amongst other bones in the body including the fibula, radius, ulna, ribs, jaw, spine, etc. It should also be noted, that despite being very rare, the possibility of extraosseous osteosarcoma also exists [10]. However, these extraskeletal lesions are somewhat controversial, as some may be misdiagnosed forms of other soft tissue sarcomas.

4   Etiology

The true etiology of osteosarcoma remains unknown. It appears to be multifactorial with both genetic and environmental components. While other sarcomas like Ewing's have demonstrated consistent chromosomal translocations and abnormalities, the majority of osteosarcomas are aneuploid [11]. However, there seems to be a molecular basis for the development of osteosarcoma, as certain genetic diseases with known mutations of tumor suppressor genes have an increased incidence and reports exist of siblings developing osteosarcomas [12]. Despite this, most cases appear to be the result of sporadic mutations.

Inherited retinoblastoma is the result of a genetic defect of the RB1 gene located on chromosome 13q14.2. This causes tumors of the retina in young children predominantly. The role of the *RB* gene is to help regulate the transition between G_0/G_1 and the S phase of the cell cycle [13]. When mutated, cell growth continues unchecked leading to tumor development. These patients have been found to have a 500 times increased risk of osteosarcoma compared to the normal population [14]. Also, mutations in the *RB1* gene have also been detected in sporadic cases of osteosarcoma as well [15].

Another disease with a high incidence of osteosarcoma is Li-Fraumeni syndrome. This is a syndrome characterized by a variety of different types of cancers including, breast, sarcomas, adrenocortical, brain, and leukemias [16]. It is autosomal dominant in inheritance and results in the inactivation of the p53 tumor suppressor gene which helps regulate progression in the cell cycle in the presence of DNA damage. It has also been shown that mutation in other genes involved in the p53 pathway such as MDM2, p14^{ART}, and CDK4 may predispose a person to developing osteosarcoma [11].

Finally, DNA helicase abnormalities have also been associated with osteosarcomas. In Rothman-Thomas syndrome, which is an autosomal recessive disease associated with skin changes, short stature, alopecia, cataracts, and osteosarcoma there is a defect of the *RECQL4* gene which codes for a DNA helicase. Similar DNA helicase abnormalities are found in Werner syndrome where the WRN or *RECQL2* gene is defective causing soft tissue sarcomas, melanomas, and osteosarcomas and Bloom syndrome where BLM or *RECQL3* gene defects cause patients to be predisposed to many types of cancer at a young age [13].

Osteosarcoma in the adult population seems to have a different behavior compared to those in children and young adults. As mentioned previously, patients with Paget's disease are at an increased risk of developing secondary osteosarcoma. A genetic association with Paget's has been shown based on a mutation of the *SQSTM1* gene which is involved in the TNF and RANKL pathways during bone turnover, and this may potentially have a role in the subset of patients who later develop osteosarcomas [17]. Osteosarcoma secondary to Paget's disease accounts for almost 20 % of the cases in patients over 40 years of age, and are high-grade with a poor prognosis [18]. Similar to Paget's disease, osteosarcoma has been associated with other preexisting benign processes of bone including bone infarcts, enchondromas, fibrous dysplasia, and osteomyelitis [19–21].

The most common and delineated environmental cause of osteosarcoma is ionizing radiation. It has been shown that high-dose therapeutic radiation is associated with the development of secondary osteosarcomas, especially in patients with Ewing's sarcoma treated with radiation, since they require high therapeutic doses [22]. However, it is interesting to note that studies have not shown an increased incidence of osteosarcoma in the populations exposed to the atomic bomb fallout in Japan [23].

5   Gross and Histologic Subtypes

Osteosarcoma is typically further subdivided. As mentioned in the etiology section, it may be classified as a primary or secondary lesion depending on whether it arose from a preexisting bone lesion. They may also be classified based on their location in relation to the bone as well as their histologic characteristics. The different subtypes are known to have distinctive natural histories and behaviors. In general, they are differentiated as intramedullary versus surface lesions. The intramedullary subtypes include conventional, telangiectatic, small cell and low-grade. The surface subtypes include parosteal, periosteal, and high-grade surface lesions [24–26].

Conventional osteosarcoma is the archetypal form of osteosarcoma and is what most of the literature and statistics are based upon. It presents as a high-grade intramedullary tumor most commonly in the metaphyseal regions of long bones.

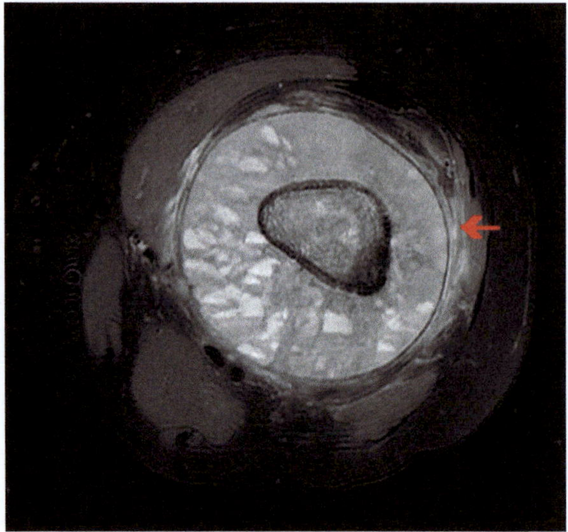

Fig. 2 An axial STIR sequence MRI of the same osteosarcoma is shown in Fig. 1. The large soft tissue mass is evident circumferentially surrounding the cortical bone

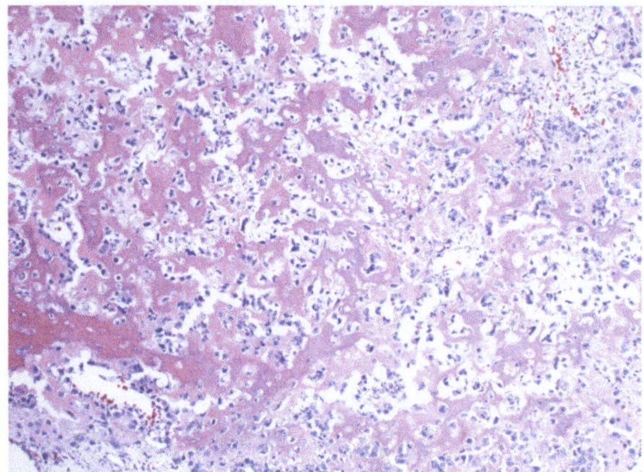

Fig. 3 An H&E histology slide of osteoblastic osteosarcoma showing high-grade malignant cells producing the characteristic *pink colored* osteoid

It is aggressive in nature and has usually broken through the cortex with an associated soft tissue mass at the time of diagnosis as seen in Fig. 2. Since it is osteogenic, the bone may appear sclerotic or radiodense on X-rays, as described in the imaging section. Histologically, it will show pleomorphic spindle type cells with significant amounts of cellular atypia, but most importantly the malignant cells must be producing osteoid to fit the diagnosis of osteosarcoma as seen in Fig. 3. Conventional osteosarcoma is histologically further subdivided into the osteoblastic, fibroblastic, or chondroblastic type based on the appearance of the background matrix. The osteoblastic form is twice as common as the other two, and the distinction is mainly histologic as the treatments and prognosis are similar between them [24]. Osteosarcomas may also demonstrate unusual histologic forms which appear similar to other bone lesions such as osteoblastomas, chondromyxoid fibromas, clear-cell sarcoma, giant cell tumor, or epithelioid tumors. The behavior of these histologic variants is similar to that of conventional osteosarcoma, so they are considered to be subtypes [24, 26].

Telangiectatic osteosarcoma has very unique characteristics compared to the conventional subtype. Although also found in the metaphysis of long bones, it deceptively resembles the radiographic appearance of an aneurysmal bone cyst (ABC) with large lucent lesions and fluid–fluid levels on MRI [27]. Although the presence of malignant bone matrix within the lesion may help differentiate from an ABC, most often it is not detectable [26]. The two entities may be distinguished based on pathology since the telangiectatic osteosarcoma will have cellular atypia and osteoid formation within the lining [26]. These are one of the most locally and systemically aggressive types of osteosarcoma [28]. Given their extensive bony destruction, many patients present with a pathologic fracture at the time of diagnosis [24]. Overall, the treatment and prognosis is similar to conventional osteosarcoma.

Small cell osteosarcoma is a rare intramedullary subtype, comprising about 1 % of osteosarcomas [29]. Its unique feature is that it has many similarities to Ewing's sarcoma. Like conventional osteosarcoma, it is typically found in the metaphyseal region of long bones. However, they are often lytic and are associated with large soft tissue masses similar to Ewing's [27, 29]. On biopsy, they contain many small round blue cells, however their distinguishing feature in addition to osteoid, is the presence of spindling within the tumor which differentiates them as osteosarcomas [29]. However, it is interesting that they typically stain for CD99 and have demonstrated t(11;22) translocations as seen in Ewing's sarcoma. Since these features are not found in other types of osteosarcomas, some have proposed they are actually a part of the Ewing's/PNET family of tumors. This is controversial since the treatment protocols are different between the two types of tumors [26].

Low-grade central osteosarcoma is the only intramedullary subtype which is low-grade histologically and more indolent in terms of progression. Typically it presents in the femur and tibia, similar to conventional osteosarcoma. Its radiographic features are variable and it may present with a sclerotic rim alluding to its slow progression. It may have a "ground glass" appearance similar to fibrous dysplasia, but the presence of cortical disruption can provide a clue that it is a malignant process [27]. Histologically, the cells have less atypia than most other osteosarcomas and there is usually a fibrous stroma present. Despite their indolent nature, these tumors should be treated with wide resection as they have a high incidence of recurrence when inadequately resected [26].

Surface osteosarcomas include parosteal, periosteal, and high-grade surface tumors. They are distinct in that often times they sit on the surface of the bone and are not contiguous with the medullary canal like conventional osteosarcomas. They also tend to be more indolent and are treated differently, usually with wide surgical excision alone, high-grade surface osteosarcomas being an exception.

Parosteal or juxtacortical osteosarcomas were first described by Geschickter and Copeland in 1951 [30]. They are slow growing lesions found on the surface of the bone. While they have been found on many different bones of the appendicular

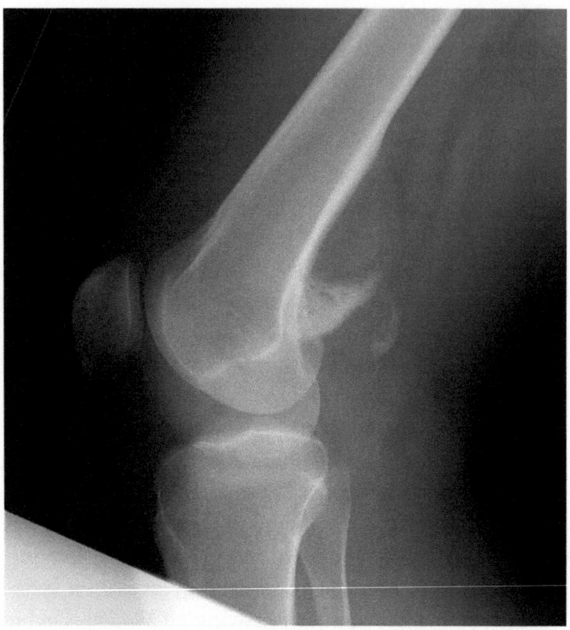

Fig. 4 A lateral X-ray of the knee demonstrating a posterior distal femur parosteal osteosarcoma

skeleton, they are most commonly found on the posterior distal femur as seen in Fig. 4, and a lesion in this area is almost pathognomonic for this type of tumor [31]. Clinically, the patients notice a painless slow growing mass in their posterior knee region. Radiographs commonly reveal a sclerotic, smooth, well-marginated lesion which has a characteristic, "stuck on bone" appearance. The lesion may appear to be attached to the bone in a small portion and be separated from the bone elsewhere by a thin radiolucent line. If large enough, they may grow both longitudinally and circumferentially around the bone [32]. While some may eventually invade the medullary canal, most do not, and this is an important distinction in order to differentiate them from benign osteochondromas. Histologically, they demonstrate mature bony trabeculae arranged in a parallel fashion similar to periosteal new bone formation. They may have osteoblastic rimming, but the bone is not organized in a lamellar pattern. Also, there will be some evidence of spindle cells with slight cellular atypia. Like an osteochondroma, there may be evidence of a cartilage cap, but there will not be evidence of continuity with marrow elements [26]. Cytogenetically, these tumors are associated with extranumerary ring chromosomes, most commonly chromosome 12 [24]. These indolent tumors are typically treated with wide surgical resection and reconstruction with good results. However, there does exist a dedifferentiated subtype with increased cellular atypia that has a higher recurrence and metastasis rate requiring it to be treated similar to conventional osteosarcoma [31, 33].

Periosteal osteosarcomas are another unique surface variant. They present more commonly along the diaphysis of the long bones with a predilection for the tibia. They have a similar clinical presentation as parosteal osteosarcomas with slow growing painless masses. Radiographically, they are distinct in that they cause marked periosteal elevation and thus a sunburst pattern with perpendicular bony spicules to the long axis of the bone. They are mixed lytic/blastic [32]. On histology they are predominantly cartilage and appear as intermediate-grade chondroblastic osteosarcomas [26]. They also are treated with wide surgical resection.

The final surface variant is high-grade surface osteosarcoma. These tumors are found on the surface of long bones and given their high grade, may grow more rapidly and cause more pain compared to the other surface lesions. Their radiographic appearance is variable and often a mixture of lytic/blastic regions. There may be a large soft tissue mass with outer rim mineralization [27]. Histologically, they demonstrate the cellular atypia associated with high-grade tumors [26]. While they are mainly on the surface of the bone, they are more likely to erode the cortical surface compared to the more indolent surface osteosarcomas. Treatment is the same as that for conventional osteosarcoma with wide resection and chemotherapy.

It should be noted that while extremely rare, extraskeletal osteosarcomas have been described within soft tissues [34]. Most commonly they present in the extremities, but have been reported in the breast, heart, and colon amongst other visceral organs [10, 34–36]. There may be an association with prior radiation. They are of mesenchymal origin, high-grade, and produce the characteristic osteoid histologically. Treatment is similar to other soft tissue sarcomas and includes resection and possible radiation, but is beyond the scope of this paper [10].

6   Patient Presentation

The most common reason why osteosarcoma patients present is pain at the site of the tumor. When small, many of the tumors are painless. However, as they grow and disrupt the bony architecture pain becomes more evident. Most patients describe it as a dull, aching, persistent pain. It may be exacerbated with activity, but it is also present at rest or at night when the patient is trying to sleep. While not typically associated with trauma, many patients may associate the pain with some unrelated minor traumatic event from the past. Patients may also report noticing a mass if a sufficiently large soft tissue mass is present. As a result, there may be a delay in diagnosis in patients with deep tumors such as those found in the pelvis. In terms of systemic symptoms, most patients do not report fevers or significant weight loss unless the disease is quite advanced.

Laboratory values have not been shown to be helpful in the diagnosis of osteosarcoma. However, it is prudent to obtain them to establish baseline levels, specifically a complete blood count, metabolic profile, alkaline phosphatase, and serum lactate dehydrogenase. Alkaline phosphatase and serum lactate dehydrogenase can be trended during the treatment and some studies have suggested a negative prognosis if they are elevated at baseline [37, 38].

7   Imaging

Imaging plays a key role in the diagnosis, treatment, and surveillance of bone tumors such as osteosarcoma. While advanced imaging has significantly improved our ability to detect metastatic disease and better determine the extent of bony and soft tissue tumor margins, plain radiographs continue to be the first line in detection and observation.

At the time of presentation, the majority of osteosarcomas are evident on plain radiographs. As mentioned previously, most are found in the metaphyseal regions of the long bones, mainly the distal femur, proximal tibia, and proximal humerus [39]. Conventional osteosarcomas will commonly demonstrate both lucent and sclerotic features as the tumors destroy normal bone and lay down osteoid. Given their aggressive behavior, they will demonstrate evidence of rapid growth on X-ray, such as elevated periosteum and a wide zone of transition. Codman described this phenomenon whereby subperiosteal bone formation will occur at the point where the tumor elevates the periosteum off normal bone, creating a triangle of subperiosteal bone, known as "Codman's triangle" as demonstrated in Fig. 1 [7]. Similarly, as the periosteum is elevated, new bone will form perpendicular to the shaft of the bone creating spicules that give what has been described as a sunburst appearance. Since many osteosarcomas have broken through the cortex at the time of diagnosis, there is often a large soft tissue mass. This mass is usually mineralized, which is characteristic of osteosarcoma. Interestingly, after chemo-therapy, this soft tissue mass usually demonstrates increased ossification [40, 41]. The amount of bony destruction makes patients susceptible to pathologic fracture, and up to 15–20 % may demonstrate a fracture at the time of diagnosis [42].

Once there is reasonable evidence to suggest osteosarcoma on plain radio-graphs, it is important to use advanced and nuclear imaging techniques to better evaluate the tumor itself, and to look for other sites of metastasis. At a minimum, every patient with an osteosarcoma needs an MRI of the entire involved bone, a whole body bone scan, and a chest CT.

MRI is critical in the staging and surgical management of osteosarcoma as it accurately demonstrates the tumor's intramedullary extent, the size of the soft tissue mass, and the surrounding structures. This is crucial for surgeons in their planning of bony resection levels and in obtaining adequate margins at the time of resection. It can also demonstrate intra-articular tumor involvement or invasion of neurovascular structures which may limit limb sparing options for reconstruction. It is important to image the entire involved bone with MRI to evaluate for the presence of skip metastases. Skip metastases are small foci of discontiguous tumor usually within the proximal intramedullary canal of the involved bone and are demonstrated in Fig. 5. While large lesions may be visible on plain radiographs, MRI has been shown to be the most sensitive method for detecting their presence [43]. The detection of skip metastases is important for two main reasons. First, that portion of the bone needs to be included in the surgical resection. Second, even

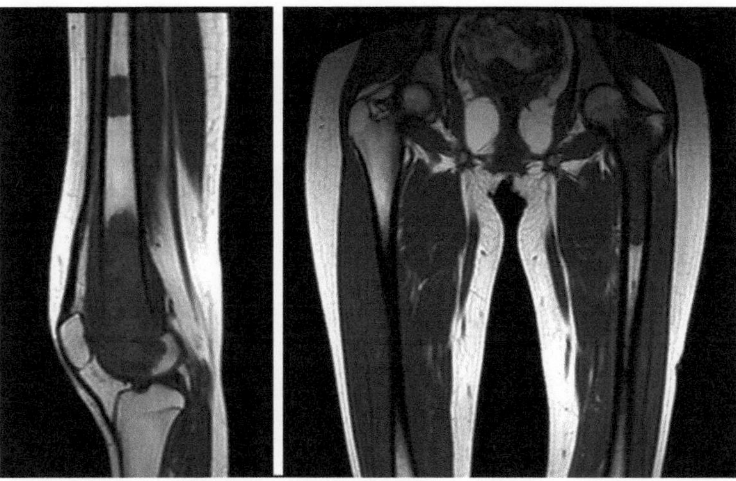

Fig. 5 Sagittal and coronal T1 weighted MRI images of a patient with skip lesions. The distal femur was probably the primary site with discontiguous lesions developing in the diaphysis and proximal femur. This patient required resection of the entire femur and reconstruction with a total femur endoprosthesis

though the lesion is within the same bone, it is considered a site of distant metastasis in terms of staging and it has negative prognostic implications [44].

Like other sarcomas, the lungs are the most common site of distant metastasis in osteosarcoma. While 80 % of patients have metastatic disease at the time of diagnosis, we are only able to detect metastatic lesions in approximately 20 % of patients with our current imaging modalities [45, 46]. This is due to the fact that the vast majority of patients have micro-metastatic disease at presentation. Since the lung is the most common site of metastatic disease, it is important to obtain a CT scan of the chest at the time of diagnosis and in follow-up. It should be noted that there is poor correlation between the presence of overt pulmonary metastasis and lesions seen on imaging. Many lesions which are palpable based on manual exam at the time of thoracotomy are not seen on the preoperative CT and likewise, many nodules noted on CTs have been demonstrated to not be metastatic [47]. Despite this, CT scan remains the gold standard imaging technique for the lungs.

The final technique of routine work-up in osteosarcoma patients is a whole body technetium bone scan (Fig. 6). This test provides a reliable means of imaging the entire body to look for other sites of osseous and nonosseous disease. The bone scan demonstrates areas of high bone turnover and given the osteoblastic nature of most osteosarcomas, the majority show increased uptake at sites of disease. The bone scan may show distant sites of uptake from the known primary tumor which can be further investigated with MRI or CT depending on their location.

There are additional imaging techniques such as positron emission technology (PET) scans and dynamic contrast-enhanced MRI's (DCE-MRI), which are more recent in their development. Although they are not part of the current routine

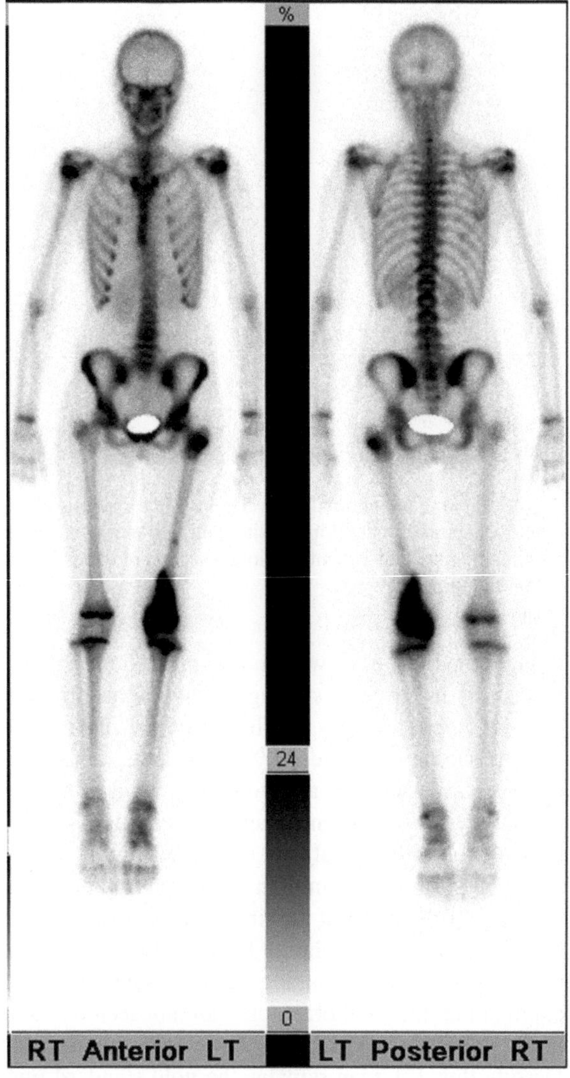

Fig. 6 Whole body technetium bone scan of the patient in Fig. 5, demonstrating osteosarcoma skip lesions within the left femur

imaging protocol for osteosarcoma, investigators are currently trying to determine what role they may play in the future regarding diagnosis, monitoring treatment response, or detecting recurrence.

For clinical practice, the most commonly used radiolabel in PET scanning is (^{18}F) fluorodeoxyglucose (FDG). The glucose molecule is taken up preferentially in areas of increased metabolic activity where glucose is being consumed at an increased rate, such as in tumors. When combined with whole body CT or MRI scans, this can provide not only a sensitive method for detecting cancers, but also the signal intensity can be quantitatively compared over time to determine tumor growth or response to treatment [48]. Recent studies have suggested that increased sarcoma signals on PET scans correlate with a worse histologic grade on pathology [49]. Also, PET scans can be used to monitor a patient's response to chemotherapy, with an improvement in the PET signal suggesting increased tumor necrosis and subsequent improved prognosis [49]. Despite these promising early findings, many medical insurance companies in the United States do not currently cover PET scans for use in sarcoma treatment due to their high cost and unestablished role. Also, there is an evidence to suggest that PET scans are not as sensitive in the detection of osseous disease as whole body bone scans [50].

DCE-MRI is another dynamic imaging modality that can be used to assess tumor function. It relies on the principle that tumors depend on angiogenesis and increased vascularity to support their rapid growth. This vascularity is disorganized and more permeable than normal tissue. On a standard MRI, this is appreciated by enhancement when intravenous gadolinium contrast is injected. However, a standard MRI is only a single snapshot of the contrast. In comparison, the DCE-MRI takes rapid images before, during, and after contrast injection to measure the difference in contrast uptake and washout in the tissue. Tumors demonstrate intense uptake and rapid washout due to the permeability of its vasculature [51]. Similar to PET, increased signal on DCE-MRI has been shown to correlate with worse histologic grade and prognosis [52]. It has also been used to measure response to chemotherapy and was found to be as effective as bone scan [53]. However, the role of this modality in the treatment of osteosarcomas has yet to be determined, and is mainly experimental at this point.

8 Staging

Cancer staging provides a method of determining the extent of the tumor within the body and its chance for spreading. It therefore provides a method for predicting prognosis. As Enneking described, a good staging system should allow practitioners to easily communicate the extent of a patient's disease, imply prognosis, guide surgical management, and suggest appropriate adjuvant treatments [54]. At this time, the two most widely used surgical staging systems for osteosarcomas and malignant bone sarcomas are the Enneking/MSTS and the AJCC systems.

In order to determine the stage based on either system, it is first important to characterize the tumor and its spread. As mentioned in the imaging section, this is first achieved by ordering the necessary imaging studies. For osteosarcoma this begins with plain radiographs of the involved bone. The amount of local spread and extent of the tumor is then better characterized with an MRI that includes the involved bone in its entirety. This is critical in the evaluation of skip metastases which may be discontiguous with the primary tumor and have negative prognostic implications. In order to evaluate for distant spread of the tumor, it is necessary to perform a whole body technetium bone scan to evaluate for bony metastasis as well as a chest CT to look for pulmonary spread. In addition, the staging systems rely on the histologic grade of the tumors which is determined based on a biopsy.

Many of the first cancer staging systems were devised by the American Joint Committee on Cancer and pertained to carcinomas. The unique aspects of sarcomas made them initially difficult to stage. However, Enneking et al. devised the first comprehensive system for use with sarcomas which is still widely used today, the Surgical Staging System of Musculoskeletal Tumors in 1980 [54]. The AJCC later created their own sarcoma system based on an adaptation of Enneking's, which corresponds more directly with their other systems [55]. Despite some minor differences between these systems, many of the basic concepts are the same as they each rely on the tumors grade, size, and the presence of metastases.

Tumor grade is predominately determined based on histologic analysis. Cells are considered a higher grade and at a higher risk of spread if there is poor differentiation, increased mitotic activity, necrosis, cellular atypia, microvascular invasion, and a high cell/matrix ratio. The Enneking system is considered a surgical staging system and allows grade to be influenced by the aggressiveness of the tumor as seen on imaging [54]. Most classic intramedullary osteosarcomas are considered high-grade, with some surface osteosarcomas being low-grade.

Tumor size and location are also important factors as they suggest how aggressive the tumor is in its growth and spread. Like other sarcomas, osteosarcomas tend to respect tissue barriers such as fascia, cartilage, synovium, and initially periosteum. However as the tumor spreads, most will break through the cortex and periosteum resulting in a soft tissue mass. Once the tumor breaks through the anatomic constraints of its compartment, it may spread rapidly within that compartment.

The Enneking system is composed of three different stages. Stage I tumors are low-grade and have a lower risk of disease spread. Stage II tumors are considered high-grade. These stages are each divided into A or B subcategories with A being intracompartmental tumors and B being extracompartmental. Finally, tumors are Stage III when there are any skip or distant metastases. It has been shown that prognosis is related to the stage, with Stage I tumors having the best survival regardless of whether they are intra or extracompartmental. This is followed by Stage IIA, then IIB, and III which have progressively worse survival rates [54].

The current AJCC staging system for bone is different in that there are four different stages, similar to its systems for other types of cancers. It is based on a TNM system, where T relates to the size of the tumor, N the presence of lymph node involvement, and M relating to distant metastasis. In its basic principles, it is very similar to the Enneking system. Stage I tumors are lower grade and Stage II are higher grade. They are subcategorized as A or B based on whether the tumor is larger or smaller than 8 cm. Stage III is high-grade with skip metastases. Stage IV contains distal metastases and is further divided into A with pulmonary metastasis and B containing lymph node or other metastases [55].

9 Treatment

The prognosis in terms of overall survival and postoperative functional status for osteosarcoma patients has improved dramatically over the past 50 years in response to major advances in chemotherapy as well as surgical resection and reconstruction options. Currently, most cancer centers treat osteosarcoma patients with neoadjuvant chemotherapy and subsequent wide surgical resection of the tumor followed by additional adjuvant chemotherapy for high-grade lesions. Low-grade lesions, such as surface lesions, are commonly treated with surgical resection alone. Patients with resectable pulmonary metastatic lesions undergo thoracotomies and metastectomies. This regimen has improved survival from less than 20 % to around 70 % at 5 years for patients who present without known metastases [56–60]. In addition, most patients currently are able to avoid amputation and retain their involved extremity through the use of limb sparing reconstructions [57].

9.1 Chemotherapy

Prior to the 1970s, the outlook for patients diagnosed with osteosarcoma was especially bleak. For those who did not present with metastases at the time of diagnosis, the 5-year survival was a consistent 20 % amongst major cancer centers [56, 61]. Even despite quick diagnosis and aggressive surgical resections, most patients developed pulmonary metastases within 6–12 months following amputation [61]. This suggested that in 80 % of the cases, osteosarcoma had already metastasized in these patients, even though no lesions were clinically detected. Therefore, simply removing the primary tumor was proving to be ineffective. In order to address the systemic spread of the disease, a systemic treatment was needed. Chemotherapy had previously been shown to be effective in other childhood cancers including leukemia and there was hope that it could provide help in the treatment of osteosarcoma. Initial attempts were discouraging as the chemotherapeutic agents used in other cancers, such as vincristine, were found to be relatively ineffective in the treatment of osteosarcoma [62].

However, the tides began to turn with the discovery of methotrexate (MTX) as a chemotherapeutic agent. MTX functions as a folic acid antagonist to suppress cell replication and was found to be effective in the treatment of leukemias. In the 1970s Jaffe et al. showed that treating osteosarcoma patients with MTX reduced the amount and size of pulmonary metastases and could be used as a postoperative adjuvant treatment. In order to prevent myelosuppression when it is given, it is combined with a leucovorin rescue where leucovorin is infused with each cycle. Subsequent studies during that time showed that the addition of other chemotherapeutic agents to MTX such as doxorubicin, cisplatin, or cyclophosphamide could increase disease free survival from 20 to upto 65 % [63, 64].

Despite these promising improvements in survival, chemotherapy in the treatment of osteosarcoma remained controversial into the 1980s. The Mayo Clinic had demonstrated an increase in survival from 20 to 40 % without the use of chemotherapy during the same time period [65]. It was their opinion that improvements in diagnosis, imaging, and surgery explained the improvement in survival that was being observed, rather than chemotherapy as other studies suggested. They subsequently performed a randomized trial which showed that survival remained about 40 % with or without the use of MTX, suggesting that adjuvant chemotherapy offered no advantage [66]. With increasing uncertainty regarding the role of chemotherapy, two major randomized clinical trials were performed in the United States in the 1980s.

The Multi-Institutional Osteosarcoma Study (MIOS) by Link et al. showed that the use of a multidrug adjuvant chemotherapy regimen increased survival from 17 to 66 % over a 2 year period [58]. The results were so striking that the study was terminated prematurely. Concurrent work by Eilber et al. had similar findings, thereby confirming the critical importance of chemotherapy in the treatment of osteosarcoma at that time [60]. More recent long-term follow-up studies have since confirmed these findings [57, 59].

Currently, the best chemotherapy regimen for osteosarcoma remains unknown and the specific agents used is somewhat dependent on whether the patient is involved in a clinical trial or is at the discretion of the treating institution. The most commonly used agents include high-dose methotrexate, doxorubicin, cisplatin, and ifosfamide, but other agents such as vincristine, bleomycin, and cyclophosphamide are sometimes used as well [67]. Interestingly, at this time survival rates remain somewhat consistent regardless of the regimen used with studies showing no definite advantage of one regimen over another. For example, ifosfamide has been shown to be a good agent for recurrent disease, however, when added to the standard regimen of high-dose methotrexate, doxorubicin, and cisplatin (MAP regimen) for primary disease, a clear advantage has not been shown, suggesting it should be reserved for poor responders [68]. Other examples include no significant survival advantage being found between doxorubicin and cisplatin versus vincristine, MTX, doxorubicin, and bleomycin or between doxorubicin and cisplatin with or without the addition of MTX [69, 70].

Regarding the timing of chemotherapy, most centers currently do neoadjuvant therapy before surgery and a course of adjuvant chemotherapy after. While the critical importance of adjuvant therapy has been demonstrated, the same cannot be said for neoadjuvant therapy [57–60]. In the early days of limb sparing surgery, neoadjuvant therapy was important as a means of preventing disease progression until custom made implants or size matched allografts could be obtained for surgical reconstruction [71]. However, with the availability of these items today, this waiting period is often unnecessary. Studies have shown that while delaying surgery for neoadjuvant therapy does not worsen survival, it does not necessarily improve it either [45, 62, 72–74]. However, there are benefits to neoadjuvant therapy beyond survival. One benefit is that certain tumors may demonstrate good response to the chemotherapy thereby decreasing their size or consolidating them which assists in the surgical resection and may improve the patient's chances of avoiding amputation [71, 75]. Similarly, by performing neoadjuvant therapy, it is possible to determine the extent of tumor necrosis at the time of resection. Pathologists will examine the resected specimen to determine the amount of tumor necrosis. Tumors with greater than 90 % necrosis are considered good responders and those with less than 90 % are poor responders. Good responders have been shown to have an improved prognosis long-term [45, 59, 73]. If the patient is found to be a poor responder, most centers will alter their postoperative chemotherapy regimen.

In terms of the future, current research is focusing on alternative methods of impairing osteosarcoma outside of cytotoxic chemotherapy. One field which has shown promise is the use of mifamurtide. Mifamurtide is an immumostimulant which is thought to stimulate the immune system to attack the malignant cells. Studies have shown improved survival when it is added to chemotherapy regimens and it is currently approved for use in Europe for the treatment of osteosarcoma, but not yet in the United States [76, 77]. Other options include the use of targeted molecular therapies, such as monoclonal antibodies to deliver chemotherapeutic drugs selectively to cancer cells [78]. Also, certain poor responders to chemotherapy have been found to have a mutation to the MDR or multidrug resistance gene which encodes for a p-glycoprotein pump in the cell that has been implicated in the export of doxorubicin from the cells, decreasing its effectiveness. As a result, studies are underway to attempt to block this pump making chemotherapy more successful [79].

9.2 Surgical Treatment

While chemotherapy has been shown to dramatically increase the survival in patients with osteosarcoma by treating micrometastases, its effectiveness is dependent on the surgical resection of any known tumors in the bones or elsewhere. Resection of osteosarcoma in the extremities is a two-part endeavor including both the resection of the tumor as well as the reconstruction of the resulting anatomic defect (Fig. 7). Surgical planning begins with the imaging and subsequent biopsy. In general, the orthopedic oncologist should be performing the biopsy, or be in communication with the interventional radiologist who may use image-guided methods. This ensures that oncologic principles are maintained during the procedure as outlined in the section on biopsy principles. Also, it ensures that the biopsy site can be incorporated into the surgical resection at the time of definitive surgery.

Currently, most resections of osteosarcoma are considered wide rather than radical resections. Radical resections involve removing the entire involved compartment and are significantly more anatomically disabling without an improvement in survival. Wide resections include the removal of the tumor with a circumferential cuff of healthy normal surrounding tissue. The exact margin required is debatable and somewhat variable depending on which structures are nearby. It is often preferable to have a smaller margin if it means saving important

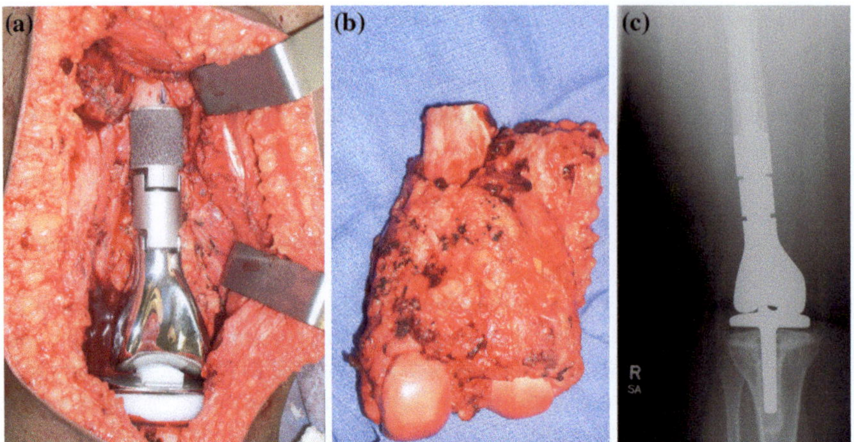

Fig. 7 **a** Intraoperative photograph of a distal femur endoprosthesis. **b** The resected distal femur osteosarcoma specimen. **c** Postoperative X-ray of the same distal femur endoprosthesis

neurovascular structures. If a wide margin is obtained, local disease is controlled 95 % of the time and has been shown to improve both prognosis and survival [80].

In the past, nearly all cases of extremity osteosarcoma were surgically treated with amputation, as viable limb sparing techniques did not exist. However, currently, more than 80 % of patients are treated with limb sparing reconstructions [57]. In order for limb preservation to be considered, it is important that a wide resection can be performed so there is no increased risk of recurrence. Similarly, the patient should be left with a limb that is durable and functional, at least in comparison to amputation. When determining this, it is important to examine the location of the tumor, its relationship to neurovascular structures and soft tissues, and the age and activity level of the patient. Pathologic fracture is also not a contraindication to limb preservation if an adequate resection is possible. If performed according to these principals, limb preservation has not been shown to decrease survival or increase recurrences when compared to amputation [57, 80, 81].

In terms of the functional differences between limb preservation and amputation, multiple studies have looked at functional outcomes as well as measures of energy expenditure and efficiency. In general, limb preservation has been shown to demonstrate improved functional scores and requires decreased energy expenditure in the lower extremity. The drawback is that it is associated with an increased number of surgeries and complications compared with amputation [82–86]. It should be noted that as prosthetic technology continues to evolve, the functional differences may become even more minimal. Regarding the psychological impact of limb sparing versus amputation, there does not appear to be a significant difference between the two [87].

The most frequently used options for limb preservation include endoprosthetic megaprostheses, bulk allografts, and allograft prosthetic composites which are a combination of the two. Each of these comes with specific indications, advantages, and disadvantages.

In the past, an endoprosthetic reconstruction required the development of a custom implant for each patient. Currently, most implants are modular and thus can be stocked and constructed to fit the size of a bony defect at the time of reconstruction. The most commonly used endoprosthetics include distal femur, proximal femur, proximal tibia, and proximal humerus devices [88]. They are typically used for metaphyseal tumors where the articular surface or joint must be resected. Intercalary endoprosthesis implants do exist, but their use is limited. The benefit of endoprostheses is that they allow immediate weight bearing and functional range of motion since they do not rely on bony healing for stability. In addition to being susceptible to infection, the major drawback is that they are a prosthetic device and prone to wear, fatigue, and loosening over time. As one would expect, given the extensive surgeries, immunocompromised patients, and oncologic basis for the reconstruction, the complications for these implants are much higher than a standard total joint replacement. Henderson et al. looked at modes of endoprosthetic failure in a large multi-institutional study with over 2,000 patients. They were the first to define five modes of failure to include soft tissue failure, aseptic loosening, structural failure, infection, and tumor progression. In their study, infection was the most common cause of failure and varied depending on the anatomic location with an average of 8 %. Larger implants such as a total femur and humerus had higher infection rates (12 and 19 %, respectively) compared to smaller implants. Also, implants with good soft tissue coverage such as the proximal femur had a much lower infection rate (3 %) compared to superficial implants such as the proximal tibia (15–23 %). Time to failure also depended on anatomic site with the shortest being the distal humerus implants at 11 months and the longest being the proximal humerus implants at 53 months. Regarding aseptic loosening, this was higher around constrained joints such as the knee, but averaged about 5 % [88]. Other studies looking at endoprosthesis survival have demonstrated 5-year implant survival greater than 80 %, which drops to 60–70 % at the 10-year mark [89, 90].

Bulk allografts are another commonly used reconstruction method. Prior to the availability of endoprostheses, they were one of the only means for reconstructing large bony defects as pioneered by Phemister [8]. In recent times, they have become more available with the proliferation of bone banks to provide size matched samples. The benefit to allografts is that after a period of time, typically 3–5 years, they theoretically incorporate into the body [91]. They also have the advantage of coming with attached tendons and ligaments which provides a reliable way of reconstructing the soft tissue envelope, especially around the shoulder and knee. Despite this, there are many complications associated with allografts including infection, fracture, nonunion, and graft resorption. Studies have shown infection rates of greater than 10 % in the first year and fracture rates of 15–20 % within the first 3 years following surgery [91–93]. These fractures are typically slow to heal and may require additional surgeries.

Unlike endoprostheses, allografts do not allow immediate weight bearing as the graft-host junctions require healing first. This can take anywhere from 6 to 12 months and nonunions are common, especially at diaphyseal junctions. Similarly, osteoarticular allografts are associated with subchondral collapse resulting in joint arthritis and subsequent revision [94, 95].

Allograft prosthetic composites (APCs) are a reconstructive option that serves to combine the benefits of both endoprostheses and allografts. They typically involve reconstructing the metaphyseal segment with allograft and its associated soft tissue attachments, and replacing the joint with a more standard prosthesis. This allows some bony incorporation with the stability and durability of a joint replacement. However the same complications of infection, fracture, nonunion, and graft resorption exist. Despite this, they have been shown to be an effective option in the shoulder, elbow, hip, and knee [96–101].

Since most osteosarcomas occur in adolescents and young adults, some patients may have a significant amount of growth left at the time of their resection. If the tumor does not involve the physis, great care is taken to avoid injuring it, and reconstructions commonly involve intercalary allografts. However with the metaphysis commonly involved, it is often necessary to resect the physis, which may create large limb length inequalities at the time of maturity. This continues to be problematic without a good solution. The standard means of controlling this has been through the use of contralateral epiphysiodeses. However, this may significantly stunt patient growth, especially if they are diagnosed at a young age. The modular endoprostheses can usually be lengthened surgically through the addition of a segment. The minimal addition is usually 2 cm of length, which is difficult to achieve without escharectomy and is associated with infection, neurovascular injury, and severe postoperative joint stiffness and pain. In order to circumvent this, expandable endoprostheses have been developed with the hope of providing a means of slow, gradual, minimally invasive lengthening. While the concept of these devices is enticing, in practice they have been associated with many problems due to mechanical complications and failures [102]. Their use continues to be somewhat controversial amongst orthopedic oncologists [103].

Overall, despite a multitude of associated complications, limb preservation surgery has become the mainstay of treatment in osteosarcoma patients. With technological advances in external prosthetics and endoprostheses, the indications and functional results will continue to improve. One area of particular interest is developing a better means of attaching soft tissues to metal components. Also promising is the use of computer navigation during surgery to assist the surgeon in making more complex geometric resection cuts or in scenarios in which the joint can be preserved (Fig. 8). An osteosarcoma in the pelvis is an example in which computer-assisted surgery will help navigate precise bone cuts due to the complex three-dimensional anatomy and preserve critical structures [104–106].

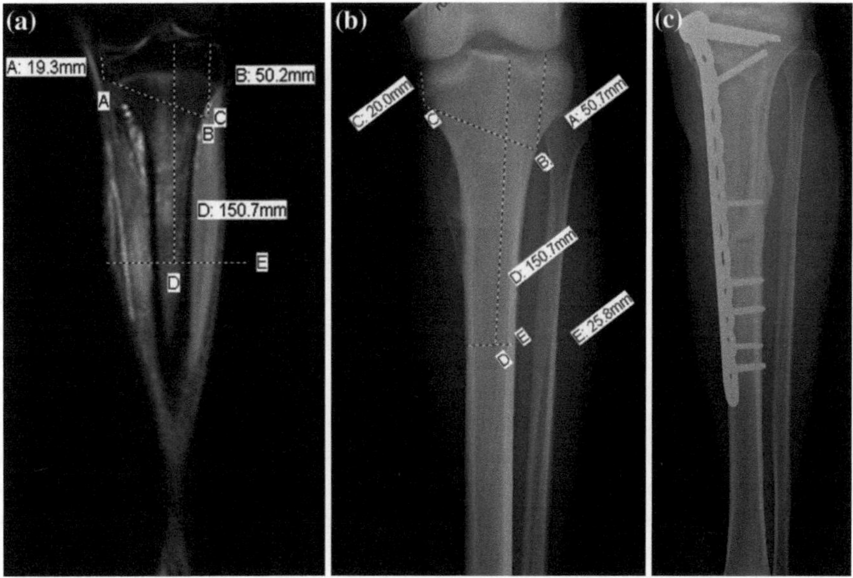

Fig. 8 **a** and **b** MRI and X-ray of a proximal tibia osteosarcoma and the planned computer navigation osteotomy sites are shown. **c** Postoperative X-ray of the same patient showing successful incorporation of an intercalary bulk allograft

10 Prognosis

For classic high-grade osteosarcomas, the prognosis has significantly improved since the use of chemotherapy was pioneered from less than 20 % survival to up to 70–80 % in patients without clinically evident metastatic disease at the time of presentation [56–60, 73]. The outcomes are even better for those patients with low-grade lesions such as parosteal or periosteal surface lesions, with about 90 % survival at 5 years, due to the low propensity of metastasis with these lesions [31, 107, 108].

Patients who present with metastases have a worse prognosis, as would be expected. The 5-year survival for these patients vary between 20–40 % with these patients often requiring multiple thoracotomies for metastectomies [109]. A similar decrease in survival is seen in patients who present with skip metastases at the time of presentation [46]. For those who are unfortunate enough to develop a recurrence after primary tumor resection, the overall survival drops to around 15 % at 5 years, with most patients eventually dying as a result of pulmonary failure from metastases [110].

Patients who experience a pathologic fracture are also at increased risk of local recurrence and have an overall lower survival of 55 % at 5 years compared to those who do not [81]. Positive prognostic factors include low-grade tumors, resections with a negative margin, and greater than 90 % necrosis after chemotherapy [31, 59, 80]. Negative prognostic factors include large tumors, those in the axial skeleton, the presence of metastases, increased patient age, and secondary osteosarcomas such as in the setting of Paget's disease [72, 111, 112].

11 Summary

In summary, osteosarcoma is a malignant tumor arising from osteoid producing mesenchymal cells. Most tumors are high-grade and found in the metaphyseal regions of long bones in young adults and adolescents. Pain is the primary complaint of the patient and imaging will show evidence of an aggressive bone tumor and may show evidence of soft tissue extension with mineralization. The appropriate imaging includes plain X-rays, MRI with contrast of the entire involved bone, whole body bone scan, and chest CT to evaluate for metastasis. Definitive diagnosis is based on biopsy, which demonstrates sarcomatous cells with cellular atypia in an osteoid matrix. Typical treatment regimens include neoadjuvant chemotherapy, followed by surgical resection and limb preservation surgery if possible, and an additional course of adjuvant chemotherapy. With modern treatment up to 70 % of patients are able to preserve their limbs and survive longterm. The hope is that these numbers will continue to improve with continued research, new medical therapies, and improved surgical reconstructive options.

References

1. Enneking WF (2009) History of orthopedic oncology in the United States. In: Pediatric and adolescent osteosarcoma. Cancer treatment and research. Springer, New York, pp 531–534
2. Boyer Alexis (1805) The lectures of Boyer upon disease of the bone. James Humphreys, Philadelphia
3. Dupuytren Guillaume (1847) On injuries and diseases of bones. Sydenham Society, London
4. Lebert H (1845) Physiologie pathologiques des recherches cliniques, on experimentales et microscopiques, etc. JB Bailliere, Paris
5. Virchow Rudolf (1867) Die Krankenhaften Gewulstewulste. Hirschwald, Berlin
6. Gross SW (1879) Sarcoma of the long bones: based on a study of one hundreed sixty-five cases. Am J Med Sci 8:338–377
7. Codman E (1909) The use of the X-ray and radiation in surgery. In: Surgery, its principles and practice by various authors. WB Saunders, Philadelphia, p 1170
8. Phemister DB (1940) Conservative surgery in the treatment of bone tumors. Surg Gynecol Obstet 70:355–364
9. Mirabello L, Troisi RJ, Savage SA (2009) Osteosarcoma incidence and survival rates from 1973 to 2004: data from the surveillance, epidemiology, and end results program. Cancer 115(7):1531–1543. doi:10.1002/cncr.24121
10. Iannaci G, Luise R, Sapere P, Costanzo RMA, Rossiello R (2013) Extraskeletal osteosarcoma: a very rare case report of primary tumor of the colon-rectum and review of the literature. Pathol Res Pract 209(6):393–396. doi:10.1016/j.prp.2013.03.010
11. Kansara M, Thomas DM (2007) Molecular pathogenesis of osteosarcoma. DNA Cell Biol 26(1):1–18. doi:10.1089/dna.2006.0505

12. Ottaviani G, Jaffe N (2002) Clinical and pathologic study of two siblings with osteosarcoma. Med Pediatr Oncol 38(1):62–64
13. Wang LL (2005) Biology of osteogenic sarcoma. Cancer J Sudbury Mass 11(4):294–305
14. Hansen MF, Koufos A, Gallie BL et al (1985) Osteosarcoma and retinoblastoma: a shared chromosomal mechanism revealing recessive predisposition. Proc Natl Acad Sci USA 82(18):6216–6220
15. Wadayama B, Toguchida J, Shimizu T et al (1994) Mutation spectrum of the retinoblastoma gene in osteosarcomas. Cancer Res 54(11):3042–3048
16. Li FP, Fraumeni JF Jr, Mulvihill JJ et al (1988) A cancer family syndrome in twenty-four kindreds. Cancer Res 48(18):5358–5362
17. Laurin N, Brown JP, Morissette J, Raymond V (2002) Recurrent mutation of the gene encoding sequestosome 1 (SQSTM1/p62) in Paget disease of bone. Am J Hum Genet 70(6):1582–1588. doi:10.1086/340731
18. Ottaviani G, Jaffe N (2009) The etiology of osteosarcoma. Cancer Treat Res 152:15–32. doi:10.1007/978-1-4419-0284-9_2
19. Rockwell MA, Enneking WF (1971) Osteosarcoma developing in solitary enchondroma of the tibia. J Bone Joint Surg Am 53(2):341–344
20. Huvos AG, Higinbotham NL, Miller TR (1972) Bone sarcomas arising in fibrous dysplasia. J Bone Joint Surg Am 54(5):1047–1056
21. Johnston RM, Miles JS (1973) Sarcomas arising from chronic osteomyelitic sinuses. A report of two cases. J Bone Joint Surg Am 55(1):162–168
22. Le Vu B, de Vathaire F, Shamsaldin A et al (1998) Radiation dose, chemotherapy and risk of osteosarcoma after solid tumours during childhood. Int J Cancer 77(3):370–377
23. Shigematsu I (1994) Health effects of atomic bomb radiation. Rinsho Byori 42(4):313–319
24. Fletcher CDM, Unni KK, World Health Organization, International Agency for Research on Cancer(2002) Pathology and genetics of tumours of soft tissue and bone. IARC Press, Lyon
25. Messerschmitt PJ, Garcia RM, Abdul-Karim FW, Greenfield EM, Getty PJ (2009) Osteosarcoma. J Am Acad Orthop Surg 17(8):515–527
26. Klein MJ, Siegal GP (2006) Osteosarcoma: anatomic and histologic variants. Am J Clin Pathol 125(4):555–581. doi:10.1309/UC6K-QHLD-9LV2-KENN
27. Yarmish G, Klein MJ, Landa J, Lefkowitz RA, Hwang S (2010) Imaging characteristics of primary osteosarcoma: nonconventional subtypes. Radiogr Rev Publ Radiol Soc North Am Inc 30(6):1653–1672. doi:10.1148/rg.306105524
28. Sangle NA, Layfield LJ (2012) Telangiectatic osteosarcoma. Arch Pathol Lab Med 136(5):572–576. doi:10.5858/arpa.2011-0204-RS
29. Nakajima H, Sim FH, Bond JR, Unni KK (1997) Small cell osteosarcoma of bone. Review of 72 cases. Cancer 79(11):2095–2106
30. Jacobson SA (1958) Early juxtacortical osteosarcoma (parosteal osteoma). J Bone Joint Surg Am 40-A(6):1310–1328
31. Okada K, Frassica FJ, Sim FH, Beabout JW, Bond JR, Unni KK (1994) Parosteal osteosarcoma. A clinicopathological study. J Bone Joint Surg Am 76(3):366–378
32. Raymond AK (1991) Surface osteosarcoma. Clin Orthop 270:140–148
33. Wold LE, Unni KK, Beabout JW, Sim FH, Dahlin DC (1984) Dedifferentiated parosteal osteosarcoma. J Bone Joint Surg Am 66(1):53–59
34. Allan CJ, Soule EH (1971) Osteogenic sarcoma of the somatic soft tissues. Clinicopathologic study of 26 cases and review of literature. Cancer 27(5):1121–1133
35. Kallianpur AA, Gupta R, Muduly DK, Kapali A, Subbarao KC (2013) Osteosarcoma of breast: a rare case of extraskeletal osteosarcoma. J Cancer Res Ther 9(2):292–294. doi:10.4103/0973-1482.113392
36. Karagöz Özen DS, Oztürk MA, Selcukbiricik F, et al (2013) Primary osteosarcoma of the heart: experience of an unusual case. Case Reports Oncol 6(1):224–228. doi:10.1159/000351123

37. Adamkova Krakorova D, Vesely K, Zambo I, et al (2012) Analysis of prognostic factors in osteosarcoma adult patients, a single institution experience. Klin Onkol Cas Ceské Slov Onkol Spolecnosti 25(5):346–358
38. Durnali A, Alkis N, Cangur S et al (2013) Prognostic factors for teenage and adult patients with high-grade osteosarcoma: an analysis of 240 patients. Med Oncol Northwood Lond Engl 30(3):624. doi:10.1007/s12032-013-0624-6
39. Dahlin DC, Unni KK (1986) Bone tumors: general aspects and data on 8,542 cases, 4th edn. Charles C. Thomas, Springfield
40. Fox MG, Trotta BM (2013) Osteosarcoma: review of the various types with emphasis on recent advancements in imaging. Semin Musculoskelet Radiol 17(2):123–136. doi:10.1055/s-0033-1342969
41. Chuang VP, Benjamin R, Jaffe N et al (1982) Radiographic and angiographic changes in osteosarcoma after intraarterial chemotherapy. AJR Am J Roentgenol 139(6):1065–1069. doi:10.2214/ajr.139.6.1065
42. Jaffe N, Spears R, Eftekhari F et al (1987) Pathologic fracture in osteosarcoma. Impact of chemotherapy on primary tumor and survival. Cancer 59(4):701–709
43. Kager L, Zoubek A, Kastner U et al (2006) Skip metastases in osteosarcoma: experience of the Cooperative Osteosarcoma Study Group. J Clin Oncol Off J Am Soc Clin Oncol 24(10):1535–1541. doi:10.1200/JCO.2005.04.2978
44. Sajadi KR, Heck RK, Neel MD et al (2004) The incidence and prognosis of osteosarcoma skip metastases. Clin Orthop 426:92–96. doi:10.1097/01.blo.0000141493.52166.69
45. Bacci G, Briccoli A, Rocca M et al (2003) Neoadjuvant chemotherapy for osteosarcoma of the extremities with metastases at presentation: recent experience at the Rizzoli Institute in 57 patients treated with cisplatin, doxorubicin, and a high dose of methotrexate and ifosfamide. Ann Oncol Off J Eur Soc Med Oncol ESMO. 14(7):1126–1134
46. Kager L, Zoubek A, Pötschger U et al (2003) Primary metastatic osteosarcoma: presentation and outcome of patients treated on neoadjuvant Cooperative Osteosarcoma Study Group protocols. J Clin Oncol Off J Am Soc Clin Oncol 21(10):2011–2018. doi:10.1200/JCO.2003.08.132
47. Kayton ML, Huvos AG, Casher J, et al (2006) Computed tomographic scan of the chest underestimates the number of metastatic lesions in osteosarcoma. J Pediatr Surg 41(1):200–206; discussion 200–206. doi:10.1016/j.jpedsurg.2005.10.024
48. Eary JF, Mankoff DA (1998) Tumor metabolic rates in sarcoma using FDG PET. J Nucl Med Off Publ Soc Nucl Med 39(2):250–254
49. Eary JF, O'Sullivan F, Powitan Y et al (2002) Sarcoma tumor FDG uptake measured by PET and patient outcome: a retrospective analysis. Eur J Nucl Med Mol Imaging 29(9):1149–1154. doi:10.1007/s00259-002-0859-5
50. Franzius C, Sciuk J, Daldrup-Link HE, Jürgens H, Schober O (2000) FDG-PET for detection of osseous metastases from malignant primary bone tumours: comparison with bone scintigraphy. Eur J Nucl Med 27(9):1305–1311
51. Choyke PL, Dwyer AJ, Knopp MV (2003) Functional tumor imaging with dynamic contrast-enhanced magnetic resonance imaging. J Magn Reson Imaging JMRI 17(5):509–520. doi:10.1002/jmri.10304
52. Guo J, Reddick WE, Glass JO et al (2012) Dynamic contrast-enhanced magnetic resonance imaging as a prognostic factor in predicting event-free and overall survival in pediatric patients with osteosarcoma. Cancer 118(15):3776–3785. doi:10.1002/cncr.26701
53. Kawai A, Sugihara S, Kunisada T, Uchida Y, Inoue H (1997) Imaging assessment of the response of bone tumors to preoperative chemotherapy. Clin Orthop 337:216–225
54. Enneking WF, Spanier SS, Goodman MA (1980) A system for the surgical staging of musculoskeletal sarcoma. Clin Orthop 153:106–120
55. American Joint Committee on Cancer (2010) AJCC cancer staging manual, 7th edn. Springer, New York

56. Dahlin DC, Coventry MB (1967) Osteogenic sarcoma. A study of six hundred cases. J Bone Joint Surg Am 49(1):101–110

57. Bacci G, Ferrari S, Bertoni F et al (2000) Long-term outcome for patients with nonmetastatic osteosarcoma of the extremity treated at the istituto ortopedico rizzoli according to the istituto ortopedico rizzoli/osteosarcoma-2 protocol: an updated report. J Clin Oncol Off J Am Soc Clin Oncol 18(24):4016–4027

58. Link MP, Goorin AM, Miser AW et al (1986) The effect of adjuvant chemotherapy on relapse-free survival in patients with osteosarcoma of the extremity. N Engl J Med 314(25):1600–1606. doi:10.1056/NEJM198606193142502

59. Bernthal NM, Federman N, Eilber FR et al (2012) Long-term results (>25 years) of a randomized, prospective clinical trial evaluating chemotherapy in patients with high-grade, operable osteosarcoma. Cancer 118(23):5888–5893. doi:10.1002/cncr.27651

60. Eilber F, Giuliano A, Eckardt J, Patterson K, Moseley S, Goodnight J (1987) Adjuvant chemotherapy for osteosarcoma: a randomized prospective trial. J Clin Oncol Off J Am Soc Clin Oncol 5(1):21–26

61. Friedman MA, Carter SK (1972) The therapy of osteogenic sarcoma: current status and thoughts for the future. J Surg Oncol 4(5):482–510

62. Ferguson WS, Goorin AM (2001) Current treatment of osteosarcoma. Cancer Invest 19(3):292–315

63. Goorin AM, Perez-Atayde A, Gebhardt M et al (1987) Weekly high-dose methotrexate and doxorubicin for osteosarcoma: the Dana-Farber Cancer Institute/the Children's Hospital-study III. J Clin Oncol Off J Am Soc Clin Oncol 5(8):1178–1184

64. Sutow WW (1980) Multidrug chemotherapy in osteosarcoma. Clin Orthop 153:67–72

65. Taylor WF, Ivins JC, Pritchard DJ, Dahlin DC, Gilchrist GS, Edmonson JH (1985) Trends and variability in survival among patients with osteosarcoma: a 7-year update. Mayo Clin Proc Mayo Clin 60(2):91–104

66. Edmonson JH, Green SJ, Ivins JC et al (1984) A controlled pilot study of high-dose methotrexate as postsurgical adjuvant treatment for primary osteosarcoma. J Clin Oncol Off J Am Soc Clin Oncol 2(3):152–156

67. Maki RG (2012) Ifosfamide in the neoadjuvant treatment of osteogenic sarcoma. J Clin Oncol Off J Am Soc Clin Oncol 30(17):2033–2035. doi:10.1200/JCO.2012.42.3285

68. Ferrari S, Ruggieri P, Cefalo G et al (2012) Neoadjuvant chemotherapy with methotrexate, cisplatin, and doxorubicin with or without ifosfamide in nonmetastatic osteosarcoma of the extremity: an Italian sarcoma group trial ISG/OS-1. J Clin Oncol Off J Am Soc Clin Oncol 30(17):2112–2118. doi:10.1200/JCO.2011.38.4420

69. Souhami RL, Craft AW, Van der Eijken JW et al (1997) Randomised trial of two regimens of chemotherapy in operable osteosarcoma: a study of the European Osteosarcoma Intergroup. Lancet 350(9082):911–917. doi:10.1016/S0140-6736(97)02307-6

70. Bramwell VH, Burgers M, Sneath R et al (1992) A comparison of two short intensive adjuvant chemotherapy regimens in operable osteosarcoma of limbs in children and young adults: the first study of the European Osteosarcoma Intergroup. J Clin Oncol Off J Am Soc Clin Oncol 10(10):1579–1591

71. Rosen G, Marcove RC, Caparros B, Nirenberg A, Kosloff C, Huvos AG (1979) Primary osteogenic sarcoma: the rationale for preoperative chemotherapy and delayed surgery. Cancer 43(6):2163–2177

72. Bielack SS, Kempf-Bielack B, Delling G et al (2002) Prognostic factors in high-grade osteosarcoma of the extremities or trunk: an analysis of 1,702 patients treated on neoadjuvant cooperative osteosarcoma study group protocols. J Clin Oncol Off J Am Soc Clin Oncol 20(3):776–790

73. Meyers PA, Heller G, Healey J et al (1992) Chemotherapy for nonmetastatic osteogenic sarcoma: the Memorial Sloan-Kettering experience. J Clin Oncol Off J Am Soc Clin Oncol 10(1):5–15

74. Bacci G, Picci P, Ruggieri P et al (1990) Primary chemotherapy and delayed surgery (neoadjuvant chemotherapy) for osteosarcoma of the extremities. The Istituto Rizzoli Experience in 127 patients treated preoperatively with intravenous methotrexate (high versus moderate doses) and intraarterial cisplatin. Cancer 65(11):2539–2553

75. Malawer M, Buch R, Reaman G et al (1991) Impact of two cycles of preoperative chemotherapy with intraarterial cisplatin and intravenous doxorubicin on the choice of surgical procedure for high-grade bone sarcomas of the extremities. Clin Orthop 270:214–222

76. Meyers PA, Schwartz CL, Krailo MD et al (2008) Osteosarcoma: the addition of muramyl tripeptide to chemotherapy improves overall survival–a report from the Children's Oncology Group. J Clin Oncol Off J Am Soc Clin Oncol 26(4):633–638. doi:10.1200/JCO.2008.14.0095

77. Meyers PA, Schwartz CL, Krailo M et al (2005) Osteosarcoma: a randomized, prospective trial of the addition of ifosfamide and/or muramyl tripeptide to cisplatin, doxorubicin, and high-dose methotrexate. J Clin Oncol Off J Am Soc Clin Oncol 23(9):2004–2011. doi:10.1200/JCO.2005.06.031

78. Sampson VB, Gorlick R, Kamara D, Anders Kolb E (2013) A review of targeted therapies evaluated by the pediatric preclinical testing program for osteosarcoma. Front Oncol 3:132. doi:10.3389/fonc.2013.00132

79. Ling V (1997) Multidrug resistance: molecular mechanisms and clinical relevance. Cancer Chemother Pharmacol 40(Suppl):S3–S8

80. Bacci G, Longhi A, Cesari M, Versari M, Bertoni F (2006) Influence of local recurrence on survival in patients with extremity osteosarcoma treated with neoadjuvant chemotherapy: the experience of a single institution with 44 patients. Cancer 106(12):2701–2706. doi:10.1002/cncr.21937

81. Scully SP, Ghert MA, Zurakowski D, Thompson RC, Gebhardt MC (2002) Pathologic fracture in osteosarcoma: prognostic importance and treatment implications. J Bone Joint Surg Am 84-A(1):49–57

82. Rougraff BT, Simon MA, Kneisl JS, Greenberg DB, Mankin HJ (1994) Limb salvage compared with amputation for osteosarcoma of the distal end of the femur. A long-term oncological, functional, and quality-of-life study. J Bone Joint Surg Am 76(5):649–656

83. Renard AJ, Veth RP, Schreuder HW, van Loon CJ, Koops HS, van Horn JR (2000) Function and complications after ablative and limb-salvage therapy in lower extremity sarcoma of bone. J Surg Oncol 73(4):198–205

84. Otis JC, Lane JM, Kroll MA (1985) Energy cost during gait in osteosarcoma patients after resection and knee replacement and after above-the-knee amputation. J Bone Joint Surg Am 67(4):606–611

85. Harris IE, Leff AR, Gitelis S, Simon MA (1990) Function after amputation, arthrodesis, or arthroplasty for tumors about the knee. J Bone Joint Surg Am 72(10):1477–1485

86. Mason GE, Aung L, Gall S et al (2013) Quality of life following amputation or limb preservation in patients with lower extremity bone sarcoma. Front Oncol 3:210. doi:10.3389/fonc.2013.00210

87. Weddington WW Jr, Segraves KB, Simon MA (1985) Psychological outcome of extremity sarcoma survivors undergoing amputation or limb salvage. J Clin Oncol Off J Am Soc Clin Oncol 3(10):1393–1399

88. Henderson ER, Groundland JS, Pala E et al (2011) Failure mode classification for tumor endoprostheses: retrospective review of five institutions and a literature review. J Bone Joint Surg Am 93(5):418–429. doi:10.2106/JBJS.J.00834

89. Horowitz SM, Glasser DB, Lane JM, Healey JH (1993) Prosthetic and extremity survivorship after limb salvage for sarcoma. How long do the reconstructions last? Clin Orthop 293:280–286

90. Malawer MM, Chou LB (1995) Prosthetic survival and clinical results with use of large-segment replacements in the treatment of high-grade bone sarcomas. J Bone Joint Surg Am 77(8):1154–1165

91. Mankin HJ, Gebhardt MC, Jennings LC, Springfield DS, Tomford WW (1996) Long-term results of allograft replacement in the management of bone tumors. Clin Orthop 324:86–97

92. Berrey BH Jr, Lord CF, Gebhard MC, Mankin HJ (1990) Fractures of allografts. Frequency, treatment, and end-results. J Bone Joint Surg Am 72(6):825–833

93. Sorger JI, Hornicek FJ, Zavatta M et al (2001) Allograft fractures revisited. Clin Orthop 382:66–74

94. Hornicek FJ, Gebhardt MC, Tomford WW et al (2001) Factors affecting nonunion of the allograft-host junction. Clin Orthop 382:87–98

95. Getty PJ, Peabody TD (1999) Complications and functional outcomes of reconstruction with an osteoarticular allograft after intra-articular resection of the proximal aspect of the humerus. J Bone Joint Surg Am 81(8):1138–1146

96. Abdeen A, Hoang BH, Athanasian EA, Morris CD, Boland PJ, Healey JH (2009) Allograft-prosthesis composite reconstruction of the proximal part of the humerus: functional outcome and survivorship. J Bone Joint Surg Am 91(10):2406–2415. doi:10.2106/JBJS.H.00815

97. Van de Sande MAJ, Dijkstra PDS, Taminiau AHM (2011) Proximal humerus reconstruction after tumour resection: biological versus endoprosthetic reconstruction. Int Orthop 35(9):1375–1380. doi:10.1007/s00264-010-1152-z

98. Morrey ME, Sanchez-Sotelo J, Abdel MP, Morrey BF (2013) Allograft-prosthetic composite reconstruction for massive bone loss including catastrophic failure in total elbow arthroplasty. J Bone Joint Surg Am 95(12):1117–1124. doi:10.2106/JBJS.L.00747

99. Donati D, Di Bella C, Frisoni T, Cevolani L, DeGroot H (2011) Alloprosthetic composite is a suitable reconstruction after periacetabular tumor resection. Clin Orthop 469(5):1450–1458. doi:10.1007/s11999-011-1799-9

100. Benedetti MG, Bonatti E, Malfitano C, Donati D (2013) Comparison of allograft-prosthetic composite reconstruction and modular prosthetic replacement in proximal femur bone tumors: functional assessment by gait analysis in 20 patients. Acta Orthop 84(2):218–223. doi:10.3109/17453674.2013.773119

101. Farfalli GL, Aponte-Tinao LA, Ayerza MA et al (2013) Comparison between constrained and semiconstrained knee allograft-prosthesis composite reconstructions. Sarcoma 2013:489652. doi:10.1155/2013/489652

102. Henderson ER, Pepper AM, Marulanda G, Binitie OT, Cheong D, Letson GD (2012) Outcome of lower-limb preservation with an expandable endoprosthesis after bone tumor resection in children. J Bone Joint Surg Am 94(6):537–547. doi:10.2106/JBJS.I.01575

103. Aboulafia AJ, Wilkerson J (2012) Lower-limb preservation with an expandable endoprosthesis after tumor resection in children: is the cup half full or half empty? Commentary on an article by Eric R. Henderson, MD, et al.: "Outcome of lower-limb preservation with an expandable endoprosthesis after bone tumor resection in children." J Bone Joint Surg Am 94(6):e39. doi:10.2106/JBJS.K.01643

104. Ritacco LE, Milano FE, Farfalli GL, Ayerza MA, Muscolo DL, Aponte-Tinao LA (2013) Accuracy of 3-D planning and navigation in bone tumor resection. Orthopedics 36(7):e942–e950. doi:10.3928/01477447-20130624-27

105. Cartiaux O, Banse X, Paul L, Francq BG, Aubin C-É, Docquier P-L (2013) Computer-assisted planning and navigation improves cutting accuracy during simulated bone tumor surgery of the pelvis. Comput Aided Surg Off J Int Soc Comput Aided Surg 18(1–2):19–26. doi:10.3109/10929088.2012.744096

106. Li J, Wang Z, Guo Z, Chen G-J, Yang M, Pei G-X (2013) Precise resection and biological reconstruction under navigation guidance for young patients with juxta-articular bone sarcoma in lower extremity: preliminary report. J Pediatr Orthop. doi:10.1097/BPO.0b013e31829b2f23

107. Rose PS, Dickey ID, Wenger DE, Unni KK, Sim FH (2006) Periosteal osteosarcoma: long-term outcome and risk of late recurrence. Clin Orthop 453:314–317. doi:10.1097/01.blo. 0000229341.18974.95
108. Grimer RJ, Bielack S, Flege S, et al (2005) Periosteal osteosarcoma–a European review of outcome. Eur J Cancer Oxf Engl 1990. 41(18):2806–2811. doi:10.1016/j.ejca.2005.04.052
109. Briccoli A, Rocca M, Salone M, Guzzardella GA, Balladelli A, Bacci G (2010) High grade osteosarcoma of the extremities metastatic to the lung: long-term results in 323 patients treated combining surgery and chemotherapy, 1985–2005. Surg Oncol 19(4):193–199. doi:10.1016/j.suronc.2009.05.002
110. Bielack SS, Kempf-Bielack B, Branscheid D et al (2009) Second and subsequent recurrences of osteosarcoma: presentation, treatment, and outcomes of 249 consecutive cooperative osteosarcoma study group patients. J Clin Oncol Off J Am Soc Clin Oncol 27(4):557–565. doi:10.1200/JCO.2008.16.2305
111. Iwata S, Ishii T, Kawai A et al (2013) Prognostic factors in elderly osteosarcoma patients: a multi-institutional retrospective study of 86 cases. Ann Surg Oncol. doi:10.1245/s10434-013-3210-4
112. Ruggieri P, Calabrò T, Montalti M, Mercuri M (2010) The role of surgery and adjuvants to survival in Pagetic osteosarcoma. Clin Orthop 468(11):2962–2968. doi:10.1007/s11999-010-1473-7

Ewing's Sarcoma of Bone

Drew D. Moore and Rex C. Haydon

Abstract

Ewing's sarcoma of bone is a primary bone sarcoma found predominantly in patients during their second decade of life. It is a high-grade aggressive small round blue cell tumor that is part of the Ewing's family of tumors. Its exact eitiology is unknown but it commonly demonstrates reproducible staining of CD99 and translocations of the EWS gene. Historically, this diagnosis was associated with near certain metastasis and subsequent mortality. However, current management consists of extensive chemotherapy in addition to local control with surgical resection and/or radiation. As a result, survival has improved to the 55–75% range in those patients who present without known metastases. Current research aims to continue this improvement by looking further into the assocated gene abnormalities and possibly targeted therapies.

Keywords

Ewing's sarcoma · Ewing · Sarcoma · Limb salvage · Bone

1   Introduction

Ewing's sarcoma of bone is a part of the Ewing's sarcoma family of tumors, which includes primitive neuroectodermal tumors, Ewing's soft tissue sarcomas, and Askins' tumors. Each shares similar molecular and histologic findings. It is found

D. D. Moore · R. C. Haydon (✉)
Department of Orthopedic Surgery and Rehabilitation Medicine,
The University of Chicago, 5841 South Maryland, MC 3079 Chicago,
IL 60637, USA
e-mail: rhaydon@surgery.bsd.uchicago.edu

T. D. Peabody and S. Attar (eds.), *Orthopaedic Oncology*,
Cancer Treatment and Research 162, DOI: 10.1007/978-3-319-07323-1_5,
© Springer International Publishing Switzerland 2014

predominantly in the diaphysis of long bones and pelvis of patients in their second decade of life. It is a high-grade aggressive lesion that most commonly originates in bone and is associated with large soft tissue masses and frequent metastases. Histologically, it presents as sheets of small round blue cells which almost universally stain for CD99 and demonstrate common translocations of the EWS gene on chromosome 22. Treatment consists of multiagent systemic chemotherapy and local control with surgery and/or radiation. Current management has improved survival to the 55–75 % range in those who present without metastases.

2   History

The sarcoma that we currently call Ewing's sarcoma was first described in detail by famed pathologist James Ewing in 1921 [1]. He noted seeing a form of bony neoplasm that did not fit with the appearance or behavior of other known lesions such as osteosarcoma or myeloma. He described his first case of a teenage girl who presented with a pathologic fracture of her forearm in which the tumor had an impressive response to radium, which was unlike osteosarcoma. Similarly, the Bence-Jones protein was never found in her urine to suggest myeloma. He goes on to report six additional cases of teenagers with permeative lesions in the shaft of long bones. Histology showed small polyhedral cells with hyperchromic nuclei, pale cytoplasm, and a lack of intercellular stromal material. All of the tumors seemed to at least temporarily resolve after radiation was administered. Given their appearance, he surmised the tumors may have originated from the endothelium, and he named them diffuse endotheliomas of bone [1]. It is impressive that with the exception of their relationship to endothelium, nearly all of the characteristics he described remain pathognomonic for Ewing's sarcoma to this day.

The application of the name Ewing's sarcoma would come 4 years later in 1925 by Ernest Codman [2]. Codman was one of the first surgeons to promote the use of registries to further the understanding of rare diseases and to promote the use of outcomes in guiding surgical practice [3]. As a result, he created the first sarcoma registry and within its description he refers to the sarcoma as described by Ewing as a Ewing's sarcoma. Of note, Codman would be probably best known for his description of the way aggressive bone tumors elevate periosteum leading to the radiographic finding of a Codman's Triangle [4].

While the understanding of Ewing's sarcoma evolved, there were other neoplasms that were felt to be clinically unique and different based on their behavior and histology that are now known to be related and part of the Ewing's sarcoma family of tumors.

The first was described in 1918 by Arthur Stout as a tumor of the ulnar nerve composed of undifferentiated round cells which formed rosettes. This later became known as a primitive neuroectodermal soft tissue tumor or PNET. Similarly, Askin et al. in 1979 described a soft tissue tumor found in the thoracopulmonary region of adolescents, which was composed of small round cells and was associated with high rates of recurrence and mortality, which would come to be known as Askin's tumor. Nonosseous forms of Ewing's sarcoma have also been documented, but are rare compared to osseous forms.

When molecular studies showed similar genetic profiles and translocations for these three tumors, they were subsequently felt to be related, as opposed to distinct entities. As a result, currently they are all considered to be a part of the Ewing's Sarcoma Family of tumors. For the purpose of this review, the focus will be on Ewing's sarcoma of bone.

3 Epidemiology and Etiology

As with other bone cancers, much of the current understanding of the epidemiology of Ewing's sarcoma in the United States comes from the Surveillance, Epidemiology, and End Results (SEER) Program from the National Institute of Health. This is a database of cancer statistics drawn from a variety of cancer centers throughout the United States in an attempt to provide an accurate cross-section of the population. Esiashvili et al. have performed the most recent review of the SEER data from 1973 to 2004 looking specifically at Ewing's sarcoma. They found an average annual incidence of about 3 per 1 million, which has been stable over the past 40 years. The incidence peaks within the second decade of life, with more than 50 % of cases being diagnosed between the ages of 10–20. Less than 23 % are found in those younger than 10 and the incidence declines rapidly as age increases beyond 20 years. Ewing's sarcoma has a slight predominance in males at 61 % of the cases diagnosed, and is found almost exclusively in Caucasians who represented 92 % of the cases [5, 6].

In terms of location within the body, Ewing's sarcoma has a predilection for the diaphysis of tubular bones and the pelvis. The most common location is the extremities at 46 % of cases, with the lower extremity being more common than the upper. This is followed by the pelvis at 25 %, trunk including ribs or spine at 22 %, and other sites including soft tissue Ewing's at 6 % [5, 6]. These epidemiological findings in the United States are similar to those of Europe based on a study by Stiller et al. who used the Automated Childhood Cancer Information System European database to demonstrate concurrent findings regarding the epidemiology of Ewing's sarcoma [7].

The etiology of Ewing's sarcoma remains unknown. Despite most cases being associated with reproducible genetic abnormalities such as translocations, most seem to be sporadic in nature as no hereditary link has been found. Similarly, an association with environmental factors has yet to be demonstrated.

4 Patient Presentation

As with other primary bone sarcomas, pain is the most common initial symptom of patients with Ewing's sarcoma of bone. As the tumor destroys bone, patients may notice a deep, dull, aching pain in the involved region or extremity [8]. While antiinflammatories and pain medicines may initially offer some relief, often their effect diminishes as the tumor grows. Although some may notice the pain to be more severe at night, this is certainly not a universal feature with only about 20 % noting it in one study [9]. If the bone is sufficiently weakened to alter its mechanical properties, it is common for pain to worsen with activities which put increased stress on the remaining bone.

Unfortunately, many patients who initially present with pain are initially misdiagnosed as having more common benign conditions such as strains or tendinitis. More than 25 % of Ewing's patients may have a delay in diagnosis of over 6 months from the time of their first appointment with a physician. Those whose tumors are sufficiently large may have a palpable mass, leading to a quicker workup and diagnosis [9].

Systemic symptoms tend to be more commonplace in Ewing's sarcoma compared to osteosarcoma. It is not uncommon for patients to present with fevers or weight loss, which in the presence of bone pain may mislead the physician into misdiagnosing the cause as osteomyelitis. Laboratory findings can promote this as many Ewing's patients will have mildly elevated inflammatory markers such as erythrocyte sedimentation rate, creactive protein, and other cytokines [9–13]. It is important to note that in general these lab values, while elevated, are lower than those in patients with true osteomyelitis.

Other abnormal laboratory findings include the presence of anemia as well as elevated markers of bone turnover such as lactate dehydrogenase (LDH) and alkaline phosphatase (AP) [10]. The trend in the LDH and AP levels may offer some indication as to treatment response, but their current utility and role in standard care is debatable.

5 Histologic and Molecular Pathology

Similar to other bone sarcomas, a definitive diagnosis of Ewing's sarcoma is based on tissue biopsy. If possible, it is preferred that the definitive treatment team participates in the biopsy or its planning in order to assure that sound oncologic principles are used in obtaining the biopsy, facilitating surgical resection, reconstruction, and ideally limb-salvage [14].

Grossly, Ewing's sarcoma has the classic grayish/fleshy appearance of other sarcomas [1]. It may occasionally be associated with necrosis.

Histologically, Ewing's sarcoma appears as sheets of homogenous densely packed small round blue cells. They have a high nuclear to cytoplasm ratio and the nucleus is associated with fine granular chromatin and pinpoint nucleoli. The cytoplasm typically has few or small organelles and abundant glycogen [15]

(Figs. 1c, 2d and 3c). Unfortunately, they appear very histologically similar to other blue cell tumors so the differential includes other diagnoses such as lymphoma, leukemia, small cell carcinoma, rhabdomyosarcoma, neuroblastoma, and others.

One of the main ways to distinguish Ewing's sarcoma from these other diagnoses is through the use of immunohistochemistry. Most Ewing's cells stain strongly for CD99 which is a cell surface glycoprotein encoded by the MIC2 gene [16]. While CD99 staining is very sensitive for Ewing's sarcoma, it is not specific as nearly all small blue cell tumors will at least partially stain for CD99. This makes it imperative to use it as part of an immunohistochemical panel in order to differentiate from diagnoses such as lymphoma or rhabdomyoscaroma [17]. Also, this is why cytogenetic and molecular findings are typically used to confirm the diagnosis.

Cytogenetically there are a small number of characteristic and reproducible translocations associated with the Ewing's sarcoma family of tumors. All of them involve the EWS gene on chromosome 22, which encodes an RNA binding protein, whose exact role in cellular function is unknown. It is subsequently upregulated through translocations with the ETS family of transcription factor genes, the most common being FLI1 on chromosome 11 [18]. This t(11;22)(q24;q12) translocation produces the EWS-FLI1 fusion gene which is found in about 85 % of Ewing's tumors [19]. The next most common is the t(21;22)(q22;q12) translocation of the EWS-ERG gene found in another 5–10 % [20]. Other translocations that are much more rare have also been reported including EWS-ETV1, EWS-FEV, and EWS-EIAF amongst other translocations and cytogenetic abnormalities [21, 22].

At present, the prognostic value of one translocation over another remains controversial. Some studies have suggested an improved prognosis with the EWS-FLI1 translocation, [23] although others have found there to be no discernable difference in terms of phenotype or prognosis [24, 25].

Currently, these translocations are determined through the use of fluorescent in situ hybridization (FISH) and reverse transcriptase polymerase chain reaction (RT-PCR) methods. Both of these methods can be employed to detect the presence of micrometastases in bone marrow biopsies obtained for staging purposes [26, 27]. The benefit to FISH is that it has been shown to be more sensitive and specific compared to RT-PCR, but the techniques are complementary [28].

While the EWS translocations remain highly sensitive and specific for the Ewing's family of tumors, it is important to note that they have been reported in other tumors as well, underscoring the importance of the consensus between the microscopic, immunohistochemical, and molecular characteristics in the diagnosis of Ewing's sarcoma [29].

6   Imaging

Imaging studies are critical in the diagnosis, staging, and surveillance of Ewing's sarcoma. Even with many advanced imaging techniques available, standard radiographs remain the first-line choice. As mentioned in the epidemiology section,

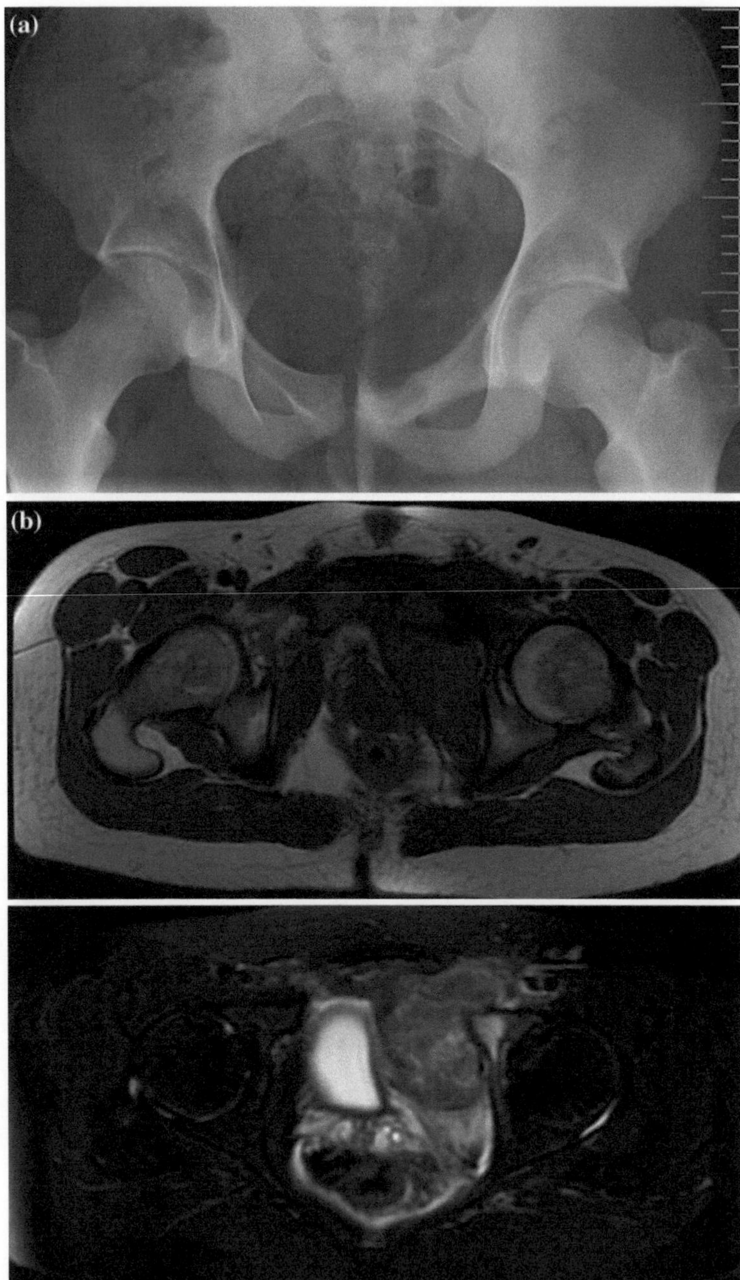

◀ **Fig. 1** Seventeen-year old male with *left* hip and groin pain. **a** Anteroposterior radiographs of the pelvis reveal a subtle, but apparent, radiolucent lesion centered on the *left* superior pubic ramus. **b** T1 and STIR Axial images on MRI reveal a large soft tissue mass centered on the *left* superior pubic ramus. **c** Representative H&E histology demonstrates sheets of small blue cells typical of Ewing's sarcoma. **d** Axial postcontrast T1 Fat Saturation image after radiation and neo-adjuvant chemotherapy reveal significant local response with a significantly reduced soft tissue mass. **e** Surgically excised specimen also reveals no discernable soft tissue mass remaining after neoadjuvant treatment. **f** Anteroposterior radiographs of the pelvis 5 years after treatment. He has remained disease free

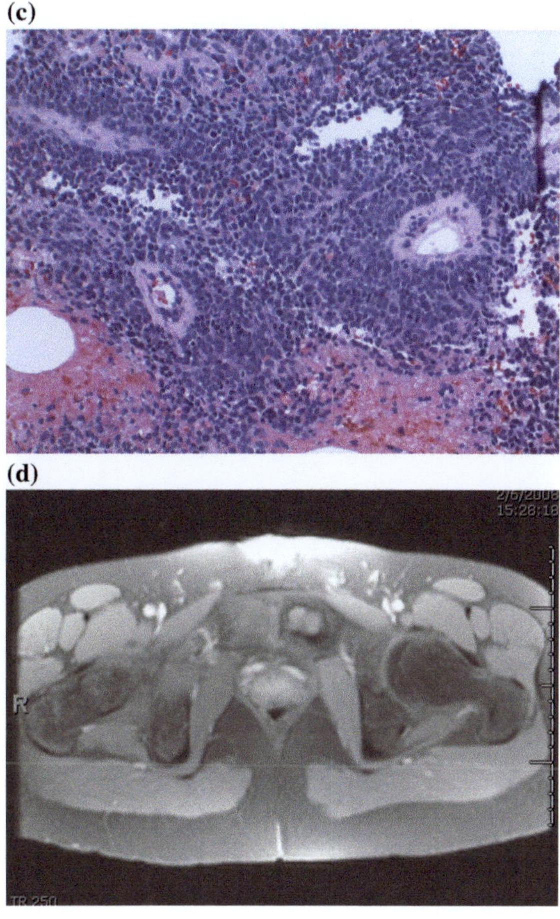

Fig. 1 (continued)

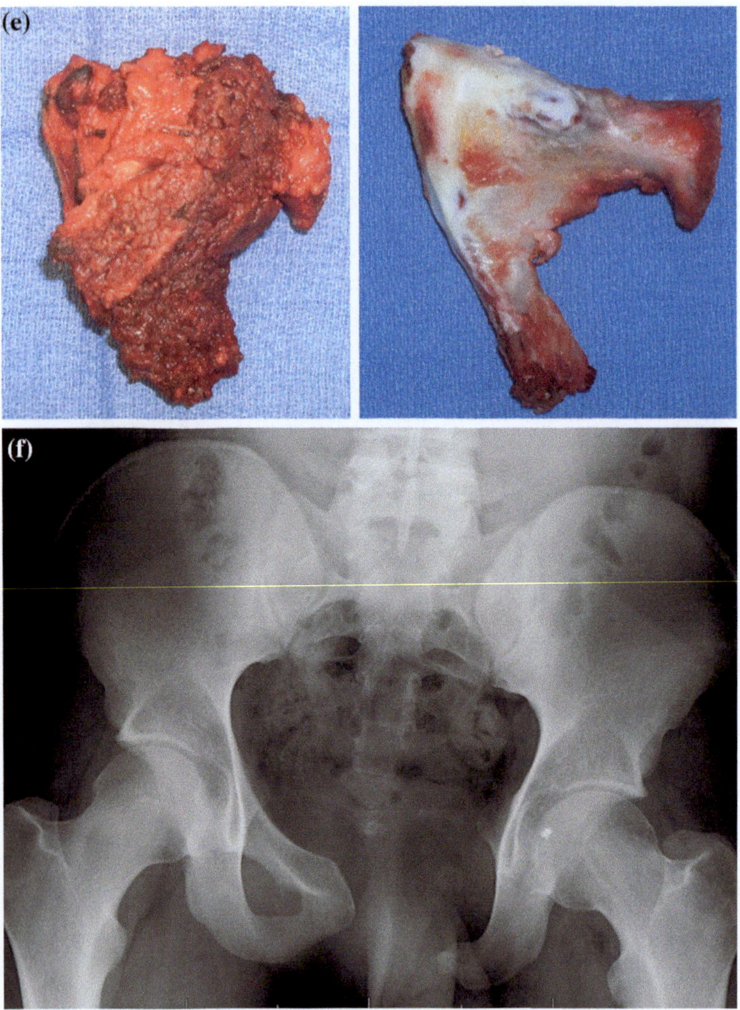

Fig. 1 (continued)

Ewing's sarcoma of bone is found predominantly in the diaphyseal region of long bones as well as the pelvis and ribs [5]. Its radiographic appearance can vary, but it will typically demonstrate aggressive features. The tumor margin is often poorly defined and permeative in nature [30]. The bone may show areas of radiulucency, or may demonstrate a mixed lytic/sclerotic appearance [31] (Figs. 1a, 2a and 3a). In the majority of patients, a soft tissue mass will be present at diagnosis, but it can be very difficult to distinguish on radiographs since it does not demonstrate ossification as is routinely seen in osteosarcoma [30]. As a result, it is not uncommon for plain radiographs to appear normal, especially when a comparison study is unavailable, leading to a delay in diagnosis [9]. In fact, an unremarkable plain X-ray of a bone

Fig. 2 Sixteen-year old female with left thigh pain. **a** Anteroposterior and lateral radiographs of the *left* femur reveal an eccentric, poorly marginated radiolucent lesion involving the mid-diaphysis of the femur. **b** T1 and STIR Axial images on MRI reveal extensive marrow changes around the lesion with a soft tissue mass not appreciated on the plain radiographs. **c** T1 and STIR Coronal images on MRI. **d** A biopsy revealed a small blue cell tumor and immunohistochemical staining that was positive for FLI-1. **e** Axial T1 and sagittal STIR imaging of the lesion after neoadjuvant chemotherapy with visible shrinkage of the soft tissue mass. **f** Intraoperative images of the surgical removal of the diaphyseal segment of the *left* femur with the tumor followed by allograft reconstruction. **g** Anteroposterior radiographs 2 years after surgery reveal healing of the allograft

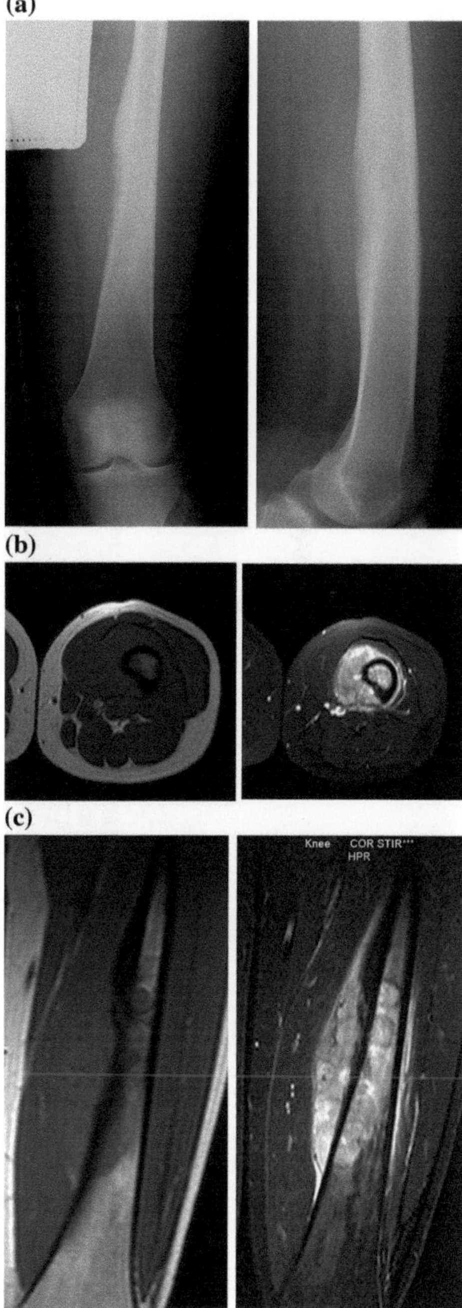

Fig. 2 (continued)

(d)

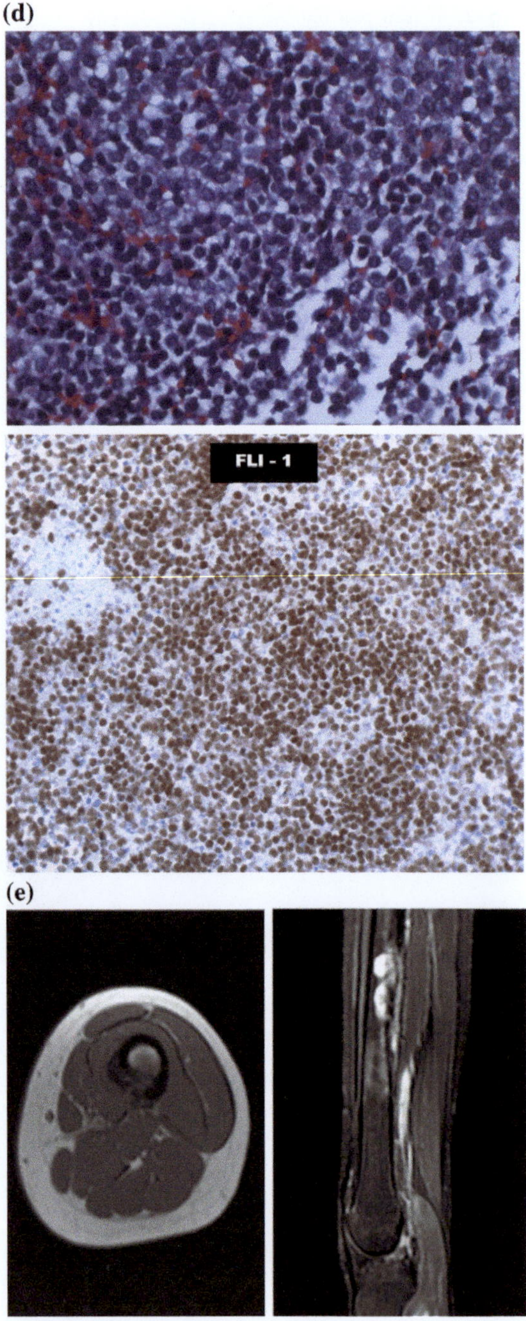

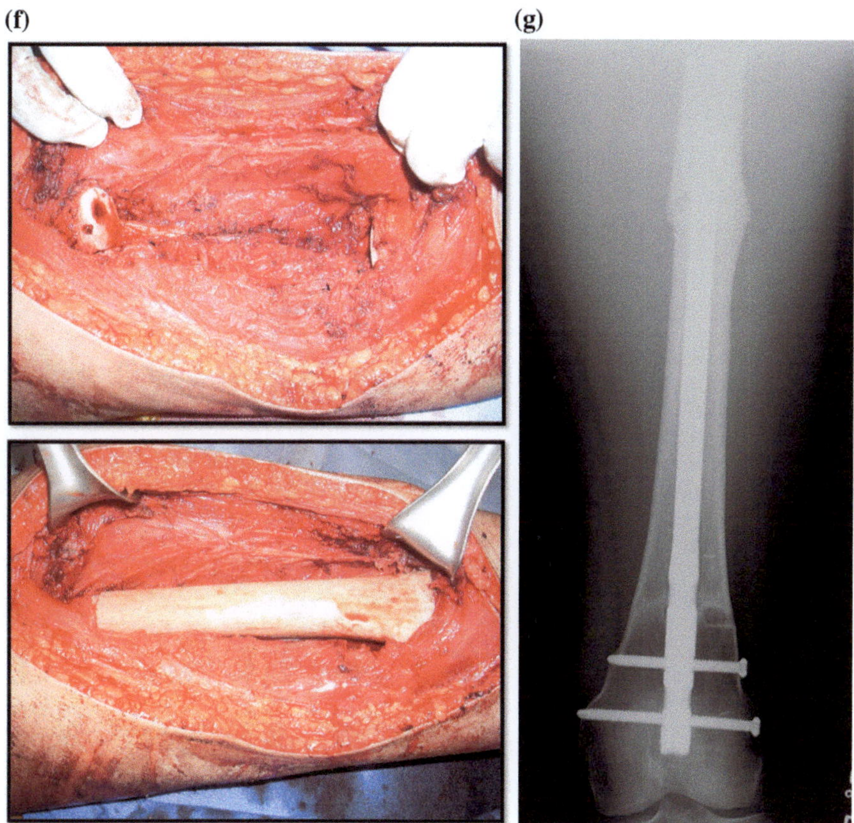

Fig. 2 (continued)

with an MRI demonstrating a bony lesion with an associated large soft tissue mass can be highly suggestive of a blue cell tumor such as Ewing's.

The soft tissue mass may be visualized on X-ray via its interaction with the periosteum. As it expands it will elevate normal periosteum which will subsequently ossify, leading to an "onion-skinning" appearance, or similarly, Codman's triangle [30–32]. Codman's triangle occurs when the soft tissue component of the tumor elevates the periosteum of the involved bone, causing new bone to form in the apex where the periosteum contacts the bone and where it has been elevated by tumor [4]. These periosteal reactions are not unique to Ewing's sarcoma, but rather demonstrate its aggressive nature.

MRI is the most sensitive imaging technique for evaluating Ewing's sarcoma, and can be especially helpful in cases where the radiographs are indeterminate. Ewing's is often heterogenous in its appearance, and is dark on T1 sequences, and mostly bright or heterogeneous on T2. It will enhance if the study is performed with gadolinium (Figs. 1b,d, 2b,c and 3b). MRI is also helpful in determining the

Fig. 3 Thirteen-year old female with *right* ankle pain and swelling.

a Anteroposterior radiographs of the *right* ankle before (*left*) and after (*right*) neoadjuvant chemotherapy. **b** T2 Axial MRI images of the *right* ankle before (*left*) and after (*right*) neoadjuvant chemotherapy. **c** A biopsy revealed a small blue cell tumor and immunohistochemical staining and subsequent FISH (not shown) revealed the 11:22 EWS-FLI-1 fusion gene. **d** Intraoperative images of the surgical removal of the *right* distal fibula with no subsequent reconstruction. **e** Anteroposterior radiographs 10 years after surgery reveal no local recurrence or ankle instability

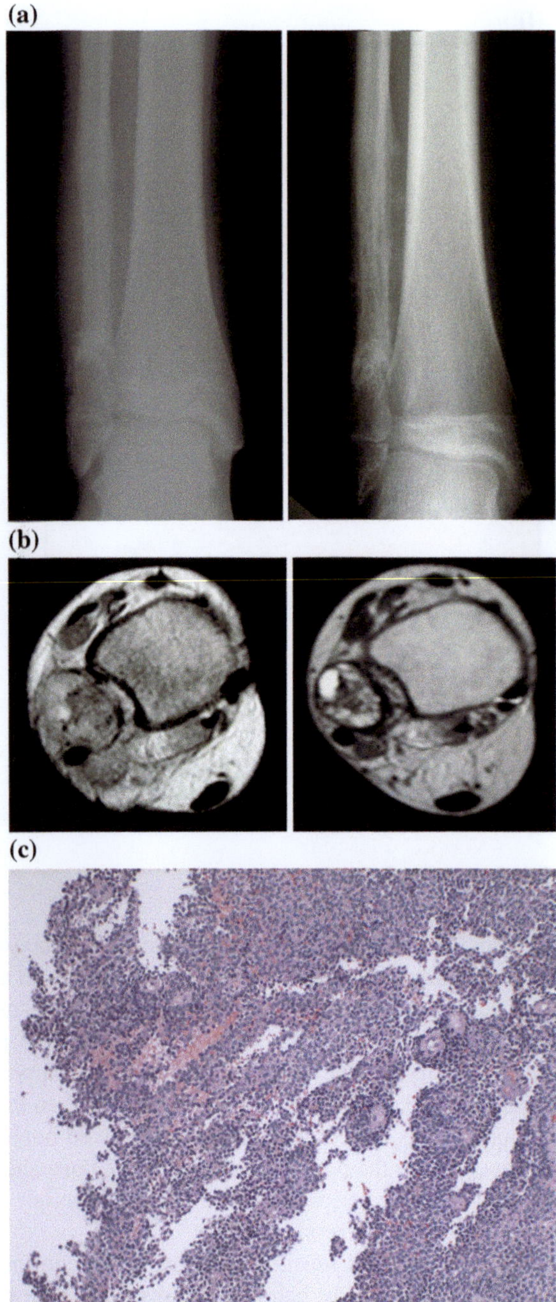

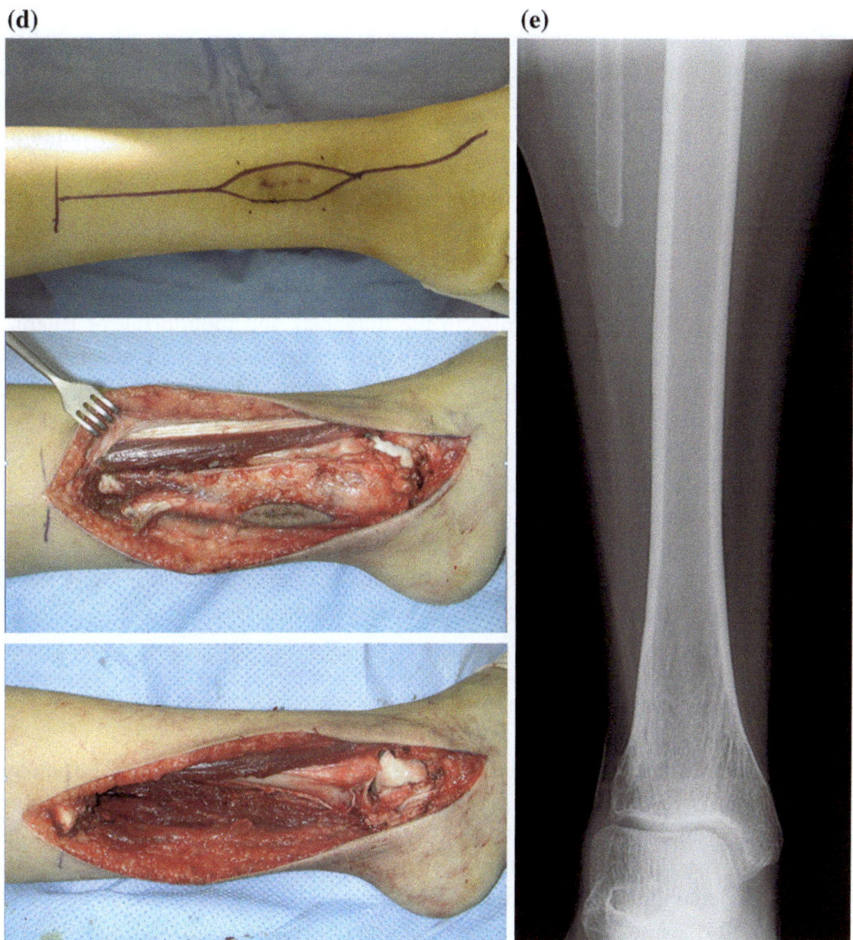

Fig. 3 (continued)

extent of the soft tissue mass and its relationship to adjacent structures. These factors become critical if a surgical resection and reconstruction is to be considered. It is important to include the entire involved bone in the MRI study to evaluate for skip metastases, which are noncontiguous tumors present within the same bone, and may be present in 10–20 % of patients [31].

While radiographs and an MRI of the involved bone are essential in the evaluation of Ewing's sarcoma, CT of the tumor is generally less helpful. Its main advantage is the ability to look at the degree of bony destruction, or if combined with angiography, to evaluate vascular structures that may be altered by the tumor.

Radiographic studies are also important to evaluate for distant sites of disease. As with other sarcomas, the most common site of Ewing's metastases are the lungs, followed by other bones or soft tissues [8].

Unfortunately, the studies used in the staging of Ewing's sarcoma are somewhat institution dependent. The National Comprehensive Cancer Network guidelines for Ewing's staging account for some of this variability [14]. They recommend that all patients should have at least an MRI of the known primary tumor, plus X-rays or a CT if indicated. For pulmonary disease, they recommend a CT scan of the chest and to evaluate for osseous metastases, either a PET scan or bone scan. In addition, they also recommend either an MRI of the spine or a bone marrow biopsy, and possibly molecular studies to look for micrometastases.

Much of the staging debate currently revolves around the role and accuracy of PET scans. Position emission tomography (PET) scanning represents a newer modality which has shown promise in the diagnosis and monitoring of Ewing's sarcoma. They rely on radio-labeled glucose molecules, which are taken up preferentially in tumors with higher metabolic rates. Increased PET uptake at diagnosis has been shown to be associated with a worse prognosis and improvement in PET uptake after treatment can be suggestive of tumor necrosis [33–35].

Many studies have been performed directly comparing the sensitivity of detecting osseous metastases of both PET and bone scans. Most support that PET scans are similar if not superior to bone scans in terms of accuracy [36–38]. However, PET scans are much more expensive, and studies also exist which demonstrate that bone scans continue to be more sensitive [39].

7   Staging and Workup

One of the first steps after a patient has been diagnosed with a Ewing's sarcoma is to determine if there are other sites of disease as this impacts both their future therapies as well as prognosis. Ewing's is similar to osteosarcoma in the sense that even though most patients do not initially present with overt metastatic disease, the majority have subclinical micrometastases that will become apparent in the future if the patient does not receive systemic treatment. This is known because prior to systemic treatments, radical surgical excision alone resulted in dismal cure rates of about 10 % [40].

The staging workup of a patient diagnosed with Ewing's sarcoma starts with a thorough history and physical exam. Baseline laboratory studies are ordered including a CBC, BMP, ESR, and LDH. There are a variety of imaging studies performed to characterize the primary tumor and look for sites of metastatic disease.

One unique staging aspect of Ewing's sarcoma compared to other primary bone sarcomas is the evaluation of micrometastatic disease. Traditionally, this has been achieved by performing either a unilateral or bilateral bone marrow biopsy or aspiration looking for malignant cells. There is little evidence to suggest the utility of this and its use is somewhat institution dependent. Some authors have recently argued that PET scans and or MRI's of the entire body may be as accurate as a bone marrow biopsy in detecting metastatic disease with much less morbidity [36, 38].

Also, molecular tests as described in the pathology section are increasingly being used in determining the presence of micrometastases.

In regards to staging systems, there is no system that is unique to Ewing's sarcoma. Rather the two most commonly used systems for Ewing's sarcoma of bone are designed for bone tumors in general. The first was created by Enneking et al. in 1980 and is the Surgical Staging System of Musculoskeletal Tumors [41]. The second was later created by the American Joint Committee on Cancer (AJCC) based on an adaptation of its system for carcinomas which relies on a TNM or tumor, node, metastasis methodology [42]. These systems are similar in that they are predominantly concerned with tumor size, grade, and the presence of metastases.

Both consider low-grade tumors to be Stage I and high-grade tumors to be at least Stage II. Ewing's sarcoma by nature is a high-grade tumor, so all are at least Stage II. These stages are further divided into A or B based on the size of the tumor with IIA/B being intra or extra-compartmental in the Enneking system or less than or greater than 8 cm in the AJCC system. In the Enneking system, Stage III implies metastatic disease; whereas, Stage III disease in the AJCC system is used to describe patients with skip metastases to the same bone, with no other sites of disease. Finally, stage IV in the AJCC implies distant metastases and is further subdivided based on the location. In general, a higher stage is suggestive of a poorer prognosis [5].

8   Treatment

Since the time of Ewing's description of Ewing's sarcoma, treatment and subsequent prognosis have improved dramatically. Surgery and radiation continue to play an important role in the control of local disease. However, major advances in survival have occurred with the addition of systemic chemotherapy. Prior to the use of systemic treatment, almost 80–90 % of patients would develop distant metastases despite the use of aggressive local control measures such as amputation [5]. Currently, the standard treatment of Ewing's sarcoma of bone involves neoadjuvant chemotherapy, followed by local treatment with either surgery and/or radiation depending on tumor characteristics such as size, proximity to critical structures, and resectability. This is then followed by a course of adjuvant chemotherapy.

8.1   Chemotherapy

Since the majority of patients who present with a localized Ewing's sarcoma will develop distant metastases with the use of local control alone, systemic chemotherapy is crucial to killing subclinical micrometastatic cells within the body in an attempt to cure.

Chemotherapy was first used to treat Ewing's sarcoma in the early 1960s, when it was discovered that cyclophosphamide therapy provided a survival benefit [43, 44]. Subsequent randomized trials throughout the 1970s and 1980s looked at the benefit of adding additional systemic agents. These studies found that survival was increased with the use of multiagent regimens incorporating vincristine, doxorubicin, cyclophosphamide, and dactinomycin (VACD), with reported 5 year survival rates in the 50–60 % range for localized disease [45–48]. VACD therapy has become the mainstay of systemic treatment to this day. Subsequent studies have examined the benefit of using additional drugs, including ifosfamide and etoposide and have shown a modest improvement in survival. For example, Grier et al. showed an improvement in 5 year event-free survival from 54 to 69 % in patients who underwent alternating cycles of ifosfamide and etoposide with VACD, compared to VACD alone for those with localized disease. Interestingly, no improvement in survival has been shown for those who presented with metastatic disease [49, 50].

Despite significant improvement in survival with the use of multiagent therapies, patients who present with known metastases continue to have poor 5 year survival figures in the 25 % range [45]. One of the methods explored to overcome this was the use of dose-intensive regimens where chemotherapy cycles were given in either higher doses or more rapidly. Included in this was the use of very high-dose treatments with a subsequent bone marrow transplant. In general, these techniques subjected patients to very high toxicities and complications with very little survival benefit [51–53]. One area which has shown some promise is the use of granulocyte colony stimulating factor in between cycles of treatment in order to offset bone marrow toxicity and restore blood counts more rapidly to decrease the time between chemotherapy cycles [54].

Like other malignancies, the latest area of interest has been the application of targeted therapies. Given that Ewing's sarcoma demonstrates common genetic translocations and abnormalities, it would seem an ideal disease for molecular therapies. However, much remains unknown about the role of the EWS fusion genes or their cellular pathways. As a result, it has been difficult to exploit the unique fusion protein in Ewing's sarcoma as a target for treatment and at this time no drugs have been approved for clinical use outside of trials [55, 56]. Certain drugs have shown promise in clinical trials, such as molecular targets for the insulin-like growth factor-I receptor. These have demonstrated the ability to decrease or stabilize some tumors, but have had little effect on others [57]. Conversely, other drugs such as the tyrosine kinase inhibitor Imatinib, which has been so efficacious in other malignancies, has demonstrated little effect in the treatment of Ewing's sarcoma [58]. Despite this, targeted therapy development continues to be an area of intense research.

8.2 Local Control

Ewing's sarcoma of bone is unique compared to other common primary bone sarcomas such as osteosarcoma or chondrosarcoma in that it is very radiosensitive. This was an observation that initially helped James Ewing distinguish it from osteosarcoma [1]. As a result, prior to the use of routine chemotherapy, it was primarily treated with external beam radiation. Radiation was often successful in halting the progression of the tumor and even causing it to shrink. However, most patients eventually succumbed to metastatic disease. Since chemotherapy has significantly improved overall survival, the complications of radiation have become more apparent, especially since patients are treated at a young age.

Most patients who receive radiation therapy will receive a total dose of about 60 Gy fractionated over 6 weeks [59]. The main advantage of radiation is that it avoids the morbidity associated with surgical intervention. However, it is associated with many complications both short-term and long-term. The short-term side-effects are often transient and include dermatitis, fatigue, and nausea. The long-term effects include fracture, growth arrest, joint stiffness, and secondary malignancies, all of which can have devastating effects on function and are particularly concerning in skeletally immature patients [59–61].

In the past, surgical resection was recommended for "expendable" bones. With more data on the long-term effects of radiation, this opinion has evolved. Controversy has developed over what defined an "expendable" bone as well as which local treatment, radiation or surgery, results in improved survival and local control. Most of the data regarding this comes from the pelvis, since its anatomic location makes it difficult to resect with negative margins and equally difficult to reconstruct.

A multitude of studies have examined outcomes in pelvic Ewing's sarcomas and they generally demonstrate improved survival and local control rates when surgical resection is performed compared to radiation alone [45, 62–67]. Yang et al. found that the overall survival in pelvic cases was 51 % with surgical resection compared to 18 % with radiation alone [62]. Similarily Frassica et al. showed 5 year overall survival was 75 % with surgery versus 25 % for radiation [63]. Local control also appears improved with surgery at 83 % compared to 67 % [66]. Surgical resection also has been shown to be superior to radiation alone with improved survival in the extremities [67, 68, 69].

However, caution should be used when interpreting these studies as there is definite selection bias in their design. All of them are retrospective, nonrandomized studies where radiation alone was often reserved for those cases where surgical resection with negative margins would be unlikely. Unfortunately, a randomized clinical trial evaluating this would be difficult to justify in light of existing data.

Therefore, the current treatment strategy employed by most orthopedic oncologists is to surgically resect Ewing's sarcoma of bone when adequate margins are obtainable and the reconstructive result will leave the patient with a satisfactorily functional limb. If there are positive margins after resection, then postoperative radiation should be considered. Radiation alone is typically reserved for tumors where the resection offers no meaningful reconstructive options necessitating amputation, or in certain cases of certain pelvic or spinal tumors.

In terms of postresection reconstruction, modern techniques make limb-salvage feasible in the majority of cases. Common reconstructive options include the use of large endoprostheses, bulk allografts, and allograft-prosthetic composites (APCs).

While endoprostheses required custom manufacturing in the past, most are currently modular and can be assembled at the time of surgery using off-the-shelf components. These endoprostheses are typically reserved for tumors involving the metaphyseal or epiphyseal sections of bones in which the articular surface must be resected with the tumor. Therefore, these devices can be used to reconstruct the joint. Like all implants, they are prone to wear and failure over time and have high rates of infection depending on surgical and anatomic factors such as soft tissue coverage [70–72].

Bulk allografts are commonly employed for tumors in the diaphysis of long bones, where resection can be performed and an intercalary allograft can be put in its place (Figs. 2f,g). The advantage with this technique is that is spares the patient's articular surfaces and once it is incorporated can allow for full activities. However, they also have high rates of complications including resorption, non-unions, fractures, and infections [73–75]. Another option employed at some centers, primarily in Asia, is to resect the involved bone, submit it to high extracorporeal doses of radiation to kill the tumor cells, and subsequently use this autograft bone to reconstruct the defect. This has been shown to result in good local control, but is associated with many of the same complications associated with cadaveric allografts [76].

Allograft-prosthetic composites are felt to be a compromise between allografts and endoprosthetics, in which articular segments are reconstructed with an allograft junction at the metaphysis and a prosthetic joint. These are most commonly employed in Ewing's sarcomas of the pelvis whereby the bone is reconstructed with allograft and the hip is replaced with a total hip prosthesis. While they have advantages, they suffer from similar complications unique to both allografts and prostheses [77, 78].

8.3   Metastatic Disease

Patients with who present with metastatic disease or who develop it later have much worse survival outcomes. However, their survival can be improved with aggressive management of metastatic lesions, especially if there is only a single site. The most common sites of metastasis are the lungs, bone, and soft tissues [5, 6]. Lung metastases can be treated with thoracotomy if there is a single lesion, or whole lung radiation if there are multiple lesions [79]. Similarly, a single bony metastasis should be treated as if it is a primary tumor with radiation or surgery depending on its location.

9   Prognosis

Overall the prognosis of a patient diagnosed with Ewing's sarcoma of bone has improved dramatically since it was first described. Prior to the use of systemic chemotherapy and local control, the overall survival was minimal at best. However, modern methods have increased the 5 year event-free survival statistics for those who present without metastases to the 55–75 % range, with overall survival being slightly less [45, 61, 62, 80–82]. Those who present with metastases or who subsequently develop a recurrence have much worse survival in the 20 % range. Also, not all metastases are equal, as metastases to the lungs have shown a survival advantage compared to those in bone [61].

In regards to negative prognostic factors, advanced age, large tumor volume, axial skeleton involvement, and lack of surgical resection have all been associated with worse outcomes [61, 80–82].

10 Summary

In summary, since first described by James Ewing almost 95 years ago, there has been a dramatic increase in our understanding and treatment of Ewing's sarcoma. Despite major improvements in survival with systemic chemotherapy and local control with surgery and/or radiation, there continues to be much room for improvement, especially in those patients who present with metastases or develop a recurrence. Current research aims to characterize and target the EWS fusion protein in order to develop new treatments that will improve survival and reduce the toxicity and morbidity associated with current treatment options.

References

1. Ewing J (1921) Diffuse endothelioma of bone. Proc NY Pathol Soc. 21:17–24
2. Codman E (1925) Bone sarcoma: an interpretation of the nomenclature used by the committee on the Registry of Bone Sarcomas of the American College of Surgeons. Paul B. Hoeber, Inc., New York
3. Codman EA (2009) The Classic: The Registry of Bone Sarcomas as an example of the End-Result Idea in Hospital Organization. Clin Orthop Relat Res 467(11):2766–2770. doi:10.1007/s11999-009-1048-7
4. Codman E (1909) The use of the x-ray and radiation in surgery. In: Keen WB (ed) Surgery. Its principles and practice by various authors, vol 1909. WB Saunders, Philadelphia, p. 1170
5. Esiashvili N, Goodman M, Marcus RB Jr (2008) Changes in incidence and survival of Ewing sarcoma patients over the past 3 decades: Surveillance Epidemiology and End Results data. J Pediatr Hematol Oncol 30(6):425–430. doi:10.1097/MPH.0b013e31816e22f3
6. Dorfman HD, Czerniak B (1995) Bone cancers. Cancer 75(1 Suppl):203–210
7. Stiller CA, Desandes E, Danon SE et al (2006) Cancer incidence and survival in European adolescents (1978–1997). Report from the Automated Childhood Cancer Information System project. Eur J Cancer Oxf Engl 1990 2(13):2006–2018. doi:10.1016/j.ejca.2006.06.002
8. Patricio MB, Vilhena M, Neves M et al (1991) Ewing's sarcoma in children: twenty-five years of experience at the Instituto Portuguếs de Oncologia de Francisco Gentil (I.P.O.F.G.). J Surg Oncol 47(1):37–40
9. Widhe B, Widhe T (2000) Initial symptoms and clinical features in osteosarcoma and Ewing sarcoma. J Bone Joint Surg Am 82(5):667–674
10. Bacci G, Balladelli A, Forni C et al (2007) Ewing's sarcoma family tumours. Differences in clinicopathological characteristics at presentation between localised and metastatic tumours. J Bone Joint Surg Br 89(9):1229–1233. doi:10.1302/0301-620X.89B9.19422
11. Rutkowski P, Kamińska J, Kowalska M, Ruka W, Steffen J (2003) Cytokine and cytokine receptor serum levels in adult bone sarcoma patients: correlations with local tumor extent and prognosis. J Surg Oncol 84(3):151–159. doi:10.1002/jso.10305

12. Nakamura T, Grimer RJ, Gaston CL, Watanuki M, Sudo A, Jeys L (2013) The prognostic value of the serum level of C-reactive protein for the survival of patients with a primary sarcoma of bone. Bone Jt J 95-B(3):411–418. doi:10.1302/0301-620X.95B3.30344

13. Ilić I, Manojlović S, Cepulić M, Orlić D, Seiwerth S (2004) Osteosarcoma and Ewing's sarcoma in children and adolescents: retrospective clinicopathological study. Croat Med J 45(6):740–745

14. Biermann JS, Adkins DR, Agulnik M et al (2013) Bone cancer. J Natl Compr Cancer Netw JNCCN 11(6):688–723

15. Suh C-H, Ordóñez NG, Hicks J, Mackay B (2002) Ultrastructure of the Ewing's sarcoma family of tumors. Ultrastruct Pathol 26(2):67–76. doi:10.1080/01913120252959236

16. Fellinger EJ, Garin-Chesa P, Triche TJ, Huvos AG, Rettig WJ (1991) Immunohistochemical analysis of Ewing's sarcoma cell surface antigen p30/32MIC2. Am J Pathol 139(2):317–325

17. Folpe AL, Goldblum JR, Rubin BP et al (2005) Morphologic and immunophenotypic diversity in Ewing family tumors: a study of 66 genetically confirmed cases. Am J Surg Pathol 29(8):1025–1033

18. Delattre O, Zucman J, Plougastel B et al (1992) Gene fusion with an ETS DNA-binding domain caused by chromosome translocation in human tumours. Nature 359(6391):162–165. doi:10.1038/359162a0

19. Delattre O, Zucman J, Melot T et al (1994) The Ewing family of tumors—a subgroup of small-round-cell tumors defined by specific chimeric transcripts. N Engl J Med 331(5):294–299. doi:10.1056/NEJM199408043310503

20. Peter M, Mugneret F, Aurias A, Thomas G, Magdelenat H, Delattre O (1996) An EWS/ERG fusion with a truncated N-terminal domain of EWS in a Ewing's tumor. Int J Cancer J Int Cancer 67(3):339–342. doi:10.1002/(SICI)1097-0215(19960729)67:3<339:AID-IJC6>3.0.CO;2-S

21. Wang L, Bhargava R, Zheng T et al (2007) Undifferentiated small round cell sarcomas with rare EWS gene fusions: identification of a novel EWS-SP3 fusion and of additional cases with the EWS-ETV1 and EWS-FEV fusions. J Mol Diagn JMD 9(4):498–509. doi:10.2353/jmoldx.2007.070053

22. Shulman SC, Katzenstein H, Bridge J et al (2012) Ewing sarcoma with 7;22 translocation: three new cases and clinicopathological characterization. Fetal Pediatr Pathol 31(6):341–348. doi:10.3109/15513815.2012.659397

23. De Alava E, Kawai A, Healey JH et al (1998) EWS-FLI1 fusion transcript structure is an independent determinant of prognosis in Ewing's sarcoma. J Clin Oncol Off J Am Soc Clin Oncol 16(4):1248–1255

24. Ginsberg JP, Alava E de, Ladanyi M et al (1999) EWS-FLI1 and EWS-ERG gene fusions are associated with similar clinical phenotypes in Ewing's Sarcoma. J Clin Oncol 17(6):1809

25. Le Deley M-C, Delattre O, Schaefer K-L et al (2010) Impact of EWS-ETS fusion type on disease progression in Ewing's sarcoma/peripheral primitive neuroectodermal tumor: prospective results from the cooperative Euro-E.W.I.N.G. 99 trial. J Clin Oncol Off J Am Soc Clin Oncol 28(12):1982–1988. doi:10.1200/JCO.2009.23.3585

26. Wagner LM, Smolarek TA, Sumegi J, Marmer D (2012) Assessment of minimal residual disease in Ewing sarcoma. Sarcoma 2012:780129. doi:10.1155/2012/780129

27. Dubois SG, Epling CL, Teague J, Matthay KK, Sinclair E (2010) Flow cytometric detection of Ewing sarcoma cells in peripheral blood and bone marrow. Pediatr Blood Cancer 54(1):13–18. doi:10.1002/pbc.22245

28. Bridge RS, Rajaram V, Dehner LP, Pfeifer JD, Perry A (2006) Molecular diagnosis of Ewing sarcoma/primitive neuroectodermal tumor in routinely processed tissue: a comparison of two FISH strategies and RT-PCR in malignant round cell tumors. Mod Pathol Off J U S Can Acad Pathol Inc 19(1):1–8. doi:10.1038/modpathol.3800486

29. Thorner P, Squire J, Chilton-MacNeil S et al (1996) Is the EWS/FLI-1 fusion transcript specific for Ewing sarcoma and peripheral primitive neuroectodermal tumor? A report of four cases showing this transcript in a wider range of tumor types. Am J Pathol 148(4):1125–1138

30. Kuleta-Bosak E, Kluczewska E, Machnik-Broncel J et al (2010) Suitability of imaging methods (X-ray, CT, MRI) in the diagnostics of Ewing's sarcoma in children—analysis of own material. Pol J Radiol Pol Med Soc Radiol 75(1):18–28
31. Peersman B, Vanhoenacker FM, Heyman S et al (2007) Ewing's sarcoma: imaging features. JBR-BTR Organe Société R Belge Radiol SRBR Orgaan Van K Belg Ver Voor Radiol KBVR 90(5):368–376
32. Van der Woude HJ, Bloem JL, Hogendoorn PC (1998) Preoperative evaluation and monitoring chemotherapy in patients with high-grade osteogenic and Ewing's sarcoma: review of current imaging modalities. Skeletal Radiol 27(2):57–71
33. Eary JF, Mankoff DA (1998) Tumor metabolic rates in sarcoma using FDG PET. J Nucl Med Off Publ Soc Nucl Med 39(2):250–254
34. Eary JF, O'Sullivan F, Powitan Y et al (2002) Sarcoma tumor FDG uptake measured by PET and patient outcome: a retrospective analysis. Eur J Nucl Med Mol Imaging 29(9):1149–1154. doi:10.1007/s00259-002-0859-5
35. Sharma P, Khangembam BC, Suman KCS et al (2013) Diagnostic accuracy of 18F-FDG PET/CT for detecting recurrence in patients with primary skeletal Ewing sarcoma. Eur J Nucl Med Mol Imaging 40(7):1036–1043. doi:10.1007/s00259-013-2388-9
36. Newman EN, Jones RL, Hawkins DS (2013) An evaluation of [F-18]-fluorodeoxy-D-glucose positron emission tomography, bone scan, and bone marrow aspiration/biopsy as staging investigations in Ewing sarcoma. Pediatr Blood Cancer 60(7):1113–1117. doi:10.1002/pbc.24406
37. Treglia G, Salsano M, Stefanelli A, Mattoli MV, Giordano A, Bonomo L (2012) Diagnostic accuracy of ^{18}F-FDG-PET and PET/CT in patients with Ewing sarcoma family tumours: a systematic review and a meta-analysis. Skeletal Radiol 41(3):249–256. doi:10.1007/s00256-011-1298-9
38. Kumar J, Seith A, Kumar A et al (2008) Whole-body MR imaging with the use of parallel imaging for detection of skeletal metastases in pediatric patients with small-cell neoplasms: comparison with skeletal scintigraphy and FDG PET/CT. Pediatr Radiol 38(9):953–962. doi:10.1007/s00247-008-0921-y
39. Franzius C, Sciuk J, Daldrup-Link HE, Jürgens H, Schober O (2000) FDG-PET for detection of osseous metastases from malignant primary bone tumours: comparison with bone scintigraphy. Eur J Nucl Med 27(9):1305–1311
40. Chan RC, Sutow WW, Lindberg RD, Samuels ML, Murray JA, Johnston DA (1979) Management and results of localized Ewing's sarcoma. Cancer 43(3):1001–1006
41. Enneking WF, Spanier SS, Goodman MA (1980) A system for the surgical staging of musculoskeletal sarcoma. Clin Orthop 153:106–120
42. American Joint Committee on Cancer (2010) AJCC cancer staging manual, 7th edn. Springer, New York
43. Sutow WW, Sullivan MP (1962) Cyclophosphamide therapy in children with Ewing's sarcoma. Cancer Chemother Rep 23:55–60
44. Pinkel D (1962) Cyclophosphamide in children with cancer. Cancer 15:42–49
45. Donaldson SS, Torrey M, Link MP et al (1998) A multidisciplinary study investigating radiotherapy in Ewing's sarcoma: end results of POG #8346. Pediatric Oncology Group. Int J Radiat Oncol Biol Phys 42(1):125–135
46. Bacci G, Toni A, Avella M et al (1989) Long-term results in 144 localized Ewing's sarcoma patients treated with combined therapy. Cancer 63(8):1477–1486
47. Bacci G, Ferrari S, Avella M et al (1991) Non-metastatic Ewing's sarcoma: results in 98 patients treated with neoadjuvant chemotherapy. Ital J Orthop Traumatol 17(4):449–465
48. Nesbit ME Jr, Gehan EA, Burgert EO Jr et al (1990) Multimodal therapy for the management of primary, nonmetastatic Ewing's sarcoma of bone: a long-term follow-up of the First Intergroup study. J Clin Oncol Off J Am Soc Clin Oncol. 8(10):1664–1674

49. Grier HE, Krailo MD, Tarbell NJ et al (2003) Addition of ifosfamide and etoposide to standard chemotherapy for Ewing's sarcoma and primitive neuroectodermal tumor of bone. N Engl J Med 348(8):694–701. doi:10.1056/NEJMoa020890
50. Miser JS, Krailo MD, Tarbell NJ et al (2004) Treatment of metastatic Ewing's sarcoma or primitive neuroectodermal tumor of bone: evaluation of combination ifosfamide and etoposide—a Children's Cancer Group and Pediatric Oncology Group study. J Clin Oncol Off J Am Soc Clin Oncol. 22(14):2873–2876. doi:10.1200/JCO.2004.01.041
51. Laurence V, Pierga J-Y, Barthier S et al (2005) Long-term follow up of high-dose chemotherapy with autologous stem cell rescue in adults with Ewing tumor. Am J Clin Oncol 28(3):301–309
52. Kushner BH, Meyers PA (2001) How effective is dose-intensive/myeloablative therapy against Ewing's sarcoma/primitive neuroectodermal tumor metastatic to bone or bone marrow? The Memorial Sloan-Kettering experience and a literature review. J Clin Oncol Off J Am Soc Clin Oncol 19(3):870–880
53. Navid F, Santana VM, Billups CA et al (2006) Concomitant administration of vincristine, doxorubicin, cyclophosphamide, ifosfamide, and etoposide for high-risk sarcomas: the St Jude Children's Research Hospital experience. Cancer 106(8):1846–1856. doi:10.1002/cncr.21810
54. Womer RB, Daller RT, Fenton JG, Miser JS (2000) Granulocyte colony stimulating factor permits dose intensification by interval compression in the treatment of Ewing's sarcomas and soft tissue sarcomas in children. Eur J Cancer Oxf Engl 1990 36(1):87–94
55. Ludwig JA (2008) Ewing sarcoma: historical perspectives, current state-of-the-art, and opportunities for targeted therapy in the future. Curr Opin Oncol 20(4):412–418. doi:10.1097/CCO.0b013e328303ba1d
56. Lissat A, Chao MM, Kontny U (2012) Targeted therapy in Ewing sarcoma. ISRN Oncol 2012:609439. doi:10.5402/2012/609439
57. Olmos D, Postel-Vinay S, Molife LR et al (2010) Safety, pharmacokinetics, and preliminary activity of the anti-IGF-1R antibody figitumumab (CP-751, 871) in patients with sarcoma and Ewing's sarcoma: a phase 1 expansion cohort study. Lancet Oncol 11(2):129–135. doi:10.1016/S1470-2045(09)70354-7
58. Bond M, Bernstein ML, Pappo A et al (2008) A phase II study of imatinib mesylate in children with refractory or relapsed solid tumors: a Children's Oncology Group study. Pediatr Blood Cancer 50(2):254–258. doi:10.1002/pbc.21132
59. Donaldson SS (2004) Ewing sarcoma: radiation dose and target volume. Pediatr Blood Cancer 42(5):471–476. doi:10.1002/pbc.10472
60. Dalinka MK, Edeiken J, Finkelstein JB (1974) Complications of radiation therapy: adult bone. Semin Roentgenol 9(1):29–40
61. Cotterill SJ, Ahrens S, Paulussen M et al (2000) Prognostic factors in Ewing's tumor of bone: analysis of 975 patients from the European Intergroup Cooperative Ewing's Sarcoma Study Group. J Clin Oncol Off J Am Soc Clin Oncol 18(17):3108–3114
62. Yang RS, Eckardt JJ, Eilber FR et al (1995) Surgical indications for Ewing's sarcoma of the pelvis. Cancer 76(8):1388–1397
63. Frassica FJ, Frassica DA, Pritchard DJ, Schomberg PJ, Wold LE, Sim FH (1993) Ewing sarcoma of the pelvis. Clinicopathological features and treatment. J Bone Joint Surg Am 75(10):1457–1465
64. Thorpe SW, Weiss KR, Goodman MA, Heyl AE, McGough RL (2012) Should aggressive surgical local control be attempted in all patients with metastatic or pelvic Ewing's sarcoma? Sarcoma 2012:953602. doi:10.1155/2012/953602
65. Puri A, Gulia A, Jambhekar NA, Laskar S (2012) Results of surgical resection in pelvic Ewing's sarcoma. J Surg Oncol 106(4):417–422. doi:10.1002/jso.23107
66. Donati D, Yin J, Di Bella C et al (2007) Local and distant control in non-metastatic pelvic Ewing's sarcoma patients. J Surg Oncol 96(1):19–25. doi:10.1002/jso.20752

67. Sucato DJ, Rougraff B, McGrath BE et al (2000) Ewing's sarcoma of the pelvis. Long-term survival and functional outcome. Clin Orthop 373:193–201

68. Bacci G, Ferrari S, Longhi A et al (2004) Role of surgery in local treatment of Ewing's sarcoma of the extremities in patients undergoing adjuvant and neoadjuvant chemotherapy. Oncol Rep 11(1):111–120

69. Sluga M, Windhager R, Lang S et al (2001) The role of surgery and resection margins in the treatment of Ewing's sarcoma. Clin Orthop 392:394–399

70. Henderson ER, Groundland JS, Pala E et al (2011) Failure mode classification for tumor endoprostheses: retrospective review of five institutions and a literature review. J Bone Joint Surg Am 93(5):418–429. doi:10.2106/JBJS.J.00834

71. Horowitz SM, Glasser DB, Lane JM, Healey JH (1993) Prosthetic and extremity survivorship after limb salvage for sarcoma. How long do the reconstructions last? Clin Orthop 293:280–286

72. Malawer MM, Chou LB (1995) Prosthetic survival and clinical results with use of large-segment replacements in the treatment of high-grade bone sarcomas. J Bone Joint Surg Am 77(8):1154–1165

73. Mankin HJ, Gebhardt MC, Jennings LC, Springfield DS, Tomford WW (1996) Long-term results of allograft replacement in the management of bone tumors. Clin Orthop 324:86–97

74. Berrey BH Jr, Lord CF, Gebhardt MC, Mankin HJ (1990) Fractures of allografts. Frequency, treatment, and end-results. J Bone Joint Surg Am 72(6):825–833

75. Getty PJ, Peabody TD (1999) Complications and functional outcomes of reconstruction with an osteoarticular allograft after intra-articular resection of the proximal aspect of the humerus. J Bone Joint Surg Am 81(8):1138–1146

76. Hong AM, Millington S, Ahern V et al (2013) Limb preservation surgery with extracorporeal irradiation in the management of malignant bone tumor: the oncological outcomes of 101 patients. Ann Oncol Off J Eur Soc Med Oncol ESMO 24(10):2676–2680. doi:10.1093/annonc/mdt252

77. Benedetti MG, Bonatti E, Malfitano C, Donati D (2013) Comparison of allograft-prosthetic composite reconstruction and modular prosthetic replacement in proximal femur bone tumors: functional assessment by gait analysis in 20 patients. Acta Orthop 84(2):218–223. doi:10.3109/17453674.2013.773119

78. Donati D, Di Bella C, Frisoni T, Cevolani L, DeGroot H (2011) Alloprosthetic composite is a suitable reconstruction after periacetabular tumor resection. Clin Orthop 469(5):1450–1458. doi:10.1007/s11999-011-1799-9

79. Bölling T, Schuck A, Paulussen M et al (2008) Whole lung irradiation in patients with exclusively pulmonary metastases of Ewing tumors. Toxicity analysis and treatment results of the EICESS-92 trial. Strahlenther Onkol Organ Dtsch Röntgenges Al 4(4):193–197. doi:10.1007/s00066-008-1810-x

80. Rodríguez-Galindo C, Navid F, Liu T, Billups CA, Rao BN, Krasin MJ (2008) Prognostic factors for local and distant control in Ewing sarcoma family of tumors. Ann Oncol Off J Eur Soc Med Oncol ESMO 19(4):814–820. doi:10.1093/annonc/mdm521

81. Ahrens S, Hoffmann C, Jabar S et al (1999) Evaluation of prognostic factors in a tumor volume-adapted treatment strategy for localized Ewing sarcoma of bone: the CESS 86 experience. Cooperative Ewing Sarcoma Study. Med Pediatr Oncol 32(3):186–195

82. Lee J, Hoang BH, Ziogas A, Zell JA (2010) Analysis of prognostic factors in Ewing sarcoma using a population-based cancer registry. Cancer 116(8):1964–1973. doi:10.1002/cncr.24937

Chondrosarcoma of Bone

Lee R. Leddy and Robert E. Holmes

Abstract

Chondrosarcoma is a cartilage forming neoplasm, which is the second most common primary malignancy of bone. Clinicians who treat chondrosarcoma patients must determine the grade of the tumor, and must ascertain the likelihood of metastasis. Acral lesions are unlikely to metastasize, regardless of grade, whereas axial, or more proximal lesions are much more likely to metastasize than tumors found in the distal extremities with equivalent histology. Chondrosarcoma is resistant to both chemotherapy and radiation, making wide local excision the only treatment. Local recurrence is frequently seen after intralesional excision, thus wide local excision is sometimes employed despite significant morbidity, even in low-grade lesions. Chondrosarcoma is difficult to treat. The surgeon must balance the risk of significant morbidity with the ability to minimize the chance of local recurrence and maximize the likelihood of long-term survival.

Keywords

Chondrosarcoma · Bone sarcoma · Cartilage tumors

1   Introduction

Chondrosarcoma is a cartilage forming malignant tumor of bone. It is the second most commonly seen primary malignancy of bone, with osteosarcoma being the most common. It can be distinguished from other primary bone tumors by

L. R. Leddy (✉) · R. E. Holmes
Medical University of South Carolina, Charleston, SC, USA
e-mail: Leddyl@musc.edu

T. D. Peabody and S. Attar (eds.), *Orthopaedic Oncology*,
Cancer Treatment and Research 162, DOI: 10.1007/978-3-319-07323-1_6,
© Springer International Publishing Switzerland 2014

identification of cartilage forming malignant cells without direct osteoid formation. Chondrosarcomas are frequently recognized by orthopedic oncologists as difficult to diagnose and treat. Much of this difficulty stems from the fact that patients may have a heterogeneous constellation of symptoms, radiographic findings, and distant disease potential. The biologic behavior of these tumors is variable with certain types of chondrosarcoma presenting as highly malignant and aggressive, while others behave in a more benign manner and may never metastasize. Histology is often a poor surrogate for biologic behavior. The critical determination that the treating physician must establish is the potential for the development of distant disease.

Even with adequate imaging and histology, it is often difficult to differentiate between tumors that will behave aggressively and those that will not because the histologic differences between tumor grades are often quite subtle, and because the biopsy specimen may not have captured the portion of tissue representative of the malignant potential of the tumor. It is also difficult to correlate distant disease potential with cytologic features under the microscope.

Chondrosarcomas can form in the medullary cavity of normal bone (conventional chondrosarcoma) or may form as the result of malignant transformation of a benign cartilaginous tumor such as an osteochondroma or an enchondroma (secondary chondrosarcoma). Chondrosarcomas may be further classified as either exostotic (outside bone) or enostotic. Variants of chondrosarcoma outside the conventional type are rare and include juxtacortical, clear cell, dedifferentiated, and mesenchymal chondrosarcomas.

In addition to being difficult to diagnose, chondrosarcoma presents a challenging therapeutic dilemma for orthopedic oncologists. These tumors have not been shown to be sensitive to chemotherapy or radiation [43–45]. Currently, surgical excision is the only therapy proven to be effective. The challenge for the treating surgeon is to balance the amount of surgical morbidy with the risk of recurrence and potential metastatic disease. This can prove problematic particularly in the case of large tumors [32], tumors with sensitive surrounding structures, or when significant loss of limb function is anticipated, such as in tumors of the proximal humerus [26]. For clinicians, chondrosarcoma represents a challenging diagnostic and therapeutic challenge, with patients frequently experiencing significant morbidity.

2   Diagnosis

2.1   Clinical Characteristics

There are a few general characteristics that make a lesion more likely to be malignant. These include:
1. Tumor size, as larger lesions carry a greater risk of malignancy.
2. Central (medullary).

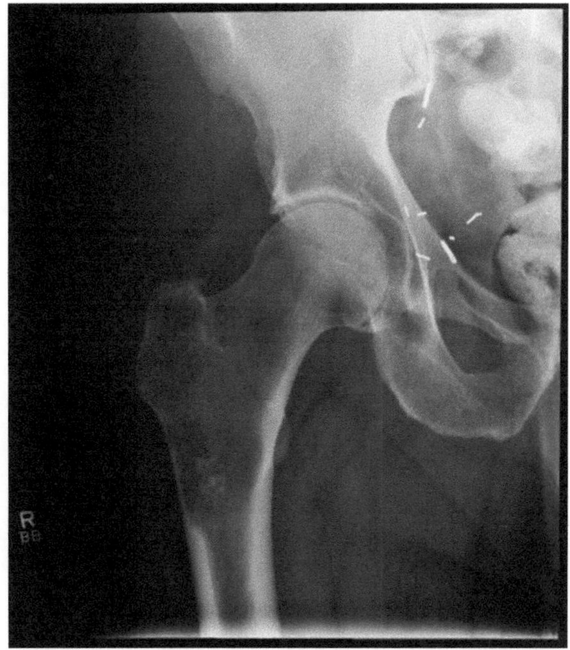

Fig. 1 X-ray of the proximal femur showing a permeative change from a mineralized lesion

3. More proximal location.
4. Age of the patient greater than 50.

Since patients with chondrosarcoma may present with a wide variety of clinical symptoms of differing severity and biologic behavior, it is important to define characteristics for which a malignant tumor is more likely. These tumors can often be found incidentally in the proximal humerus or distal femur when these areas are imaged for other reasons such as shoulder impingement or knee pain (Figs. 1 and 2). Often, the decision to work up the lesion or to observe is made on the basis of clinical presentation and the presence or absence of symptoms.

Pain is the most common symptom reported on presentation. The presence of night pain should raise concern of a possible malignancy, particularly if the pain worsens at night. It should be noted, however, that some patients with chondrosarcoma can have no pain and may have tumors which are found incidentally. Patients may present with a pathologic fracture. Fractures occurring from a low energy mechanism should warrant further workup.

In general, patients presenting with larger cartilaginous tumors have a higher risk of malignancy than patients with smaller tumors. In addition, lesions of the pelvis and axial skeleton are more likely to be malignant than lesions of peripheral origin [40]. Specifically, lesions in the pelvis, proximal femur, scapula, and proximal humerus may behave more aggressively than tumors arising in the distal extremities [8] (Figs. 1 and 2) [1–6].

Patients can also be stratified for risk of malignancy based on their age. In general, conventional chondrosarcoma is a disease more commonly found in adults

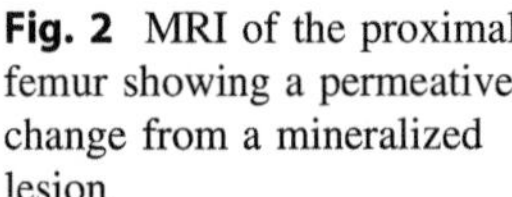

Fig. 2 MRI of the proximal femur showing a permeative change from a mineralized lesion

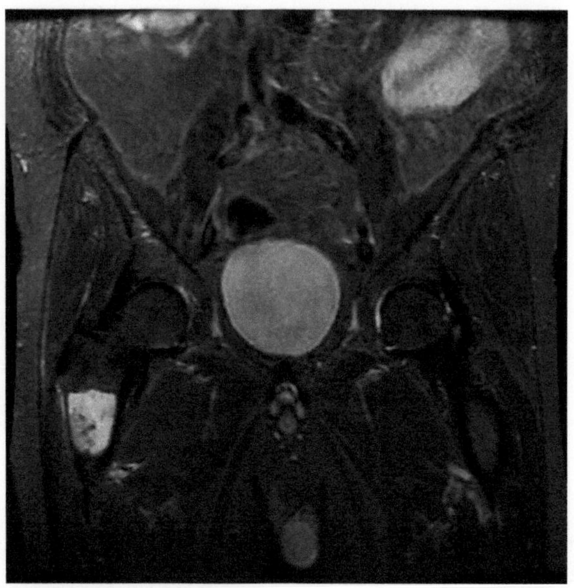

and those of older age, most commonly in those from 40 to 60 years of age. Patients younger than 25 are at significantly lower risk than older patients to have a malignant cartilage tumor [23, 27–28]. In addition, the presence of multiple lesions, such as with Ollier's disease or multiple hereditary exostosis should raise the suspicion of a possible chondrosarcoma, whereas the presence of a solitary lesion may be more likely indicative of a benign process [48, 49]. The presence of multiple medullary lesions should also cause the clinician to consider hereditary conditions such as Ollier's disease or Mafucci's syndrome. These conditions increase the risk of a malignant lesion, particularly in the case of Mafucci's syndrome, where the likelihood of chondrosarcoma has been found to be close to 50 %. There is also a risk of visceral malignancy in these patients. While the risk is less for Ollier's disease (5–20 %), the risk is certainly higher than in the general population.

2.2 Imaging

Radiographically, chondrosarcomas have a heterogenous appearance with cortical thickening, expansion, or thinning, and most showing some cartilaginous mineralization (Fig. 3). Lower grade lesions are frequently smaller and most often intraosseous, without evidence of soft tissue extension. In contrast, higher grade chondrosarcomas are frequently found to be large, destructive lesions with cortical expansion, and a soft tissue mass. In addition, these lesions may show features of bone destruction, along with cartilaginous mineralization, and may frequently be accompanied by a soft tissue mass. In patients with higher grade, central

Fig. 3 X-ray of the distal
femur showing a mineralized
lesion with evidence of
cortical thinning

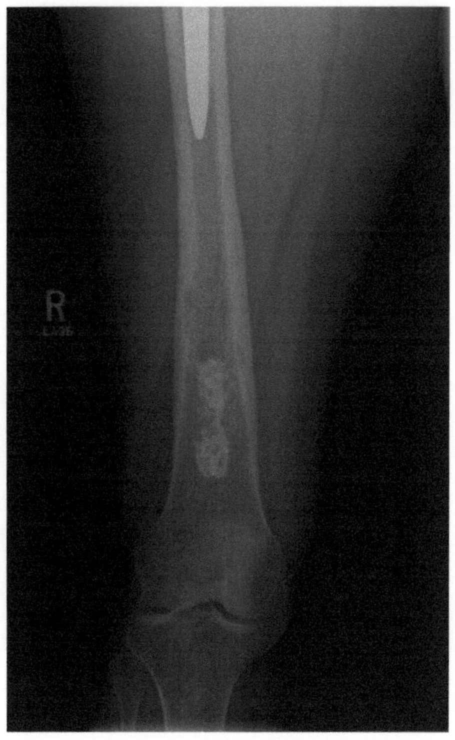

chondrosarcoma, plain films are usually diagnostic when bone destruction, thickening or thinning of the cortex and intralesional mineralization consistent with cartilage formation are seen (Figs. 4 and 5). In lower grade lesions, or when plain films are nondiagnostic, MRI is indicated to further elucidate intraosseous and extraosseous characteristics and to evaluate the extent of soft tissue extension. Chondrosarcomas are typically low signal intensity on T1-weighted images and high signal on T2-weighted images.

For further evaluation of bony abnormalities, particularly the endosteal surface or cortical integrity, a CT scan may be helpful, especially in the pelvis or other flat bones. A CT scan may also help to visualize lytic changes adjacent to a mineralized lesion, which is suggestive of a chondrosarcoma which has undergone transformation from a benign cartilage tumor [22, 29, 34].

For exostotic lesions, the soft tissue component may be mineralized, and can be identified on plain films. An MRI is also indicated to determine the extent of the soft tissue involvement and a CT may be indicated to define the full extent of intra- and extraosseous involvement (Fig. 6).

Technetium bone scan can also be a useful tool when negative. The positive predictive value of the bone scan is somewhat low, however, as both benign and malignant tumors can produce a "hot" lesion. The negative predictive value of the test is much more useful, since a "cold" lesion is very unlikely to be malignant.

Fig. 4 X-ray of the humerus showing a mineralized lesion with evidence of cortical expansion

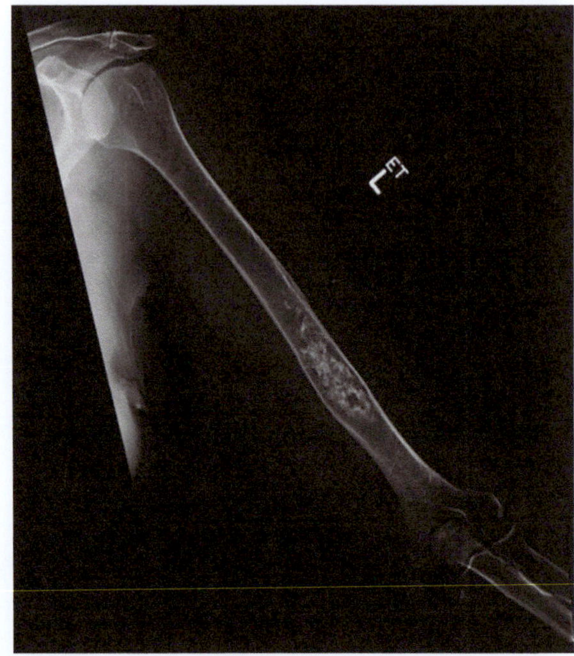

Fig. 5 Wide excision specimen from the patient from Fig. 4. Specimen shows intramedullary cartilage formation, cortical expansion, and endosteal scalloping

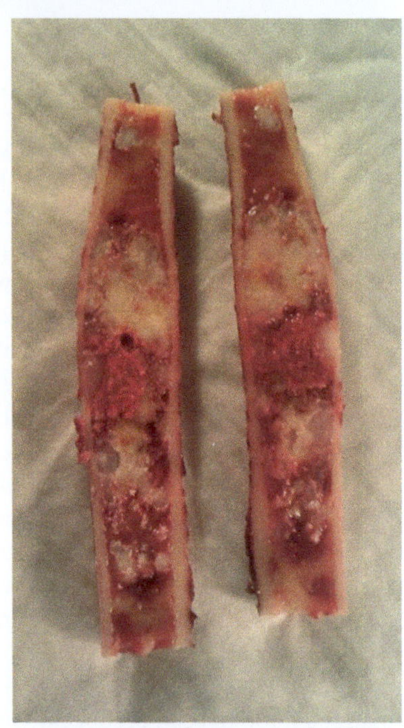

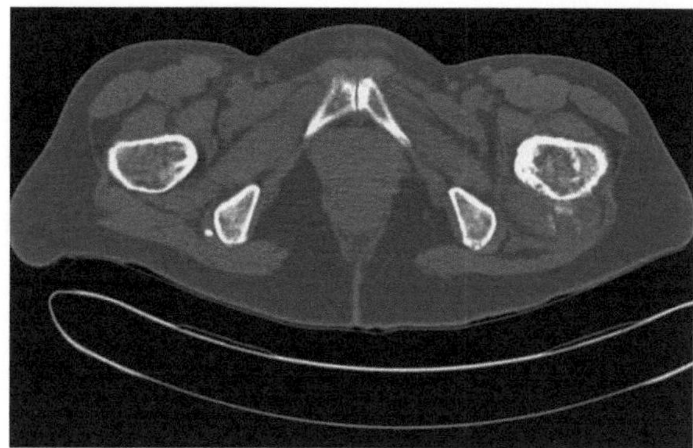

Fig. 6 CT of proximal femur with evidence of a mineralizing soft-tissue mass posterior to the left proximal femur

2.3 Histology

Histologic basis for differentiating benign cartilage tumors from chondrosarcoma is difficult. Furthermore, histology is often a poor surrogate for biologic behavior in cartilaginous neoplasms. This is evident in cartilaginous lesions in the small bones of the hand. There are two different grading systems for chondrosarcoma. Pathologists disagree as to which grading scheme is superior. Some define these tumors as grades 1–3, whereas others grade these tumors as grades 1–4. More important to the clinician, is the description of the tumor as either high grade or low grade. Intermediate grade often provides little information for the clinical decision making process. On the 1–3 scale, grade 1 would be considered low grade, whereas grades 1 and 2 would be low grade on the 1–4 scale. All chondrosarcomas regardless of grade show malignant characteristics such as hypercellularity, pleomorphism, mitotic nuclei, myxoid intracellular matrix, binucleate lacunae, and cellular atypia. Low-grade tumors typically are well differentiated, with moderate cellularity, and little pleomorphism or atypia. Other features such as host bone entrapement are more indicative of a malignant process [41, 42, 46, 47]. The grading system progresses in degrees from low grade to high, depending on the appearance of the above characteristics. The higher grade tumors are markedly hypercellular, atypical, and pleomorphic, with many mitotic figures [17, 19, 20]. The principal histologic characteristic of malignancy is the presence of host bone lamellae entrapped by the tumor. This may include areas of bony destruction, as opposed to a benign appearing tumor which is abutting the bone, but not entrapping or destroying the host bone. Ideally, the biopsy specimen should include the area of host bone entrapment (Fig. 7), and specifically the tumor-bone interface.

A unique feature of chondrosarcoma happens to be that location can suggest the chance of metastasis. For example, chondrosarcoma of the hand may look quite aggressive histologically and radiographically [21, 24, 30, 36, 39]. However, regardless of histologic grade, chondrosarcoma of the hand is rarely metastatic [8]. A chondrosarcoma of the pelvis with the exact same histology as the previous

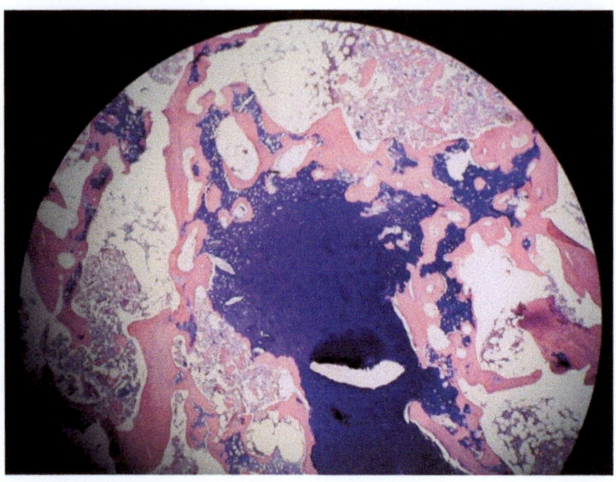

Fig. 7 Histologic specimen showing host bone entrapment

example in the hand would have a higher likelihood to metastasize [11]. For this reason, the clinician must consider location as an important predictor of prognosis and likelihood of metastasis.

2.4 Staging

WHO classification
- Central Conventional
  - Central chondrosarcomas arise within the medullary cavity of bone, most commonly, the proximal femur, ilium, and proximal humerus. These tumors are thought to arise primarily from within the bone although it has been suggested that up to 40 % of central conventional chondrosarcomas may arise from asymptomatic enchondromas.
  - Central conventional chondrosarcoma is most common in patients over 50, with a slight preponderance to the male gender. Pain is the most common presenting symptom, with an insidious onset of months to years. Pain is typically worse at night and may be accompanied by local swelling. A pathologic fracture may be present on presentation in up to 17 % of cases.
- Secondary
  - Secondary chondrosarcomas originate from a preexisting cartilaginous lesion. This may occur in patients with solitary or multiple osteochondromas, or as sequelae of a hereditary condition such as Ollier's disease or Mafucci's syndrome. Serial observation of benign surface lesions may eventually reveal rapid thickening of the cartilaginous cap, a sign of malignant transformation. Overall the prognosis is good for secondary chondrosarcoma with most tumors being low to intermediate grade, and distant metastasis being uncommon. Local recurrence can be a problem for some patients, particularly those with secondary malignant transformation occurring in the pelvis.

- Mesenchymal
  - Mesenchymal chondrosarcomas are highly malignant tumors with high likelihood of distant metastases, and a high probability of local and distant recurrence. Approximately 20 % of patients will have metastatic disease present on initial presentation. These tumors differ from other chondrosarcomas in that the patients are much younger, with an average age of 25. Approximately, one-third of mesenchymal tumors will show extraskeletal manifestations. These tumors have a high affinity for the axial skeleton, with craniofacial, vertebral and pelvic bones being mainly affected.
- Dedifferentiated
  - Dedifferentiated chondrosarcomas are also highly malignant lesions and histologically include two different components: one, a well-differentiated cartilage tumor, which is most often an enchondroma or low-grade chondrosarcoma. Second, they contain a high-grade sarcoma which is noncartilaginous [10]. Both components of the tumor share several genetic markers, leading to the conclusion that they are likely derivatives of the same cell line. Age at presentation is typically older than in conventional chondrosarcoma with the average age being 50–60 years old. These most frequently develop in the humerus, femur, and pelvis [7].
- Clear Cell
  - Clear cell chondrosarcoma is a low-grade tumor which derives its name from the clear and empty cytoplasm seen on light microscopy. It is a slow growing tumor, frequently found in the epiphysis of long bones, commonly in the proximal femur, differentiating it from the location of other types of chondrosarcoma. Long-term survival is very good despite the propensity of these tumors to metastasize late [14–16]. Long-term follow-up is required, and the treatment of choice is wide surgical excision.
- Periosteal
  - As defined in the name, periosteal sarcoma arises from the periosteal surface, most frequently of the femoral diaphysis. This tumor is extremely uncommon, but is most frequently seen in young adults, 20–40 years old. Histology reveals a well differentiated tumor which can often be mistaken for a benign lesion. The malignant potential is frequently detected by invasion of the surrounding soft tissue. While these are low-grade lesions, distant metastasis may still occur. Patients should be worked up for metastasis upon diagnosis [35].

2.5   Treatment

All chondrosarcomas without metastasis, regardless of grade or subtype, require surgery for curative potential. This stems from the fact that chondrosarcoma in general is resistant to both chemotherapy and radiation. Treatment is determined based on stage, grade, and location. For example, localized acral lesions rarely

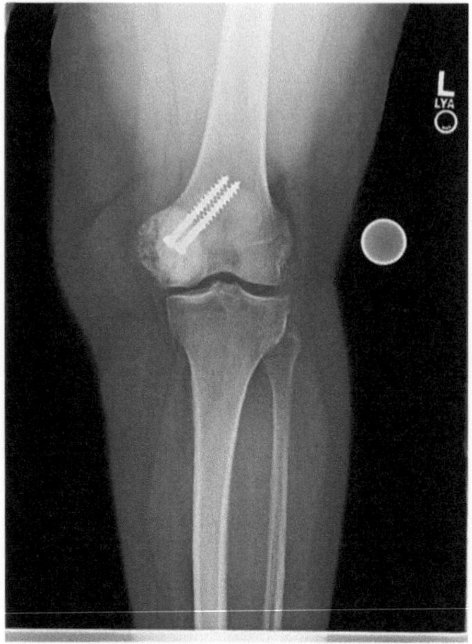

Fig. 8 X-ray of the distal femur of a patient who developed local recurrence after being treated with curettage and cement

metastasize, regardless of grade [8]. These tumors can be treated with limited excision or curettage, ensuring that margins are adequate. On the other end of the spectrum, chondrosarcoma of the pelvis is almost always treated with wide local excision, since even low-grade tumors have a high local recurrence rate [11].

The treatment of low grade, long bone chondrosarcomas, particularly Enneking Stage IA tumors, remains controversial. Many surgeons will choose to treat these tumors with intralesional excision and curettage. While low-grade chondrosarcomas rarely metastasize, they may recur after intralesional excision and curettage (Figs. 8 and 9). For this reason, wide excision is sometimes the recommended treatment for low-grade chondrosarcoma [33, 34]. Wide excision often produces functional deficits and is a more morbid procedure than intralesional treatment [50]. Therefore, when choosing between intralesional versus wide excision, one must consider the balance between the risks of surgical morbidity and risks of local recurrence [18, 25, 37, 38].

More aggressive appearing tumors of long bones should be treated with wide local excision (Fig. 5), if possible, or amputation if limb salvage is not feasible. Inadequate resection results in high rates of local recurrence for tumors of the pelvis, humerus, tibia, and femur.

Adjuvant chemotherapeutic agents have not been shown to improve survival in Grade III chondrosarcoma and dedifferentiated chondrosarcoma. Patients should be routinely followed with careful examinations to evaluate for local recurrence and/or pulmonary metastases. Regular imaging studies should be performed for up to 10 years after wide local resection.

Fig. 9 CT scan of the distal femur of a patient who developed local recurrence after being treated with curettage and cement

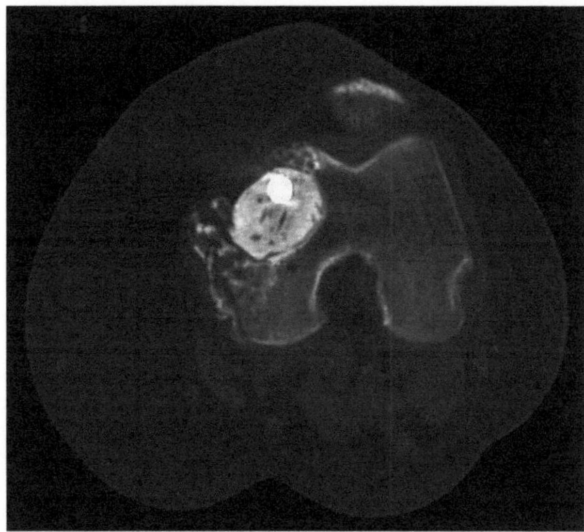

3   Summary

In conclusion, chondrosarcoma is a cartilage forming neoplasm, which is the second most common primary malignancy of bone. Clinicians who treat chondrosarcoma patients must determine the grade of the tumor, and must ascertain the likelihood of metastasis. Acral lesions are unlikely to metastasize, regardless of grade, whereas axial, or more proximal lesions are much more likely to metastasize than tumors found in the distal extremities with equivalent histology [12]. Chondrosarcoma is resistant to both chemotherapy and radiation, making wide local excision the only treatment. Local recurrence is frequently seen after intralesional excision, thus wide local excision is sometimes employed despite significant morbidity, even in low-grade lesions [13]. Chondrosarcoma is difficult to treat. The surgeon must balance the risk of significant morbidity with the ability to minimize the chance of local recurrence and maximize the likelihood of long-term survival.

References

1. Berend KR, Toth AP, Harrelson JM, Layfield LJ, Hey LA, Scully SP (1998) Association between ratio of matrix metalloproteinase-1 to tissue inhibitor of metalloproteinase-1 and local recurrence, metastasis, and survival in human chondrosarcoma. J Bone Joint Surg Am 80(1):11–17
2. Bjornsson J, McLeod RA, Unni KK, Ilstrup DM, Pritchard DJ (1998) Primary chondrosarcoma of long bones and limb girdles. Cancer 83(10):2105–2119

3. Bovee JV, Cleton-Jansen AM, Taminiau AH, Hogendoorn PC (2005) Emerging pathways in the development of chondrosarcoma of bone and implications for targeted treatment. Lancet Oncol 6(8):599–607. doi:10.1016/s1470-2045(05)70282-5

4. Brenner W, Conrad EU, Eary JF (2004) FDG PET imaging for grading and prediction of outcome in chondrosarcoma patients. Eur J Nucl Med Mol Imaging 31(2):189–195. doi:10.1007/s00259-003-1353-4

5. Brien EW, Mirra JM, Kerr R (1997) Benign and malignant cartilage tumors of bone and joint: their anatomic and theoretical basis with an emphasis on radiology, pathology and clinical biology. I. The intramedullary cartilage tumors. Skeletal Radiol 26(6):325–353

6. Campanacci M (2001) Bone and soft tissue tumors: clinical features, imaging, pathology and treatment, 2nd edn. Springer, New York (Radiology 220(1):236)

7. Capanna R, Bertoni F, Bettelli G, Picci P, Bacchini P, Present D, Campanacci M (1988) Dedifferentiated chondrosarcoma. J Bone Joint Surg Am 70(1):60–69

8. Cawte TG, Steiner GC, Beltran J, Dorfman HD (1998) Chondrosarcoma of the short tubular bones of the hands and feet. Skeletal Radiol 27(11):625–632

9. Cesari M, Bertoni F, Bacchini P, Mercuri M, Palmerini E, Ferrari S (2007) Mesenchymal chondrosarcoma. An analysis of patients treated at a single institution. Tumori 93(5):423–427

10. Dickey ID, Rose PS, Fuchs B, Wold LE, Okuno SH, Sim FH., Scully SP (2004) Dedifferentiated chondrosarcoma: the role of chemotherapy with updated outcomes. J Bone Joint Surg Am 86-A(11):2412–2418

11. Donati D, El Ghoneimy A, Bertoni F, Di Bella C, Mercuri M (2005) Surgical treatment and outcome of conventional pelvic chondrosarcoma. J Bone Joint Surg Br 87(11):1527–1530. doi:10.1302/0301-620x.87b11.16621

12. Enneking WF (1986) A system of staging musculoskeletal neoplasms. Clin Orthop Relat Res 204:9–24

13. Evans HL, Ayala AG, Romsdahl MM (1977) Prognostic factors in chondrosarcoma of bone. A clinicopathologic analysis with emphasis on histologic grading. Cancer 40(2):818–831. doi:10.1002/1097-0142(197708)40:2<818:aid-cncr2820400234>3.0.co;2-b

14. Hisaoka M, Hashimoto H (2005) Extraskeletal myxoid chondrosarcoma: updated clinicopathological and molecular genetic characteristics. Pathol Int 55(8):453–463. doi:10.1111/j.1440-1827.2005.01853.x

15. Itala A, Leerapun T, Inwards C, Collins M, Scully SP (2005) An institutional review of clear cell chondrosarcoma. Clin Orthop Relat Res 440:209–212

16. Kawaguchi S, Wada T, Nagoya S, Ikeda T, Isu K, Yamashiro K, Hasegawa T (2003) Extraskeletal myxoid chondrosarcoma: a multi-institutional study of 42 cases in Japan. Cancer 97(5):1285–1292. doi:10.1002/cncr.11162

17. Kusuzaki K, Murata H, Takeshita H, Hirata M, Hashiguchi S, Tsuji Y, Hirasawa Y (1999) Usefulness of cytofluorometric DNA ploidy analysis in distinguishing benign cartilaginous tumors from chondrosarcomas. Mod Pathol 12(9):863–872

18. Lee FY, Mankin HJ, Fondren G, Gebhardt MC, Springfield DS, Rosenberg AE, Jennings LC (1999) Chondrosarcoma of bone: an assessment of outcome. J Bone Joint Surg Am 81(3):326–338

19. Lee FY, Yu J, Chang SS, Fawwaz R, Parisien MV (2004) Diagnostic value and limitations of fluorine-18 fluorodeoxyglucose positron emission tomography for cartilaginous tumors of bone. J Bone Joint Surg Am 86-A(12):2677–2685

20. Lin C, McGough R, Aswad B, Block JA, Terek R (2004) Hypoxia induces HIF-1alpha and VEGF expression in chondrosarcoma cells and chondrocytes. J Orthop Res 22(6):1175–1181. doi:10.1016/j.orthres.2004.03.002

21. Lin PP, Moussallem CD, Deavers MT (2010) Secondary chondrosarcoma. J Am Acad Orthop Surg 18(10):608–615

22. Littrell LA, Wenger DE, Wold LE, Bertoni F, Unni KK, White LM, Sundaram M (2004) Radiographic, CT, and MR imaging features of dedifferentiated chondrosarcomas: a

retrospective review of 174 de novo cases. Radiographics 24(5):1397–1409. doi:10.1148/rg.245045009

23. Mandahl N, Gustafson P, Mertens F, Akerman M, Baldetorp B, Gisselsson D, Larsson O (2002) Cytogenetic aberrations and their prognostic impact in chondrosarcoma. Genes Chromosomes Cancer 33(2):188–200

24. Mankin HJ (1999) Chondrosarcomas of digits: are they really malignant? Cancer 86(9):1635–1637

25. Mankin HJ, Gebhardt MC, Jennings LC, Springfield DS, Tomford WW (1996) Long-term results of allograft replacement in the management of bone tumors. Clin Orthop Relat Res 324:86–97

26. Marco RA, Gitelis S, Brebach GT, Healey JH (2000) Cartilage tumors: evaluation and treatment. J Am Acad Orthop Surg 8(5):292–304

27. McGough RL, Aswad BI, Terek RM (2002) Pathologic neovascularization in cartilage tumors. Clin Orthop Relat Res 397:76–82

28. McGough RL, Lin C, Meitner P, Aswad BI, Terek RM (2002) Angiogenic cytokines in cartilage tumors. Clin Orthop Relat Res 397:62–69

29. Mitchell AD, Ayoub K, Mangham DC, Grimer RJ, Carter SR, Tillman RM (2000) Experience in the treatment of dedifferentiated chondrosarcoma. J Bone Joint Surg Br 82(1):55–61

30. Mittermayer F, Dominkus M, Krepler P, Schwameis E, Sluga M, Toma C, Kotz R (2004) Chondrosarcoma of the hand: is a wide surgical resection necessary? Clin Orthop Relat Res 424:211–215

31. Miyaji T, Nakase T, Onuma E, Sato K, Myoui A, Tomita T, Yoshikawa H (2003) Monoclonal antibody to parathyroid hormone-related protein induces differentiation and apoptosis of chondrosarcoma cells. Cancer Lett 199(2):147–155

32. Morris HG, Capanna R, Del Ben M, Campanacci D (1995) Prosthetic reconstruction of the proximal femur after resection for bone tumors. J Arthroplasty 10(3):293–299

33. Muller S, Soder S, Oliveira AM, Inwards CY, Aigner T (2005) Type II collagen as specific marker for mesenchymal chondrosarcomas compared to other small cell sarcomas of the skeleton. Mod Pathol 18(8):1088–1094. doi:10.1038/modpathol.3800391

34. Murphey MD, Walker EA, Wilson AJ, Kransdorf MJ, Temple HT, Gannon FH (2003) From the archives of the AFIP: imaging of primary chondrosarcoma: radiologic-pathologic correlation. Radiographics 23(5):1245–1278. doi:10.1148/rg.235035134

35. Nojima T, Unni KK, McLeod RA, Pritchard DJ (1985) Periosteal chondroma and periosteal chondrosarcoma. Am J Surg Pathol 9(9):666–677

36. Ogose A, Unni KK, Swee RG, May GK, Rowland CM, Sim FH (1997) Chondrosarcoma of small bones of the hands and feet. Cancer 80(1):50–59

37. Ozaki T, Lindner N, Hillmann A, Rodl R, Blasius S, Winkelmann W (1996) Influence of intralesional surgery on treatment outcome of chondrosarcoma. Cancer 77(7):1292–1297. doi:10.1002/(sici)1097-0142(19960401)77:7<1292:aid-cncr10>3.0.co;2-x

38. Pant R, Yasko AW, Lewis VO, Raymond K, Lin PP (2005) Chondrosarcoma of the scapula: long-term oncologic outcome. Cancer 104(1):149–158. doi:10.1002/cncr.21114

39. Patil S, de Silva MV, Crossan J, Reid R (2003) Chondrosarcoma of small bones of the hand. J Hand Surg Br 28(6):602–608

40. Pring ME, Weber KL, Unni KK, Sim FH (2001) Chondrosarcoma of the pelvis. A review of sixty-four cases. J Bone Joint Surg Am 83-A(11):1630–1642

41. Reith JD, Horodyski MB, Scarborough MT (2003) Grade 2 chondrosarcoma: stage I or stage II tumor? Clin Orthop Relat Res 415:45–51. doi:10.1097/01.blo.0000093895.12372.c1

42. Rosenthal DI, Schiller AL, Mankin HJ (1984) Chondrosarcoma: correlation of radiological and histological grade. Radiology 150(1):21–26

43. Sandberg AA, Bridge JA (2003) Updates on the cytogenetics and molecular genetics of bone and soft tissue tumors: chondrosarcoma and other cartilaginous neoplasms. Cancer Genet Cytogenet 143(1):1–31

44. Sawyer JR, Swanson CM, Lukacs JL, Nicholas RW, North PE, Thomas JR (1998) Evidence of an association between 6q13-21 chromosome aberrations and locally aggressive behavior in patients with cartilage tumors. Cancer 82(3):474–483

45. Shao L, Kasanov J, Hornicek FJ, Morii T, Fondren G, Weissbach L (2003) Ecteinascidin-743 drug resistance in sarcoma cells: transcriptional and cellular alterations. Biochem Pharmacol 66(12):2381–2395

46. Sheth DS, Yasko AW, Johnson ME, Ayala AG, Murray JA, Romsdahl MM (1996) Chondrosarcoma of the pelvis. Prognostic factors for 67 patients treated with definitive surgery. Cancer 78(4):745–750. doi:10.1002/(sici)1097-0142(19960815)78:4<745:aid-cncr 9>3.0.co;2-d

47. Skeletal Lesions Interobserver Correlation among Expert Diagnosticians (SLICED) Study Group (2007) Reliability of histopathologic and radiologic grading of cartilaginous neoplasms in long bones. J Bone Jt Surg 89(10):2113–2123. doi:10.2106/jbjs.f.01530

48. Terek RM (2006) Recent advances in the basic science of chondrosarcoma. Orthop Clin North Am 37(1):9–14. doi:10.1016/j.ocl.2005.09.001

49. Terek RM, Schwartz GK, Devaney K, Glantz L, Mak S, Healey JH, Albino AP (1998) Chemotherapy and P-glycoprotein expression in chondrosarcoma. J Orthop Res 16(5):585–590. doi:10.1002/jor.1100160510

50. van Loon CJ, Veth RP, Pruszczynski M, Wobbes T, Lemmens JA, van Horn J (1994) Chondrosarcoma of bone: oncologic and functional results. J Surg Oncol 57(4):214–221

Evaluation and Treatment of Spinal Metastatic Disease

Shah-Nawaz M. Dodwad, Jason Savage,
Thomas J. Scharschmidt and Alpesh Patel

Abstract

With the increased survival of oncologic patients, evaluation and management of patients with spinal metastasis is crucial to reducing morbidity and maximizing function. In this chapter, we present some guidelines for the initial systematic evaluation of patients with spinal lesions, as well as the risks, benefits, and alternatives to nonoperative and operative management of metastatic spinal disease, and the overall survival of these patients.

Keywords

Spinal metastasis · Spinal neoplasms · Anterior/posterior spine surgery for tumors · Vertebroplasty · Kyphoplasty · Staging/management for spinal tumors · Operative and nonoperative management of spinal metastasis

1   Background

According to the American Cancer Society (ACS), the United States will have approximately 1.6 million new cases of cancer diagnosed in 2013 and about 13.7 million people living with cancer. As our medical treatments improve, the life

S.-N. M. Dodwad · J. Savage · A. Patel (✉)
Northwestern Memorial Hospital, 676 N St Clair St, Suite 1350, Chicago, IL 60611, USA
e-mail: Alpesh.Patel@nmff.org

T. J. Scharschmidt
The Ohio State University Wexner Medical Center, 410 W 10th Ave, Columbus, OH 43210, USA

T. D. Peabody and S. Attar (eds.), *Orthopaedic Oncology,*
Cancer Treatment and Research 162, DOI: 10.1007/978-3-319-07323-1_7,
© Springer International Publishing Switzerland 2014

expectancy of many oncology patients is increasing. The ACS reports that the 5 year relative survival rate for all cancers diagnosed between 2002 and 2008 is 68 %, up from 49 % in 1975–1977 [1]. With this increase in survival, management of metastatic disease has become more relevant.

Bone is the third most common location for metastatic spread of cancer, following the lung and liver. The spinal column is the most common site for bone metastasis, with about 20,000 new cases per year with up to 70 % of patients with cancer developing spinal lesions [2–5]. The thoracic spine is the most common site of spinal metastasis, followed by the lumbar spine and then the cervical spine. About 10 % of oncologic patients develop symptomatic spinal disease [6–9]. Primary malignancies of the spinal column are rare, and therefore, the majority of oncologic disease in the spine is secondary to metastasis. The likely reason for this is that Batson's venous plexus communicates with the venous system of the prostate, breast, kidney, thyroid, and lung and serves as a potential route for the hematogenous spread of tumor as well as infection [10]. Of these, breast and prostate cancer are the most common cancers to spread to bone [11]. Another mechanism is through arterial embolization of tumor, for example, from the segmental arteries, which may establish metastatic deposits in the marrow of the vertebral bodies.

2   Initial Evaluation of a Spinal Lesion

The majority of patients have an identified primary tumor at the time of metastatic presentation with only about 3–4 % of patients having an unidentifiable primary. Of the patients with metastatic bone disease with an unknown primary at the time of diagnosis, 85 % were ultimately identified using a comprehensive workup as described by Rougraff et al. as summarized in Table 1 [11]. When evaluating a new bony spinal lesion, basic tumor principles must be followed. A comprehensive evaluation must be performed to determine whether the spinal lesion is primary or metastatic, as treatment options vary for each. A thorough history and physical exam is required, with a prior history of malignancy noted as the likely source of metastasis to the spine. Previous treatment, including chemotherapy and radiation, as well as the presence of any new constitutional symptoms such as fatigue, malaise, and unintentional weight loss should be documented.

The initial presentation of a patient with metastatic spine disease is often characterized by new and/or progressive back pain. These patients should be clinically and radiographically evaluated for the presence of spinal metastatic disease. This often includes advanced imaging studies, such as an MRI (with and without contrast) and a CT scan of the area of concern. It is vital to ascertain whether the pain is generating from the underlying tumor or if it is mechanical in nature as treatment options differ for each. Tumor pain is often represented by persistent pain that is worse at night. Mechanical pain, on the other hand, is worse with axial loading of the spine, such as occurs during sitting, standing, and walking and is relieved with rest. In some circumstances, pain is followed by weakness, numbness, and then bowel/bladder dysfunction [12].

Table 1 Diagnostic strategy for bone metastasis of unknown origin as described by Rougraff

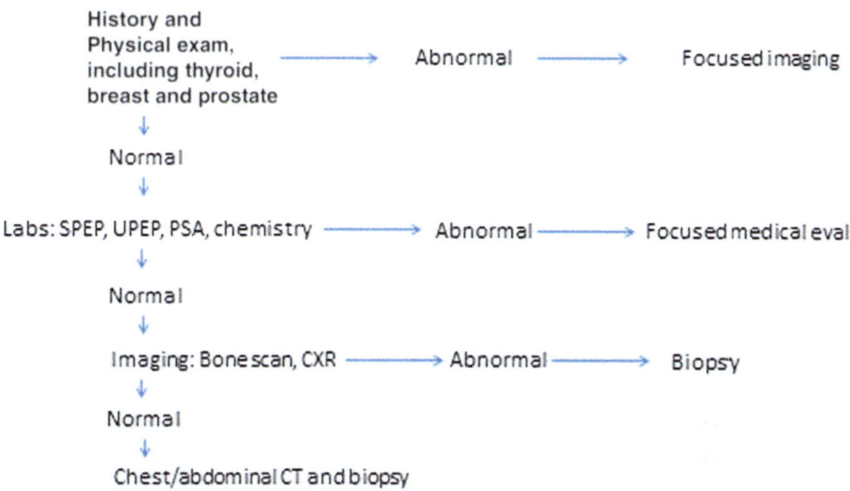

On physical exam, the entire spinal column should be palpated, as there are often noncontiguous areas involved. As mentioned, any area of concern should be evaluated radiographically. A thorough cervical, thoracic, and lumbar neurologic exam must be performed, and includes a detailed motor, sensory, reflex, and perineal (including rectal tone) examination to assess the neurologic status of the patient as defined by the American Spinal Injury Association (ASIA).

The initial evaluation of a patient with suspected metastatic spinal disease without a known primary malignancy includes laboratory and imaging studies. The tests used in an oncologic workup include complete blood count, liver enzymes, erythrocyte sedimentation rate, C-reactive protein, complete chemistry, alkaline phosphatase, serum and urine protein electrophoresis, and prostate-specific antigen [11]. Radiographic imaging includes standing plain radiographs, an MRI of the entire spinal column, whole body bone scan, CT scans of the chest, abdomen, and pelvis, and/or positron emission tomography (PET) scan. In detecting spinal metastasis, PET scan alone had a sensitivity of 74 % and PET scan registered with CT had a sensitivity of 98 % [13]. Of note, some metastatic cancers are not always identified on bone scan, including multiple myeloma (25 %), leukemia, and anaplastic carcinomas, and can cause a false-negative result [14]. Finally, tissue sampling via open or CT-guided biopsy is needed to confirm the histologic diagnosis. Oftentimes, another metastatic lesion outside of the vertebral column may be found on diagnostic imaging to biopsy with greater ease than the spine. Although tumor recurrence in biopsy tracts may occur, their incidence is low and possibly negligible in metastatic disease [15]. Knowledge of the primary lesion is critical to guide medical and surgical treatment as well as provide critical prognostic information [11].

3   Evaluation of Metastatic Spinal Disease

Once a diagnosis of spinal metastatic disease is established, one must confirm that imaging of the entire neural axis (cervical, thoracic, lumbar, and sacral segments) is completed. Similar to noncontiguous spinal lesions in the setting of trauma or infection, tumor can have multiple skip lesions throughout the spine necessitating imaging of the entire spine [16–18]. Initial X-rays often do not show bone destruction until 30–50 % of the bone has become replaced with tumor. However, pathologic compression fractures, as are common in metastatic disease, may be seen readily, yielding a detection rate of bone metastasis on plain X-ray of around 40 % [19]. CT scans delineate bone anatomy more clearly than MRI and can show evidence of bone metastasis up to 6 months prior to being seen on plain X-ray. Canal compromise can be evaluated using myelography in those patients who are unable to have an MRI scan. Although high-resolution CT provides excellent visualization of bone anatomy, lesions without significant bone destruction can be missed. In evaluating osseous metastatic disease to the spine, the sensitivity of CT was 66.2 % compared to 98.5 % with MRI [20]. On MRI, metastatic deposits are hypointense on T1-weighted images and hyperintense on T2-weighted images. Tumor and infection will have increased signal on T1 post-contrast imaging sequences. MRI with and without contrast allows assessment of mass location, soft tissue extension, vertebral destruction, and neurologic sites of compression for potential surgical planning.

The Weinstein-Boriani-Biagini (WBB) surgical staging classification system allows universal communication to define spinal tumors to aid in surgical management and outcome analysis. The WBB staging system delineates an axial image of the spine divided into 12 radiating segments similar to a clock face. The radiating segments proceed in a clockwise orientation beginning and ending at the spinous process. This system is further divided into five concentric regions progressing from extraosseous soft tissue, intraosseous superficial, intraosseous deep, extraosseous extradural, and extraosseous intradural [21]. For some tumors, en bloc resection of a spine tumor is not possible as it would require transecting the spine to have clear margins. The cerebrospinal fluid compartment travels throughout the entire spinal column and with some invasive tumors, would represent potential metastatic contamination that is not amenable to surgical resection. WBB regions allow surgeons to plan their resections accordingly and utilize the radial wedge section concept for tumor removal.

Life expectancy is a critical aspect in determining surgical versus nonsurgical management. In general, most oncologic surgeons feel that if life expectancy is equal or greater than 3 months, then surgical intervention may be beneficial. Additionally, if life expectancy is greater than 1 month, then radiation treatment is regarded as beneficial. In actual practice, these rough guidelines may be modified based on specific patient and surgeon preferences. Tokuhashi et al. described a scoring system to help predict life expectancy of cancer patients by evaluating performance status, number of metastases in extraspinal bone and vertebral bone, metastases to major internal organs, primary cancer, and neurologic status [22].

Table 2 Preoperative scoring system to evaluate indications for surgery and outcomes

Treatment options for metastatic spine disease

Tokuhashi score	Survival	Treatment
0–8	0–6 months	Conservative versus palliative
9–11	>6 months	Palliative
12–15	>1 year	Excisional

A total score of 0–8 predicts less than 6 months survival. A total score of 9–11 predicts a life expectancy of 6 months or more. A total score of 12–15 predicts life expectancy of 1 year or more as summarized in Table 2.

4 Nonoperative Management of Metastatic Spinal Disease

In general, metastatic lesions that are not associated with neurologic compromise and/or spinal instability can be treated nonoperatively. This may include radiation with or without chemotherapy depending on the histology and sensitivity of the primary lesion. Multiple myeloma is typically radiosensitive, as well as, lymphoma which also responds well to the administration of steroids and chemotherapy. Breast, lung, and prostate cancer are moderately radiosensitive, whereas renal cell carcinoma and melanoma are notoriously radioresistant. If life expectancy is short and there is concern for impending instability, pain management and bracing are palliative options that often provide some relief in symptoms.

In the setting of acute neurological compromise due to underlying metastatic disease, intravenous steroids can play a significant role in treatment and may serve to decrease the local inflammation around the spinal cord [23]. There is also some evidence of tumor lysis with steroid treatment depending on the specific type of cancer. This is particularly an effective treatment in the setting of lymphoma and, as such, should only be given after a biopsy has been performed to avoid a false-negative interpretation.

Bisphosphonate therapy is commonly used in osteoporosis management but has an important role in management of metastatic bone disease. Bisphosphonate medications inhibit osteoclast activity by inducing apoptosis. Osteoclast apoptosis slows bone resorption and has been shown to decrease the risk of fracture and skeletal morbidity [24]. There is some debate with the use of bisphosphonate therapy in the setting of achieving spinal fusion. However, when weighing the risks and benefits and given that many oncologic patients do not attain bone fusion, this issue becomes less important [25–28].

As mentioned, radiation therapy is often used in the treatment of metastatic cancer to the spine. Prostate and lymphoid cancers are often radiosensitive. Breast cancer is 70 % sensitive and 30 % resistant. Gastrointestinal and renal cell carcinomas are often radioresistant. Radiation therapy for metastatic spine disease is often given at 30 Gy in 10 fractions [29, 30]. Although radiation therapy is a pillar in treatment of metastatic spine disease, it should be performed in conjunction with surgical evaluation when appropriate. Patchell et al. studied over 100 patients with spinal cord compression caused by metastatic cancer and found that direct decompressive surgery plus postoperative radiotherapy was superior to treatment with radiotherapy alone. 84 % of the combined surgery and radiotherapy group was able to walk after treatment compared to 57 % of the radiotherapy alone group as well as they retained the ability to walk longer with 122 days versus 13 days, respectively. Additionally, the need for steroids and narcotics was significantly less in the combined group [31]. The patients not included in their study were those that had total paraplegia for greater than 48 hours, those that had very radiosensitive tumors or multiple areas of spinal cord compression. Furthermore, they recommended primary treatment as surgical intervention prior to radiation, because their study found that patients who underwent radiation treatment first and then crossed over to the surgical arm did worse in that 30 % of those patients regained the ability to walk compared to 62 % of patients who were initially treated with surgical decompression regaining their ability to walk. Additionally, 4 of the 10 patients treated with radiation first had surgical complications including infection and hardware failure.

Another radiation treatment strategy discussed in spinal metastasis is stereotactic radiosurgery, which involves using three-dimensional imaging to precisely target and deliver high-dose radiation to a specific lesion and avoid normal tissue. Compared to conventional radiotherapy, the high dose of radiation in radiosurgery is significant enough to treat even radioresistant tumors that would have otherwise not been amenable to conventional radiotherapy treatment. Separation surgery allows the spinal cord to be separated from the lesion to create a space to allow effective radiosurgery without damaging the spinal cord. Laufer et al. showed that after separation surgery for spinal cord compression secondary to metastatic disease, stereotactic radiosurgery was effective in local tumor control regardless of tumor histology-specific radiosensitivity with local recurrence rates of 5–10 % at 1 year [32, 33].

5   Operative Management of Metastatic Spinal Disease

Indications for surgical intervention include acute neurologic compromise, radioinsensitivity of the underlying tumor, spinal instability, and debilitating pain despite conservative treatment. The goals of surgical intervention are to improve or maintain function, provide pain relief and spinal stability, decompress the neural elements, as well as obtain local tumor control.

Several treatment algorithms exist for guiding the surgical decision-making process. The NOMS criteria assesses neurologic, oncologic (radiosensitivity), mechanical stability, and systemic disease factors in the decision-making tree to guide treatment between surgery and radiation [34, 35]. Another treatment algorithm is the spinal instability neoplastic score or SINS criteria. This system looks at patient symptoms and radiographic criteria to formulate a score. A score between 0 and 6 suggests stability, 7–12 suggests indeterminate stability, and 13–18 suggests instability. Patients who receive a spinal instability neoplastic score greater than 7 warrant surgical consultation [36]. Lytic lesions at junctional areas, such as occipital–cervical, cervical–thoracic, and thoracolumbar, are at the greatest risk of being associated with significant instability, and these lesions often require operative stabilization.

Interventional treatment options include surgery, kyphoplasty, and vertebroplasty. In general, actual bone fusion is unlikely in this patient population, given their compromised state in addition to the adjuvant use of chemotherapy and/or radiation. The goal in surgical intervention is, therefore, to decompress and achieve fixation and stability that will be durable and reliable for the patient. Klimo et al. concluded that decompressive laminectomy carries similar risks as invasive spinal surgery with minimal benefit unless the mass is primarily involving the posterior elements, causing posterior canal compromise [37]. In fact, decompressive laminectomy performed alone was found to be no more beneficial than radiation therapy alone [38].

Once the decision has been made to pursue surgical intervention, preoperative optimization, if possible, should be performed. In addition to medical optimization, nutritional status must be evaluated. Poor nutritional status increases the risk of surgical complications and some risk factors for nutritional deficiency include age >60, spinal cord injury, and diabetes [39]. Prealbumin and albumin levels can be used to assess and follow nutritional status. Some studies advocate for parenteral nutrition pre- and postoperatively to correct nutritional parameters [40, 41]. Well-controlled preoperative and perioperative blood glucose is also a key element to help decrease postoperative complications in spine patients [42]. General infection reduction techniques should be followed including screening and treatment protocols for Staph aureus, chlorhexidine cloths, and possibly incisional vancomycin powder and negative pressure incisional wound vacuums during closure [43].

Preoperative tumor embolization has a significant role in certain clinical scenarios. Sixty percent of spinal metastasis, 40 % of benign primary spinal neoplasms, and 85 % of all malignant primary spinal neoplasms are hypervascular [44–46]. Figures 1, 2, 3 and 4 describe a patient with a hypervascular metastatic renal cell spinal mass that was treated with embolization followed by surgical intervention. In particular, renal cell carcinoma, germ cell carcinoma, endocrine (thyroid) carcinoma, breast carcinoma, prostate carcinoma, hemangiomas, aneurysmal bone cysts, melanomas, osteoblastomas, osteosarcomas, giant cell tumors, and tumors of unknown origin tend to be hypervascular and likely benefit from preoperative embolization [47–50]. The goals of preoperative embolization are to improve visualization, decrease intraoperative bleeding and help prevent life-threatening hemorrhage and need for transfusion, as well as to potentially decrease operative time and related complications [51]. Several studies have shown decreased blood loss, surgical complication rates, and decreased operative times with the use of preoperative embolization [47, 52, 53]. In one study that evaluated treating renal cell spinal metastasis, there was an average of 1500 cc blood loss in the embolized group

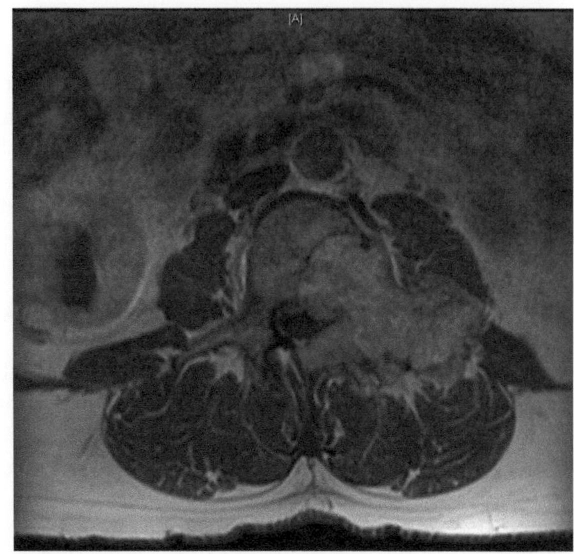

Fig. 1 Axial T1 post-contrast MRI images of a 60 year-old female with metastatic renal cell carcinoma complaining of severe left leg pain

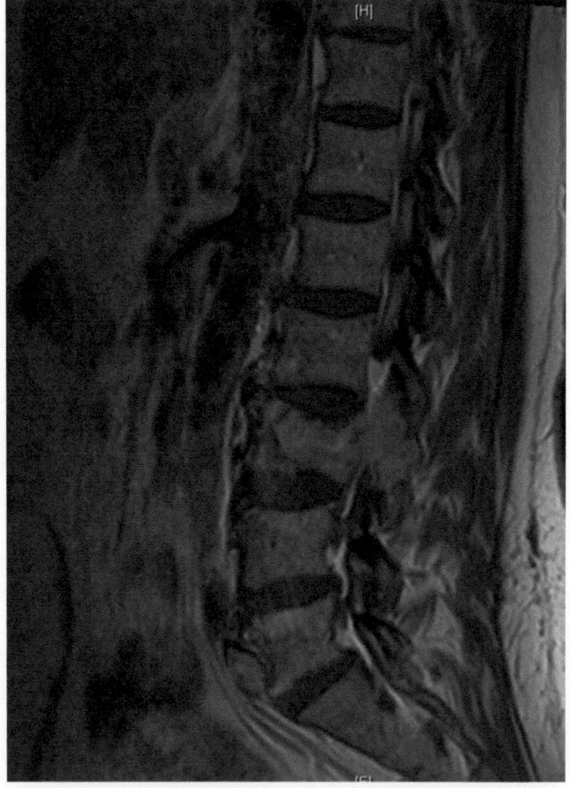

Fig. 2 Sagittal T1 post-contrast MRI of a 60 year-old female with metastatic renal cell carcinoma complaining of severe *left* leg pain

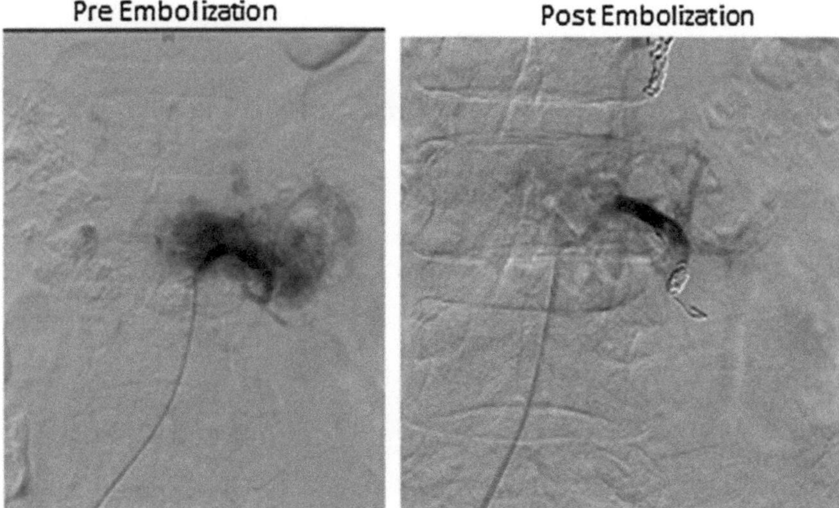

Fig. 3 Pre- and postembolization of metastastic renal cell mass depicting decrease in tumor vascular blush

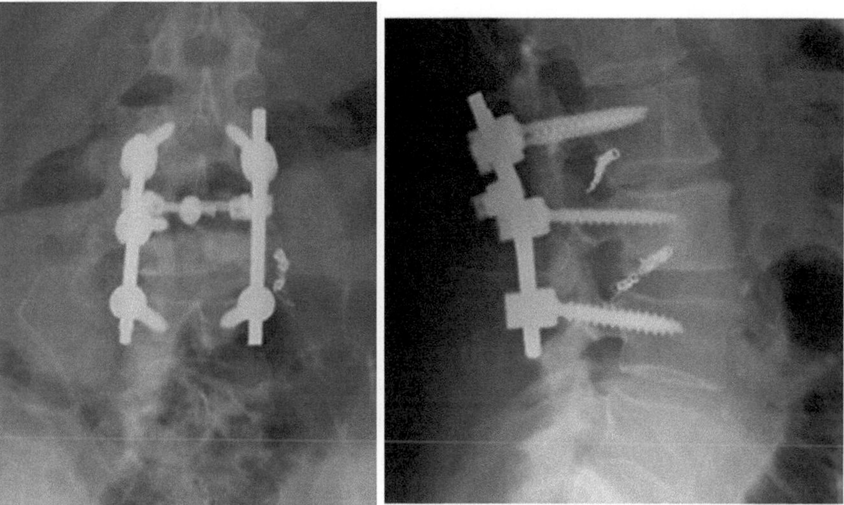

Fig. 4 Anteroposterior and lateral postoperative X-rays showing posterior decompression and fusion

compared to 5000 cc blood loss in the nonembolized group [47]. Embolization should be performed close to the operative time and within 72 h prior to the procedure as these hypervascular tumors may aggressively recanalize or collateralize blood flow [49]. Although low, reported complications of embolization include

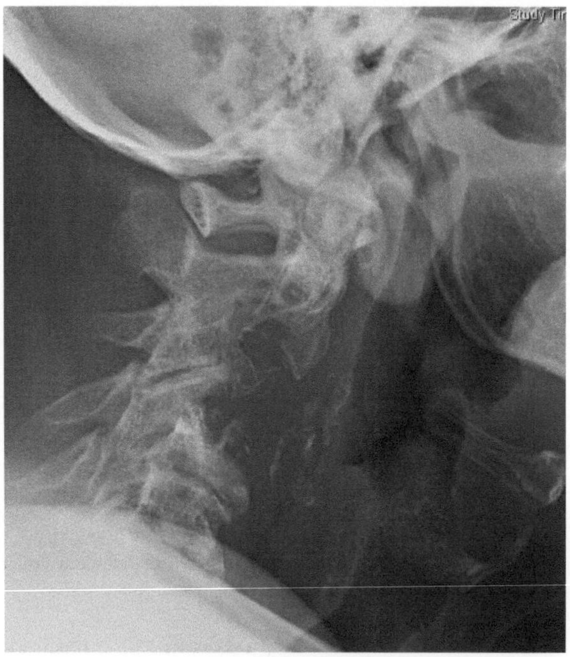

Fig. 5 Lateral cervical X-ray showing a 68 year-old male with metastatic lung adenocarcinoma involving C2–C4 with significant anterior bone destruction

death, cord ischemia, and subsequent neurologic injury, ischemia of surrounding tissue with skin and muscle necrosis in addition to the risks of angiography itself, including contrast reactions [51, 53–55].

The goals of surgical intervention in metastatic spinal disease are generally to decrease pain and improve or maintain function in this patient population. Posterior approaches to the spine allow ideal resection of posteriorly based lesions. Most vertebral metastases are within the thoracic spine and anteriorly within the vertebral body. In the cervical spine, anterior masses can cause compression of the esophagus and airway causing dysphagia and difficulty in breathing. Figures 5, 6, 7, 8 and 9 describe a patient with metastatic lung adenocarcinoma with a large anterior mass that was treated with anterior and posterior surgical decompression and fusion. Classically, one indication for anterior surgical approaches to the spine involves treating primarily anteriorly based lesions where visualization for en bloc excision is greater. However, en bloc resections are rarely required and the complications associated with the thoracotomy approach are significant, especially in an elderly, frail patient. The extracavitary posterolateral approach to these lesions, therefore, is a useful option for tumor resection, neurological decompression, and instrumented stabilization [56, 57]. This technique allows for excellent exposure of the anterior vertebral column to access anterior masses and decompress the spinal cord while sparing the patient the morbidity of an anterior approach [58]. Using the posterior

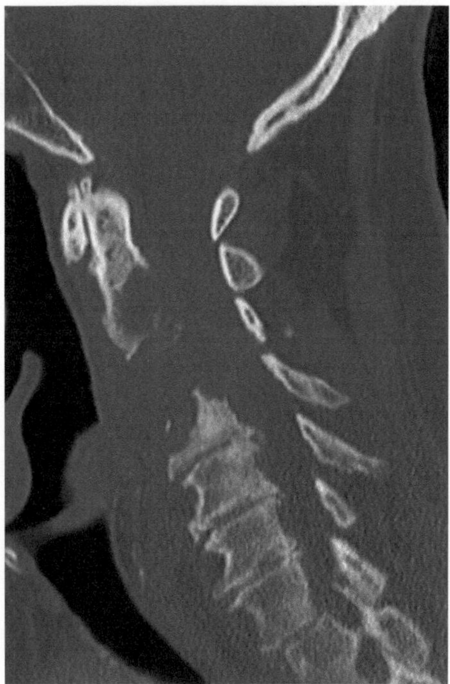

Fig. 6 Sagittal cervical CT showing a 68 year-old male with metastatic lung adenocarcinoma involving C2–C4 with significant anterior bone destruction

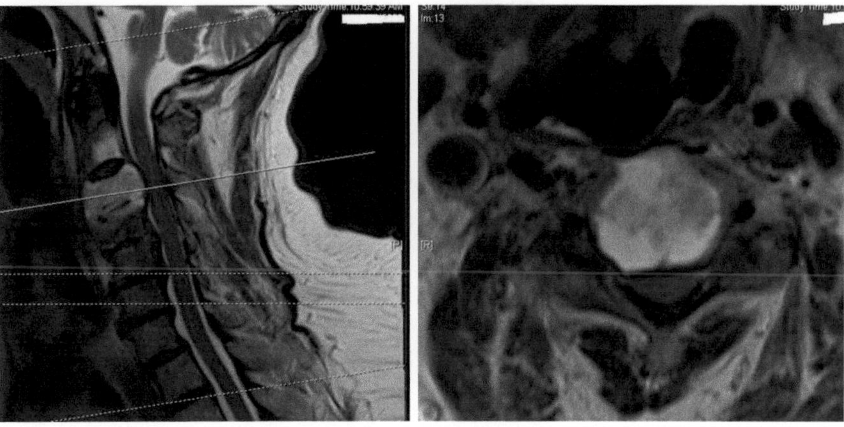

Fig. 7 Sagittal and axial MRI showing a 68 year-old male with metastatic lung adenocarcinoma involving C2–C4 anteriorly with soft tissue extension

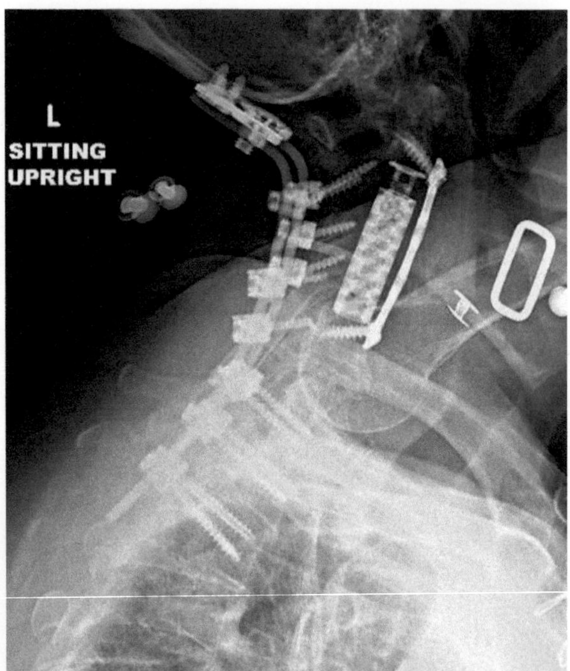

Fig. 8 Lateral X-ray of a 68 year-old male with C2–C4 metastatic lung adenocarcinoma that underwent posterior occiput—T1 fusion and instrumentation with C2–C7 laminectomy, anterior C2–C4 corpectomy with cage and C2–C5 instrumentation

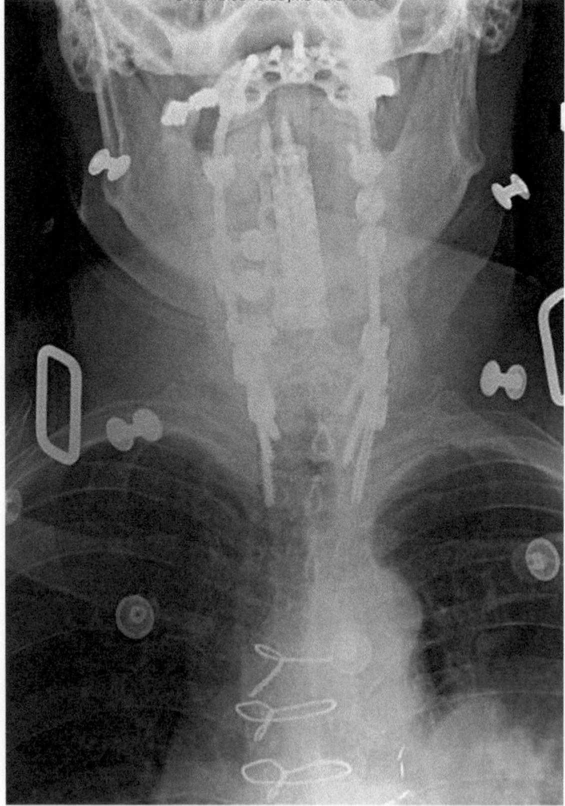

Fig. 9 Anteroposterior X-ray of the patient in Fig. 8

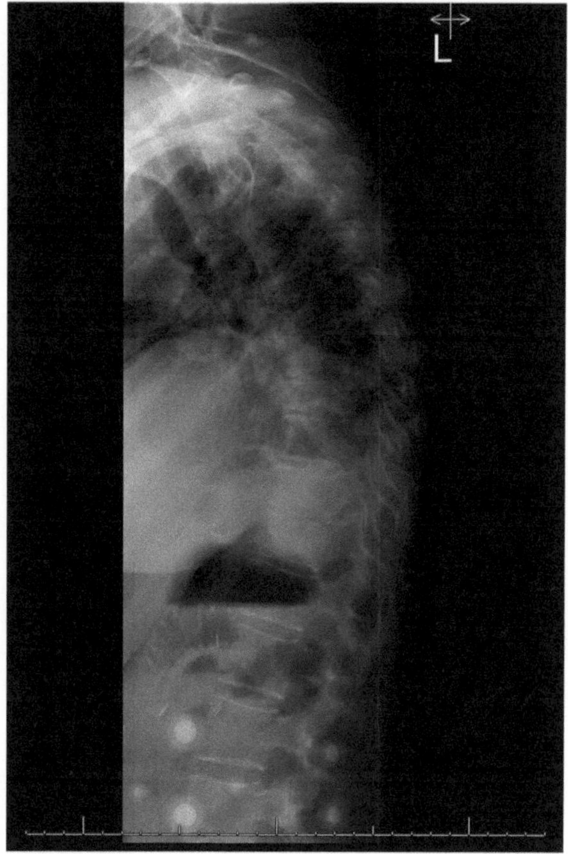

Fig. 10 Lateral thoracic X-ray of a 53 year-old female with metastatic adrenocortical carcinoma with T8 and T10 metastatic compression fractures

longitudinal ligament as a margin facilitates mass resection and protects the anterior thecal sac. Following anterior decompression or corpectomy, interbody cage or structural bone graft can be placed to create a 360° construct. In the setting of a neurologic compromise, the goal of surgery is circumferential decompression with multilevel stabilization, followed by radiation therapy as shown in Figs. 5, 6, 7, 8 and 9.

Vertebroplasty and kyphoplasty have most often been described for osteoporotic vertebral compression fractures [59, 60]. Vertebroplasty involves percutaneously injecting polymethylmethacrylate (PMMA) into the vertebral body to provide physical support to the symptomatic fracture. Kyphoplasty involves using a balloon tamp to create a small space within the vertebral body to help restore vertebral height prior to PMMA injection [61]. These techniques are being used more frequently for the treatment of painful vertebral fracture in oncologic patients that have failed conservative management as well as can be used to obtain a biopsy specimen.

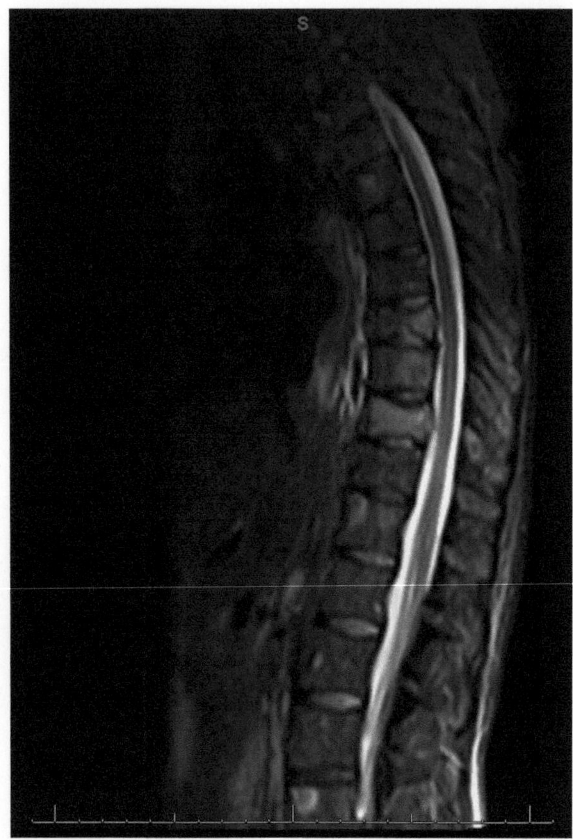

Fig. 11 Sagittal MRI shows T8 and T10 pathologic fractures in a 53 year-old female with metastatic adrenocortical carcinoma

This technique has been described with good results in the multiple myeloma population. One study looked at 55 consecutive kyphoplasty procedures performed in multiple myeloma patients and showed significant improvement in SF36 scores for bodily pain, physical function, vitality, and social functioning, as well as, they also had two complications of asymptomatic cement leakage [62]. Use of these procedures has resulted in improved pain control and reduced narcotic use [63, 64]. The CAFE trial involved a randomized, controlled, multicenter evaluation of kyphoplasty for the treatment of oncologic compression fractures and found its use effective and safe to rapidly reduce pain and improve function [65]. Cement leakage is a concern and can lead to acute neurologic deficits as depicted in Figs. 10, 11 and 12 where cement leakage necessitated emergent decompression. However, cement leakage often is asymptomatic and the risks can potentially be decreased by the use of high-viscosity cement and injecting small volumes of cement.

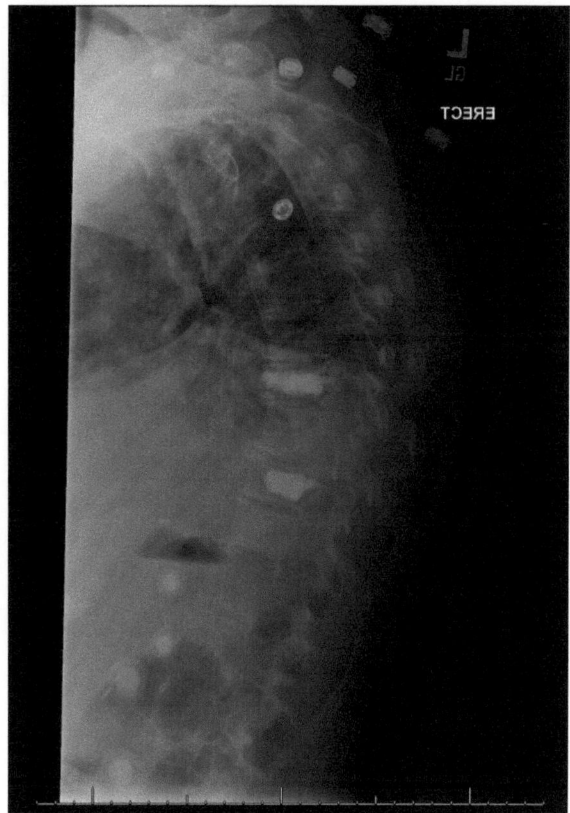

Fig. 12 Lateral X-ray of a 53 year-old female who underwent kyphoplasty at T8 and T10 for pathologic fracture but had cement extravasation at T10 necessitating emergent T8–T10 laminectomy for decompression

6 Survival

Once metastatic disease has been found in the spine, the time of survival primarily depends on the histology of the tumor and the stage of the disease process. For metastatic disease to the spine, mean survival for lung cancer is about 4–6 months, breast is about 19 months, prostate is about 18 months, renal is about 10 months, osteosarcoma is about 4.5 months, and cancer with unknown primary is about 6 months [22, 66]. Oncologic patients with spine metastases do benefit from radiation therapy and appropriate surgical intervention with improvements in quality of life including, anxiety, appetite, tiredness, nausea, well-being, drowsiness, and most notably pain [60]. Given the complex oncologic patient population, the overall complication rate in surgical management of spinal metastasis is about 25 % with the majority of these complications related to infection or wound complications [67].

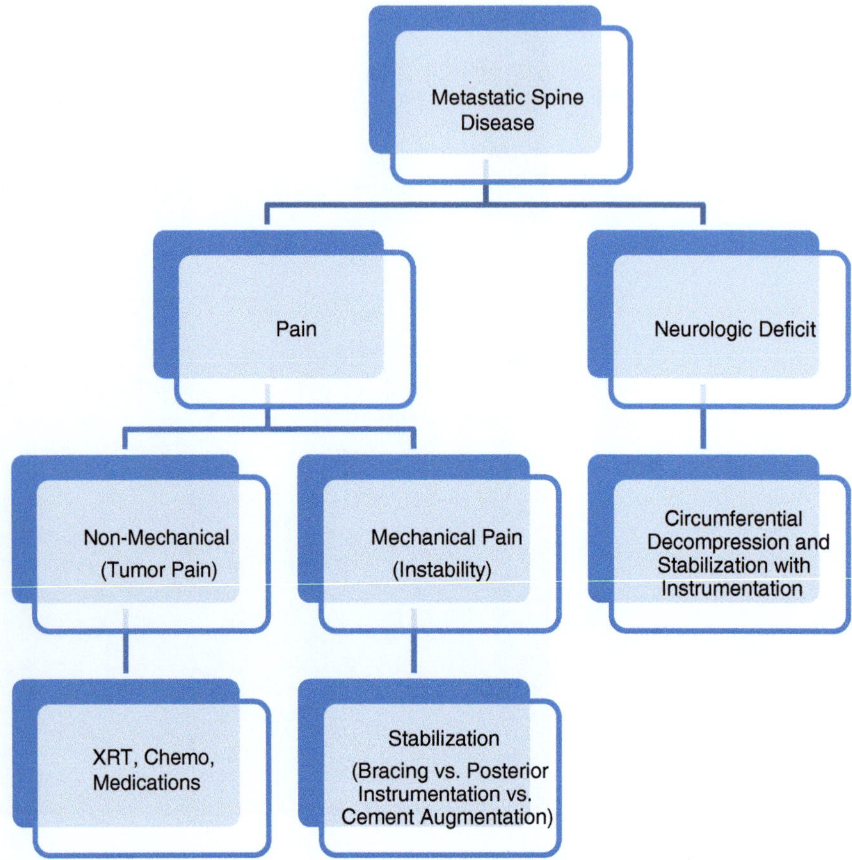

Fig. 13 General treatment algorithm for metastatic spinal disease involves a multidisciplinary approach

7 Conclusion

Management of oncologic spine disease requires a multidisciplinary approach, involving medical oncology, radiation oncology, pain management, and spine surgical services as the general treatment algorithm summarizes in Fig. 13 [68]. Several options exist for nonoperative management, including pain management, bracing, chemotherapy, and radiation. Appropriately selected patients with spinal metastases do have improved quality of life with surgical intervention. Operative intervention is often recommended in the setting of neurological compromise and/or significant spinal instability. An open discussion with the patient, oncologist, and surgeon is needed regarding life expectancy, quality of life, and surgical outcome expectations prior to undergoing surgical treatment.

References

1. American Cancer Society (2013) Cancer Facts & Figures 2013. http://www.cancer.org/acs/groups/content/@epidemiologysurveilance/documents/document/acspc-036845.pdf. Accessed June 6 2013
2. American Association of Neurologic Surgeons (2013) Patient Information. http://www.aans.org/en/Patient%20Information/Conditions%20and%20Treatments/Spinal%20Tumors.aspx. Accessed June 6 2013
3. Rougraff BT, Kneisl JS, Simon MA (1993) Skeletal metastases of unknown origin. A prospective study of a diagnostic strategy. J Bone Joint Surg Am 75(9):1276–1281
4. Sundaresan N, Digiacinto GV, Hughes JE, Cafferty M, Vallejo A (1991) Treatment of neoplastic spinal cord compression: results of a prospective study. Neurosurgery 29(5):645–650
5. Byrne TN, Benzel EC, Waxman SG (2000) Epidural tumors. In: Byrne TN, Benzel EC, Waxman SG (eds) Diseases of the spine and the spinal cord. Oxford University Press, New York, pp 166–205
6. Jaffe HL (1968) Tumors metastatic to the skeleton. In: Jaffe HL (ed) Tumors and tumorous conditions of the bones and joints. Lea and Febiger, Philadelphia, pp 589–618
7. Barron KD, Hirano A, Araki S, Terry RD (1959) Experiences with metastatic neoplasms involving the spinal cord. Neurology 9(2):91–106
8. Clarke E (1956) Spinal cord involvement in multiple myelomatosis. Brain 79(2):332–348
9. Galasko CS (1972) Skeletal metastases and mammary cancer. Ann R Coll Surg Engl 50(1):3–28
10. Nathoo N, Caris EC, Wiener JA, Mendel E (2011) History of the vertebral venous plexus and the significant contributions of Breschet and Batson. Neurosurgery 69(5):1007–1014; discussion 1014
11. Rougraff BT (2003) Evaluation of the patient with carcinoma of unknown origin metastatic to bone. Clin Orthop Relat Res 415(415 Suppl):S105–S109
12. Perrin RG, Laxton AW (2004) Metastatic spine disease: epidemiology, pathophysiology, and evaluation of patients. Neurosurg Clin N Am 15(4):365–373
13. Metser U, Lerman H, Blank A, Lievshitz G, Bokstein F, Even-Sapir E (2004) Malignant involvement of the spine: assessment by 18F-FDG PET/CT. J Nucl Med 45(2):279–284
14. Shah LM, Salzman KL (2011) Imaging of spinal metastatic disease. Int J Surg Oncol (Article ID 769753)
15. Saghieh S, Masrouha KZ, Musallam KM et al (2010) The risk of local recurrence along the core-needle biopsy tract in patients with bone sarcomas. Iowa Orthop J 30:80–83
16. Prabhu VC, Bilsky MH, Jambhekar K et al (2003) Results of preoperative embolization for metastatic spinal neoplasms. J Neurosurg 98(2 Suppl):156–164
17. Polley P, Dunn R (2009) Noncontiguous spinal tuberculosis: incidence and management. Eur Spine J 18(8):1096–1101
18. Gupta A, el Masri WS (1989) Multilevel spinal injuries. Incidence, distribution and neurological patterns. J Bone Joint Surg Br 71(4):692–695
19. Salvo N, Christakis M, Rubenstein J et al (2009) The role of plain radiographs in management of bone metastases. J Palliat Med 12(2):195–198
20. Buhmann Kirchhoff S, Becker C, Duerr HR, Reiser M, Baur-Melnyk A (2009) Detection of osseous metastases of the spine: comparison of high resolution multi-detector-CT with MRI. Eur J Radiol 69(3):567–573
21. Boriani S, Weinstein JN, Biagini R (1997) Primary bone tumors of the spine. Terminology and surgical staging. Spine (Phila Pa 1976) 22(9):1036–1044
22. Tokuhashi Y, Ajiro Y, Umezawa N (2009) Outcome of treatment for spinal metastases using scoring system for preoperative evaluation of prognosis. Spine (Phila Pa 1976) 34(1):69–73
23. Loblaw DA, Laperriere NJ (1998) Emergency treatment of malignant extradural spinal cord compression: an evidence-based guideline. J Clin Oncol 16(4):1613–1624

24. Ross JR, Saunders Y, Edmonds PM, Patel S, Broadley KE, Johnston SR (2003) Systematic review of role of bisphosphonates on skeletal morbidity in metastatic cancer. Bmj 327(7413):469
25. Huang RC, Khan SN, Sandhu HS et al (2005) Alendronate inhibits spine fusion in a rat model. Spine (Phila Pa 1976) 30(22):2516–2522
26. Lehman RA Jr, Kuklo TR, Freedman BA, Cowart JR, Mense MG, Riew KD (2004) The effect of alendronate sodium on spinal fusion: a rabbit model. Spine J 4(1):36–43
27. Nagahama K, Kanayama M, Togawa D, Hashimoto T, Minami A (2011) Does alendronate disturb the healing process of posterior lumbar interbody fusion? A prospective randomized trial. J Neurosurg Spine 14(4):500–507
28. Nakao S, Minamide A, Kawakami M, Boden SD, Yoshida M (2011) The influence of alendronate on spine fusion in an osteoporotic animal model. Spine (Phila Pa 1976) 36(18):1446–1452
29. Hartsell WF, Scott CB, Bruner DW et al (2005) Randomized trial of short- versus long-course radiotherapy for palliation of painful bone metastases. J Natl Cancer Inst 97(11):798–804
30. Gy single fraction radiotherapy for the treatment of metastatic skeletal pain: randomised comparison with a multifraction schedule over 12 months of patient follow-up (1999) Bone Pain Trial Working Party. Radiother Oncol 52(2):111–121
31. Patchell RA, Tibbs PA, Regine WF et al (2005) Direct decompressive surgical resection in the treatment of spinal cord compression caused by metastatic cancer: a randomised trial. Lancet 366(9486):643–648
32. Laufer I, Iorgulescu JB, Chapman T et al (2013) Local disease control for spinal metastases following "separation surgery" and adjuvant hypofractionated or high-dose single-fraction stereotactic radiosurgery: outcome analysis in 186 patients. J Neurosurg Spine 18(3):207–214
33. Moulding HD, Elder JB, Lis E et al (2010) Local disease control after decompressive surgery and adjuvant high-dose single-fraction radiosurgery for spine metastases. J Neurosurg Spine 13(1):87–93
34. Laufer I, Rubin DG, Lis E et al (2013) The NOMS framework: approach to the treatment of spinal metastatic tumors. Oncologist 18(6):744–751
35. Bilsky M, Smith M (2006) Surgical approach to epidural spinal cord compression. Hematol Oncol Clin North Am 20(6):1307–1317
36. Fisher CG, DiPaola CP, Ryken TC et al (2010) A novel classification system for spinal instability in neoplastic disease: an evidence-based approach and expert consensus from the Spine Oncology Study Group. Spine (Phila Pa 1976) 35(22):E1221–1229
37. Klimo P Jr, Kestle JR, Schmidt MH (2004) Clinical trials and evidence-based medicine for metastatic spine disease. Neurosurg Clin N Am 15(4):549–564
38. Young RF, Post EM, King GA (1980) Treatment of spinal epidural metastases. Randomized prospective comparison of laminectomy and radiotherapy. J Neurosurg 53(6):741–748
39. Klein JD, Hey LA, Yu CS et al (1996) Perioperative nutrition and postoperative complications in patients undergoing spinal surgery. Spine (Phila Pa 1976) 21(22):2676–2682
40. Hu SS, Fontaine F, Kelly B, Bradford DS (1998) Nutritional depletion in staged spinal reconstructive surgery. The effect of total parenteral nutrition. Spine (Phila Pa 1976) 23(12):1401–1405
41. Lapp MA, Bridwell KH, Lenke LG, Baldus C, Blanke K, Iffrig TM (2001) Prospective randomization of parenteral hyperalimentation for long fusions with spinal deformity: its effect on complications and recovery from postoperative malnutrition. Spine (Phila Pa 1976) 26(7):809–817; discussion 817
42. Halpin RJ, Sugrue PA, Gould RW et al (2010) Standardizing care for high-risk patients in spine surgery: the Northwestern high-risk spine protocol. Spine (Phila Pa 1976) 35(25):2232–2238
43. Savage JW, Anderson PA (2013) An update on modifiable factors to reduce the risk of surgical site infections. Spine J 24(13):00401–00405

44. Harrington KD (1993) Metastatic tumors of the spine: diagnosis and treatment. J Am Acad Orthop Surg 1(2):76–86

45. Nader R, Alford BT, Nauta HJ, Crow W, vanSonnenberg E, Hadjepavlou AG (2002) Preoperative embolization and intraoperative cryocoagulation as adjuncts in resection of hypervascular lesions of the thoracolumbar spine. J Neurosurg 97(3 Suppl):294–300

46. Rehak S, Krajina A, Ungermann L et al (2008) The role of embolization in radical surgery of renal cell carcinoma spinal metastases. Acta Neurochir (Wien) 150(11):1177–1181; discussion 1181

47. Manke C, Bretschneider T, Lenhart M et al (2001) Spinal metastases from renal cell carcinoma: effect of preoperative particle embolization on intraoperative blood loss. AJNR Am J Neuroradiol 22(5):997–1003

48. Broaddus WC, Grady MS, Delashaw JB Jr, Ferguson RD, Jane JA (1990) Preoperative superselective arteriolar embolization: a new approach to enhance resectability of spinal tumors. Neurosurgery. 27(5):755–759

49. Berkefeld J, Scale D, Kirchner J, Heinrich T, Kollath J (1999) Hypervascular spinal tumors: influence of the embolization technique on perioperative hemorrhage. AJNR Am J Neuroradiol 20(5):757–763

50. Finstein JL, Chin KR, Alvandi F, Lackman RD (2006) Postembolization paralysis in a man with a thoracolumbar giant cell tumor. Clin Orthop Relat Res 453:335–340

51. Truumees E, Dodwad SN, Kazmierczak CD (2010) Preoperative embolization in the treatment of spinal metastasis. J Am Acad Orthop Surg 18(8):449–453

52. Taniguchi T, Ohta K, Ohmura S, Yamamoto K, Kobayashi T (2000) Perioperative management for total en bloc spondylectomy–the effects of preoperative embolization and hypotensive anesthesia. Masui 49(2):168–171

53. Wirbel RJ, Roth R, Schulte M, Kramann B, Mutschler W (2005) Preoperative embolization in spinal and pelvic metastases. J Orthop Sci 10(3):253–257

54. Mani RL, Eisenberg RL (1978) Complications of catheter cerebral arteriography: analysis of 5,000 procedures. II. Relation of complication rates to clinical and arteriographic diagnoses. AJR Am J Roentgenol 131(5):867–869

55. Bradac GB, Oberson R (1980) CT and angiography in cases with occlusive disease of supratentorial cerebral vessels. Neuroradiology 19(4):193–200

56. Capener N (1954) The evolution of lateral rhachotomy. J Bone Joint Surg Br 36-B(2):173–179

57. Larson SJ, Holst RA, Hemmy DC, Sances A Jr (1976) Lateral extracavitary approach to traumatic lesions of the thoracic and lumbar spine. J Neurosurg 45(6):628–637

58. Jandial R, Chen MY (2012) Modified lateral extracavitary approach for vertebral column resection and expandable cage reconstruction of thoracic spinal metastases. Surg Neurol Int 3(136):136

59. Dodwad SN, Khan SN (2013) Surgical stabilization of the spine in the osteoporotic patient. Orthop Clin North Am 44(2):243–249

60. Wai EK, Finkelstein JA, Tangente RP et al (2003) Quality of life in surgical treatment of metastatic spine disease. Spine (Phila Pa 1976) 28(5):508–512

61. Spivak JM, Johnson MG (2005) Percutaneous treatment of vertebral body pathology. J Am Acad Orthop Surg 13(1):6–17

62. Dudeney S, Lieberman IH, Reinhardt MK, Hussein M (2002) Kyphoplasty in the treatment of osteolytic vertebral compression fractures as a result of multiple myeloma. J Clin Oncol 20(9):2382–2387

63. Fourney DR, Schomer DF, Nader R et al (2003) Percutaneous vertebroplasty and kyphoplasty for painful vertebral body fractures in cancer patients. J Neurosurg 98(1 Suppl):21–30

64. Pflugmacher R, Kandziora F, Schroeder RJ, Melcher I, Haas NP, Klostermann CK (2006) Percutaneous balloon kyphoplasty in the treatment of pathological vertebral body fracture and deformity in multiple myeloma: a one-year follow-up. Acta Radiol 47(4):369–376

65. Berenson J, Pflugmacher R, Jarzem P et al (2011) Balloon kyphoplasty versus non-surgical fracture management for treatment of painful vertebral body compression fractures in patients with cancer: a multicentre, randomised controlled trial. Lancet Oncol 12(3):225–235
66. Hessler C, Regelsberger J, Raimund F, Heese O, Madert J, Eggers C (2008) Prognosis after surgical treatment of spinal metastases due to lung cancer. Chirurg 79(7):671–679
67. Wise JJ, Fischgrund JS, Herkowitz HN, Montgomery D, Kurz LT (1999) Complication, survival rates, and risk factors of surgery for metastatic disease of the spine. Spine (Phila Pa 1976) 24(18):1943–1951
68. Klimo P, Jr., Kestle JR, Schmidt MH (2003) Treatment of metastatic spinal epidural disease: a review of the literature. Neurosurg Focus 15(5):E1

Evaluation and Treatment of Extremity Metastatic Disease

Aaron T. Creek, Drew A. Ratner and Scott E. Porter

Abstract

Metastases can occur as part of the natural progression of a variety of malignancies and their mode of spread, manner of presentation, and prognosis are as variable as their primary sources. The ultimate goal of musculoskeletal treatment of skeletal metastases is to get the patient in question back to his or her previous level of function as soon as possible. Skeletal metastases are seldom life threatening and their treatment will rarely render someone cured of their primary disease. Nevertheless, involvement of a musculoskeletal specialist as a part of the multidisciplinary approach can and very often does provide significant improvement in patients' qualities of life. The purpose of this chapter is to discuss the evaluation of a patient with suspected metastatic disease involving the musculoskeletal system and their pre-, intra-, and post surgical management as part of a multidisciplinary team.

Keywords

Musculoskeletal · Metastasis · Carcinoma · Bisphosphonate

1 Introduction

Metastases signify that a cancer has spread from its primary site. Similar to other metastases, bone metastases carry an inherent morbidity in that they often cause pain, inhibit patient function, and decrease quality of life. The ultimate goal of

A. T. Creek · D. A. Ratner · S. E. Porter (✉)
Department of Orthopaedic Surgery, Greenville Health System, Greenville, SC 29605, USA
e-mail: SPorter@ghs.org

T. D. Peabody and S. Attar (eds.), *Orthopaedic Oncology*,
Cancer Treatment and Research 162, DOI: 10.1007/978-3-319-07323-1_8,
© Springer International Publishing Switzerland 2014

treatment in these cases is to return the patient in question back to his or her previous level of function if possible. Secondary goals are based upon where in the life cycle of a skeletal metastasis a patient presents. Ideally, one would like to catch a metastasis early enough in its natural history to intervene and prevent progression of the local disease and all of the associated morbidities. Skeletal metastases are seldom life threatening and their treatment will rarely render someone cured of their primary disease. Nevertheless, involvement of a musculoskeletal specialist as a part of the multidisciplinary approach can and very often does provide significant improvement in patients' qualities of life. Early involvement of orthopedic surgeons can help to maximize the functional independence and the quality of the remaining life in these patients.

Recent estimates suggest that nearly 1.5 million new patients are diagnosed annually in the United States with some type of malignancy [1]. Four hundred thousand of these patients will be affected by bone metastases [2]. In fact, additional estimates would submit that 50 % of all patients with cancer have demonstrated bone metastases at autopsy and these numbers can be as high as 70 % in patients that pass away with breast and prostate cancer [3, 4]. The skeletal system is the third most common site for metastases after the liver and the lungs. The most frequently involved skeletal areas in order are the thoracic spine, the ribs, pelvis, and the proximal long bones. With these rates of involvement, skeletal metastases should be at the forefront of the minds of most healthcare providers when caring for a cancer patient. Most patients with a bone metastasis will present with pain from either a pathologic fracture or an impending pathologic fracture. A pathologic fracture is a fracture through a weakened area within the bone [5]. Pathologic fractures occur in 8 to 29 % of patients with bone metastases, with breast carcinoma causing a majority of these fractures, and the femur is the most common site for these fractures to occur [3, 6, 7]. For these reasons, musculoskeletal surgeons should be involved in a patient's care if there is any concern for possible metastasis in order to maximize the potential to prevent or delay much of the skeletal morbidity and complications caused by bone metastases.

2   Goals

Bone metastases carry a significant degree of morbidity and mortality, hence the desire of practitioners to treat in palliative, curative, as well as preventative terms. When bone metastases are present and there is concern for pathologic fracture, nerve root compression or spinal cord compression, there are four main considerations of treatment: pain relief, preservation or restoration of function, skeletal stabilization, and local tumor control [8]. Though questions may be raised concerning the aggressiveness of any treatment directed at skeletal metastases, healthcare providers should understand that the lifespan of patients once a metastasis is diagnosed continues to increase. Median survival for a breast cancer patient diagnosed with a bone metastasis, for example, ranges from 24 to 54 months. Survival for thyroid cancer and prostate cancer is 48 and 20–24 months, respectively [9].

While patients with metastatic lung cancer may have shorter survival than others, patients may enjoy relatively long life expectancies even with skeletal metastases [10].

3 Evaluation

The patient population at greatest risk for skeletal metastases is the population along the continuum of adult to elderly adult. When a patient presents with a destructive bone lesion and they are along this adult to elderly adult continuum, the most likely diagnosis is a skeletal metastasis from a carcinomatous primary followed by multiple myeloma and lymphoma. Less likely diagnoses include a primary malignant bone tumor, a destructive benign bone lesion (such as giant cell tumor), or a nonneoplastic condition (e.g., hyperparathyroidism, osteoporosis, osteomyelitis, metabolic bone disease, Gorham vanishing bone disease) [1]. In general, the workup for a bone lesion of unknown origin should start with a thorough history and physical, followed by labs and imaging, and finally, biopsy of the lesion in an effort to confirm or refute a suspected metastatic etiology.

Most patients with an appendicular bone metastasis will present with pain from either a pathologic fracture or an impending pathologic fracture. With modern imaging studies, skeletal lesions may be incidentally discovered early in their natural histories and before symptoms are likely to arise. The focus of this chapter, however, is the patient that presents with a destructive bone lesion with or without a previously diagnosed malignancy. As stated, progressive pain is the most common presentation for bone lesions caused by metastases in this patient population. The pain may be out of proportion to any inciting event, does not resolve with symptomatic treatment, and occurs with weight bearing, at rest, and even at night.

The history needs to focus on several key facts to help narrow down the differential diagnosis. When a patient presents and is discovered to have a suspicious lesion with a recent history of a known malignancy, the circumstances of their original presentation and the characteristics of the primary tumor including site, size, and grade should be investigated. A cancer patient's initial staging is very useful to quantitate the overall likelihood of metastases including those to the musculoskeletal system. For example, if a patient with a history of a 0.5-cm squamous cell carcinoma 12 years prior to their presentation of a large destructive lesion of the pelvis, the likelihood that they are related is quite low. In contrast, if that patient was diagnosed 6 months prior to the current presentation with an 8-cm renal cell carcinoma, then the chances are significantly greater that the events are related. If an evaluation discovers a lesion that is concerning for metastases in the setting of no known potential primary malignancy, the questions in the history should focus on distinguishing between the different possibilities of primary sources. A very useful mnemonic for remembering the most likely primary sites for metastatic disease to bone is "Kinds of Tumors Leaping Primarily to Bone." This mnemonic helps to recall kidney, thyroid, lung, prostate, and breast cancers as possible primaries. Helpful, probative questions may then be centered upon the following:

- Recent mammograms, pap smears, prostate exams, and colonoscopies
- Personal history of cancer radiation, chemotherapy, and Paget disease
- Smoking history, diet, and exposure to certain chemicals like asbestos
- Urinary pain/frequency or hematuria
- Change in bowel habits or rectal bleeding
- Family history of cancer

The physical exam needs to continue this theme of an investigation for a primary site of disease but should also focus on the musculoskeletal complaint in question. As stated, our goals of treatment include returning patients to his or her previous level of function and perhaps more importantly identifying a metastasis early enough in its natural history to intervene and prevent progression or the need for surgical intervention. Once the examination in pursuit of primary sites of disease concludes, healthcare providers should examine a patient to assess the likelihood of displacement of a pathologic fracture [5].

Potential laboratory workups may be rather nonspecific. A notable exception includes using serum protein electrophoresis (SPEP), which has been shown to be 92.5 % specific and 87.6 % sensitive for diagnosing multiple myeloma [11]. There are certain serum tumor markers that may help to suggest the possibility of bone metastasis in a patient with a previous history of cancer—for example, osteoprotegerin (OPG) for prostate cancer [12] or CA 15-3 for breast cancer [13]. Additional useful laboratory values may include calcium, phosphorus, and alkaline phosphatase levels in order to directly quantify the degree to which bone activity is present.

4   Imaging Studies

Generally, musculoskeletal pain and skeletal abnormalities identified on staging studies are first evaluated with simple radiographs. Metastases to the bone generally result in one of three appearances on X-ray (Fig. 1a–c). Lung, thyroid, and renal cancer metastases produce primarily radiolucent or osteolytic lesions that are best thought of as discrete areas devoid of the mineral phase of bone. Prostate cancers generally result in sclerotic or osteoblastic bone lesions on X-rays. Breast cancer skeletal metastases are unique in that they may present with an appearance anywhere on a continuum between lysis and sclerosis. In fact, they oftentimes appear to have mixed constituency with lysis and sclerosis appearing in the same lesion. Identifying a lesion as osteolytic or osteoblastic is important because osteolytic lesions and their erosion of the mineral phase and strength of bone are more likely to produce pathologic fractures, and therefore are more often acutely symptomatic than osteoblastic lesions [14].

The radiographic workup should support the stated goals of treatment. These include identifying a metastasis early enough in its natural history to intervene and prevent progression or the need for surgical intervention. To that end, if a suspicious lesion is identified in a patient with a known history of a malignancy or a patient that is suspected to have an unconfirmed primary malignancy,

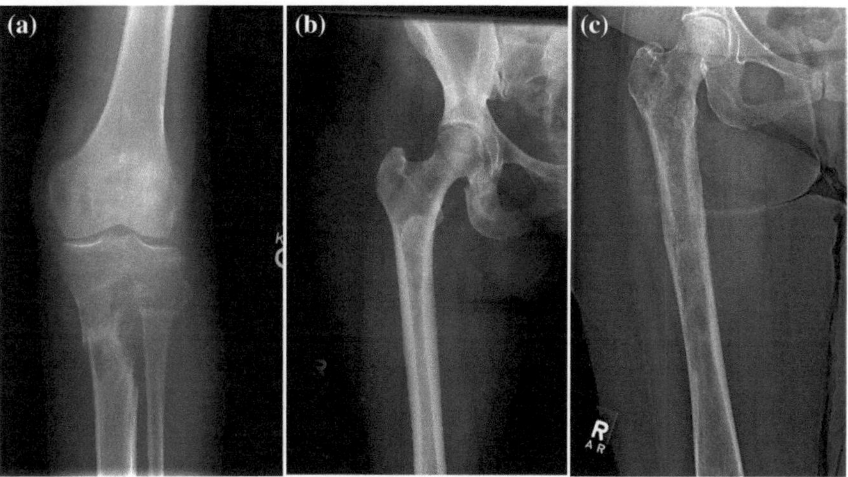

Fig. 1 AP radiograph of an osteolytic process of the proximal tibia resulting in knee pain. Note the absence of bone on the lateral side of the tibial metaphysis that has resulted in a pathological fracture. **b** AP radiograph of a classic osteoblastic metastasis to the proximal femur. Note the sclerosis present throughout the entire lesion. **c** AP radiograph of a mixed blastic and lytic lesion of the proximal and midshaft femur secondary to breast carcinoma

a Technetium-99 m-phosphonate (^{99m}Tc) scintigraphy scan should be performed to look for the presence of other lesions. Commonly referred to simply as a bone scan, it is a very efficient way to image an entire skeletal system including the remaining aspects of the bone in question (Fig. 2). This may become an important factor in the decision tree used to determine the need for and nature of any future fixation attempts. This benefit is balanced, however, by its inherent lack of specificity. Such scans detect any osteoblastic activity regardless of the etiology of that activity. They are unable to differentiate metastatic disease from increased activity due to benign conditions like osteoarthritis, healed fractures, or previously existing benign bone disease. It has been reported that 45 % of abnormal bone scans in patients with a history of carcinoma did not reflect bone metastasis, but rather trauma (25 %), infection (10 %), and other causes (10 %) [15]. Additionally, bone scans will not show a lesion with purely osteolytic activity. This is the hallmark of the lesions of multiple myeloma. In this setting, the negative predictive value of the bone scan when compared with the radiograph that prompted the healthcare provider to order it becomes equally as important. Scintigraphy has now evolved to include (18)F-Fluoride positive emission and computed tomography (PET/CT) and Fluorodeoxy-D-Glucose PET/CT. Most studies show that both (18)F-Fluoride PET/CT and Fluorodeoxy-D-Glucose PET/CT are effective in terms of sensitivity and specificity for detecting bone metastases [16].

The clinical applicability of magnetic resonance imaging (MRI) in the evaluation of skeletal metastases continues to evolve. MRI is limited, however, by its cost and its small field of view relative to the quality of its imaging. Additionally,

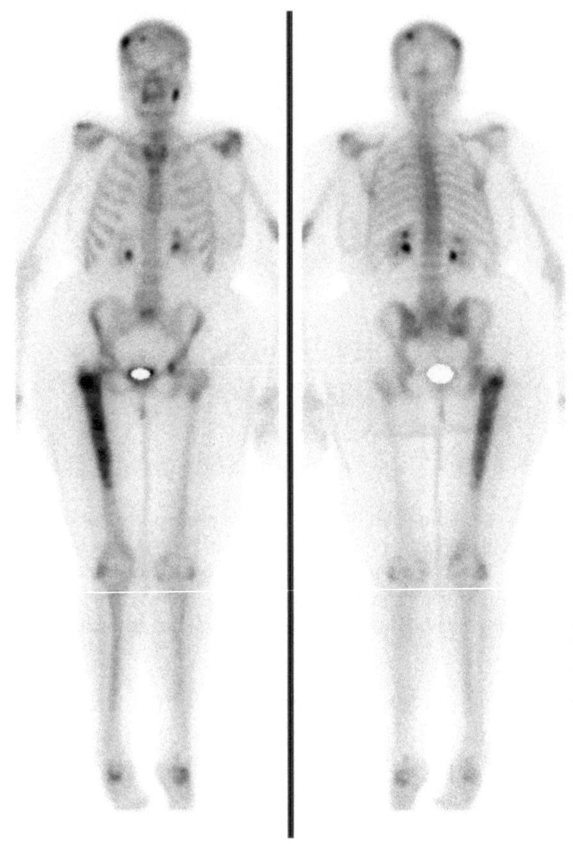

Fig. 2 Technetium-labeled bone scan of the patient presented in Fig. 1c with additional sites of active skeletal disease

outside of the spine, one can question if the additional information gleaned by MRI can justify its time and resource utilization. Notable exceptions would include evaluation of vertebral metastases in symptomatic patients and in the evaluation of patients suspected to have a skeletal lesion with an accompanying soft tissue mass (Fig. 3). This mass may be suggested by either physical exam or critical evaluation of plain radiographs that might reveal telling soft tissue densities in the vicinity of the lesion in question. In this setting, additional evaluation is strongly suggested since the differential diagnosis necessarily includes primary bone malignancies.

Computed tomography (CT) is vastly superior to radiography in the detection of trabecular and cortical bone destruction, soft tissue extension, and involvement of neurovascular structures including the spine. It may also provide this information in lieu of an MRI for patients in whom an MRI is contraindicated. CT is also useful in guiding needle biopsy of lesions. Perhaps the most important role of computed tomography is in the evaluation of a patient that has a suspicious destructive lesion but no known primary malignancy. Rougraff et al. [17] utilizing an evaluation

Fig. 3 **a** AP radiograph of a
distal femur with its coronal
magnetic resonance image
b demonstrating robust
contrast uptake and a sizable
soft tissue mass

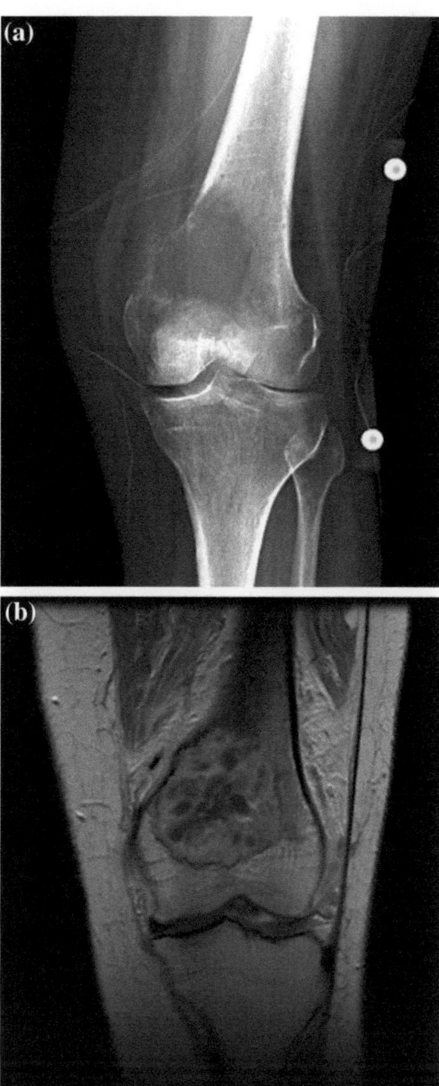

system that was anchored by CT scanning of the chest, abdomen, and pelvis, were
able to detect the primary site of disease in 85 % of their patients who had a skeletal
metastasis of unknown origin. Specifically, 28 % of the primary carcinomas were
able to be identified on CT scan but not any of the other imaging modalities.

5   Biopsy

There is debate as to the necessity of biopsying a bone lesion in a patient with a known preexisting primary carcinoma. Clayer and Duncan [18] argue that all patients who present with a new lesion should have biopsies. Their study analyzed 50 patients presenting with a new bone lesion who had preexisting breast, prostate, lung, renal, skin, or colon cancer. Their results showed that 10 of these patients' had a bone lesion caused by pathology other than the primary carcinoma. Conversely, Cronin et al. [19] argue the exact opposite. In their study, a bone lesion in a patient with known primary malignant disease was rarely something other than a metastasis from the primary tumor. The best approach may be to determine the merits of performing a biopsy before definitive treatment in each individual case. The duration of time since a patient's initial diagnosis of malignancy, the primary tumor characteristics, the preliminary staging related to a previous cancer history, the current staging results and the burden of disease, and the imaging characteristics of the new lesion in question should all help to decide whether or not a worrisome lesion should be biopsied prior to definitive treatment. In general, it is advisable to biopsy the first and only site of suspected metastatic disease to bone to avoid inadvertently treating a sarcoma as a metastatic lesion. This is less important in the face of multiple metastases to bone or viscera.

Biopsies can be done either percutaneously or through an open approach. Percutaneous fine needle aspiration biopsy (FNAB) or core biopsies are both accomplished with the aid of computed tomography for accuracy. This has become a highly preferred method for biopsies because it has been shown to have lower morbidity, lower cost, and a greater ability to biopsy more than one site if indicated when compared to open biopsy. The downsides, however, are the potential risks of the inability to provide a definitive diagnosis and even a potential error in diagnosis. Additionally, FNABs are also limited in their ability to provide pathologists with the appearance of the cellular architecture that larger biopsy samples provide [20].

Open biopsies, in contrast, yield much better accuracy rates [21]. Additionally, open biopsies are often scheduled in conjunction with a definitive fixation procedure and therefore allow the healthcare team to accomplish two goals simultaneously: confirm a diagnosis and treat an impending or displaced pathological fracture. Oncologic principles should be strictly followed when performing an open biopsy in case a lesion proves to be a primary malignancy of bone [22]. Ultimately, if a cytologic diagnosis achieved from FNAB does not match the suspected diagnosis based on history, physical, and imaging, then an open biopsy should be performed before any major surgical procedure is done [23].

6   Presurgical Considerations

Once the diagnosis of a skeletal metastasis has been confirmed or is strongly suspected by reviewing the entire clinical picture, consideration must be given to actively treating the lesion(s) in question. The two general treatment options that must be weighed are operative versus nonoperative. To determine the best possible course may be quite difficult but attention should always be paid to achieving initial goals: the detection of a metastasis early enough in its natural history to intervene and prevent progression of the local disease and all of the associated morbidities and, if the lesion results in an alteration of some type of function, returning the patient in question back to his or her previous level.

Nonoperative means of treatment for a skeletal metastasis include observation, systemic treatment of disease, bisphosphonates, radiation therapy, or any combination of these modalities. Lesions that are amenable to this line of treatment largely include small lesions, lesions that are incidentally discovered, lesions of the flat bones of the skeleton (e.g., ribs, inferior scapula, etc.), and lesions that involve non-weight-bearing bones (e.g., humerus in a patient with normal ambulatory ability). The benefits of bisphosphonates are now well established [24, 25]. Bisphosphonates halt overactive osteoclastic mechanisms via osteoclast uptake followed by osteoclast apoptosis. A large body of evidence, especially in the breast cancer literature, exists which examines the use of bisphosphonates in the treatment of metastatic disease. After 12 months of use, a significant reduction in pathologic fractures has been noted and after 24 months, a reduction in need for orthopedic surgery has been documented [26]. Additionally, economic analyses have also demonstrated bisphosphonate therapy to be cost-effective in treatment algorithms employing their use [27].

External beam radiation therapy (XRT) has long been reported to relieve bone pain and halt the progression of local disease in cancer patients with skeletal metastases. Ionizing radiation that is focused on the site of metastatic disease is thought to work by direct tumor kill followed by regeneration of bone that takes place through the well-described cycle of collagen proliferation, vascular stromal production, and osteoblastic/osteoclastic remodeling. The treatment doses that patients receive can either come in the form of single or multiple fractionations. Ultimately, the cumulative dose may differ from one primary tumor type's metastasis to another since some tumors are much more resistant to its effects [28]. Radiofrequency ablation and percutaneous cryoablation therapy have also been shown to be effective in reducing pain associated with bone metastases [29, 30]. Arguably, the most important factor in any of the nonoperative treatment algorithms is following the lesion in question to confirm improvement, stability, or worsening of disease.

With failure of nonoperative treatment or if the lesion in question meets operative indications upon its initial presentation, surgery is an option. Surgery should be considered for any lesion that is progressive despite conservative treatment, spinal lesions that present an imminent risk of mechanical failure of the vertebral column, lesions of weight-bearing bones that are at risk for fracture and displacement, and lesions that have already fractured with displacement. There are a number of published algorithms and scoring systems meant to help guide the decision to proceed with surgical stabilization of an impending fracture [31, 32]. Their common theme is their attempt to quantify the mechanical integrity of the bone in question. For long bones, Mirel's scoring system is one of the most widely used [32]. This scoring system, with a maximum of twelve points, assigns up to three points in each of the four main determinants of an impending catastrophic failure of a long bone secondary to a suspected lesion. The categories in question include the pain that the lesion causes (minimal, moderate, functional), the anatomic location of the lesion (upper extremity, lower extremity, pertrochanteric area of the femur), the radiographic pattern of the lesion (blastic, mixed, lytic), and the size of the lesion relative to the diameter of the bone in question (less than 1/3, 1/3–2/3, greater than 2/3). A total score of 8 or greater is strongly suggestive of a bone that is at risk for displacement of a pathologic fracture [30].

When the decision to proceed with surgery has been made, it is important to think about every patient individually when planning for surgery. The plan should explore the patient's preexisting comorbidities, historic or current chemotherapy regimens that may have altered a patient's cardiac function or may be currently decreasing his or her immune system, routine laboratory values specifically looking for hypercalcemia and coagulopathies, nutritional status, and the integrity of the soft tissue envelope within the proposed surgical field. Another preoperative consideration is arterial embolization of skeletal metastasis in order to decrease the risks of intraoperative hemorrhage. There are some primary tumors whose metastases are notably vascular. Renal carcinoma and thyroid carcinoma often metastasize to skeletal locations with lesions of significant size, vascularity, and soft tissue involvement (Fig. 4). Rapid and potentially life threatening volumes of blood loss can occur quickly with intralesional procedures. Robial et al. describe a universal acceptance of embolization of renal and thyroid lesions but they showed no difference in the twenty-eight breast cancer lesions and nineteen lung cancer lesions removed during spinal corpectomies and vertebrectomies [33].

7   Surgical Considerations

Routine fracture care of nonpathologic bone assumes a local environment that is rarely compromised and routinely results in healing. The environment of the metastatic focus of disease, however, is often within an immunocompromised host, and this environment may be further insulted by the use of perioperative radiation therapy. All of these are conspiring against the normal processes of healing. In addition to the rapid restoration of function, an important secondary surgical goal is to provide fixation that will last the rest of the patient's life and that does not necessarily depend upon the healing of the involved bone to do so (Fig. 5).

The surgical options that are largely available include splinting or fixation of the bone in question with plates and screws or an intramedullary device, intralesional curettage, or debulking of the tumor followed by polymethylmethacrylate (PMMA) supplementation with or without splinting of the bone as described above, resection of the bone in question with reconstruction utilizing an implant where appropriate, or amputation. Ultimately, the treatment choice depends most upon the bone that is involved, the anatomic region of involvement within the bone, the extent of disease present, and the integrity of the soft tissue envelope.

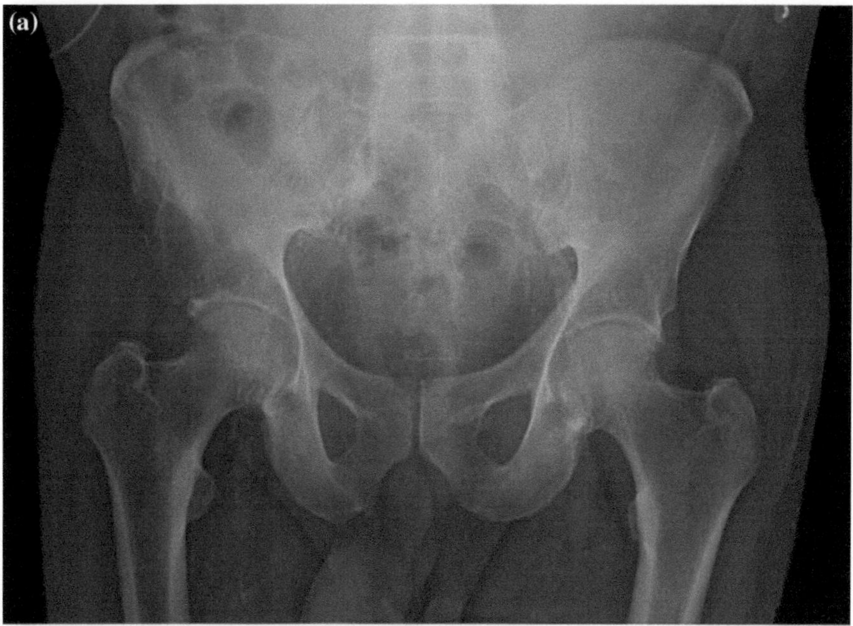

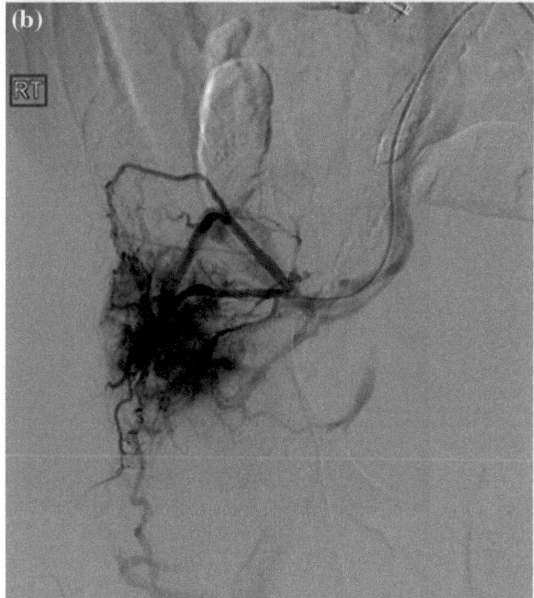

Fig. 4 **a** AP pelvis radiograph depicting a lesion in the right supra-acetabular region from a renal cell carcinoma primary. **b** represents the angiogram that was obtained prior to the embolization procedure demonstrating the vascularity of the lesion in question

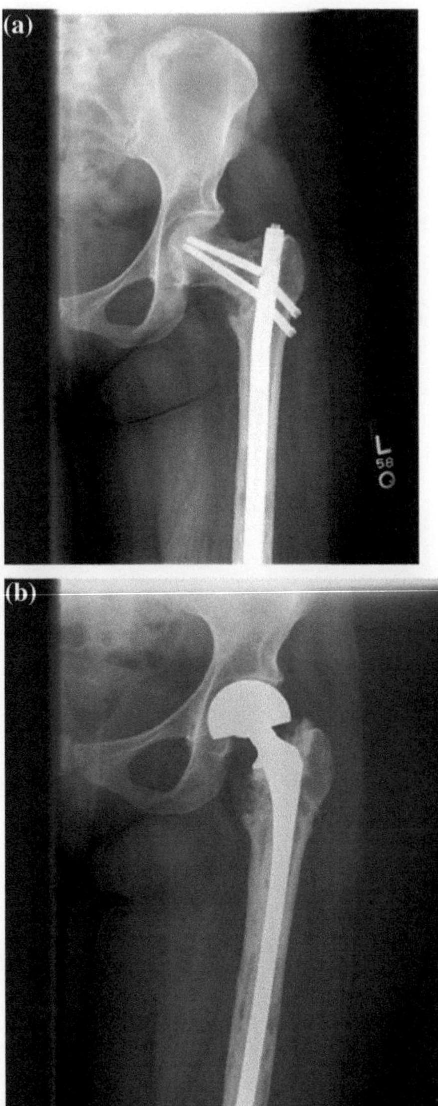

Fig. 5 **a** AP radiograph of an impending proximal femur fracture treated with cephalomedullary nail fixation. The device did not provide a rigid, fixed angle proximally and no adjuvant therapy was given. The construct ultimately failed requiring a conversion **b** to a long-stem hip hemiarthroplasty

7.1   Spine

The spine is the most common site of metastatic disease and treatment must arrest local disease given the tight anatomic confines of the vertebral column. While XRT is more commonly employed as a definitive treatment for vertebral metastases, surgery would be recommended for imminent mechanical failure of the vertebral column that may result in potentially devastating neurological compromise.

The two main surgical treatments can be broadly described as intralesional curettage with stabilization and en bloc resection of the vertebrae with stabilization. It is commonly agreed upon that en bloc resection may be reserved for patients with neurological compromise, low-grade metastases, long life expectancies, or certain cervical spine lesions due to easier surgical access to the cervical versus the thoracic or lumbar regions [34]. In patients who do not meet these criteria, intralesional curettage and stabilization is the preferred surgical technique.

7.2 Pelvis

The pelvis is the most frequent site of metastatic carcinoma after the spine. Mechanically, the pelvis plays a critical role in the weight-bearing axis and has fewer splinting options than do the long bones of the body. Metastases encountered here can be treated initially with observation and XRT or radiofrequency ablation (RFA) but when surgery is indicated, most lesions are curetted and the area in question may then be splinted with plates and screws [30]. The acetabulum can be considered to be a unique anatomic area in the pelvis. Again, metastases to the periacetabular region are often treated with observation and XRT. In situations of massive bone loss, however, extensive reconstruction of the acetabulum may be necessary in order to achieve the goal of returning a patient back to some previous level of function with a reconstruction that does not depend upon bone healing for success. Harrington popularized an approach that judiciously uses Steinman pins as rebar in conjunction with generous amounts of PMMA and conventional total hip arthroplasty. Nilsson et al. reported that this technique was effective and durable enough to relieve pain and restore function in their sample of 32 patients with advanced periacetabular metastatic destruction; while others have shown good results with different medications of the Harrington technique [35–38] (Fig. 6).

7.3 Extremity

Extremities are composed of long bones that morphologically differ from vertebrae or the flat bones of the pelvis and the surgical options exploit this difference. Once the decision for surgery has been made, the options for local control of the tumor remain identical to other skeletal sites—namely intralesional curettage or resection. The reconstruction, however, differs in that the choices routinely include prosthetic reconstruction and intramedullary nailing in addition to fixation with plates and screws. As stated previously, the choice of reconstruction ultimately depends upon the anatomic region of the bone in question and the extent of involvement but ultimately this choice adheres to the goals of returning a patient back to a desired level of function and providing fixation that will last the rest of the patient's life. To this end, most surgeons still subscribe to the tenet of splinting the entire length of the long bone in question in order to protect against disease progression or recurrent involvement of the same bone.

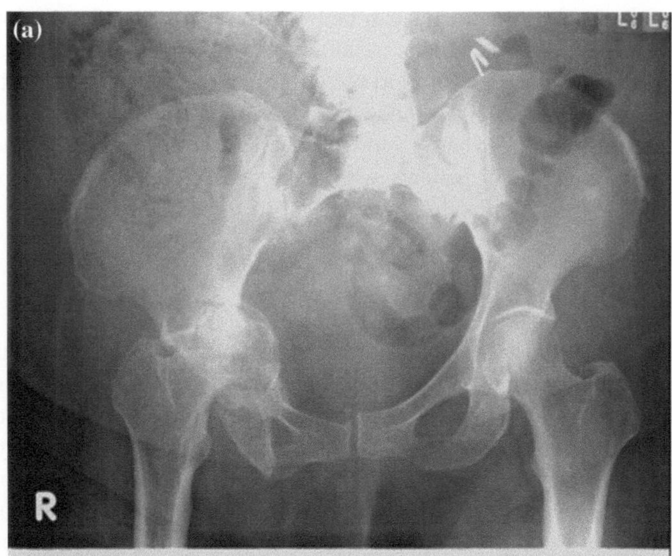

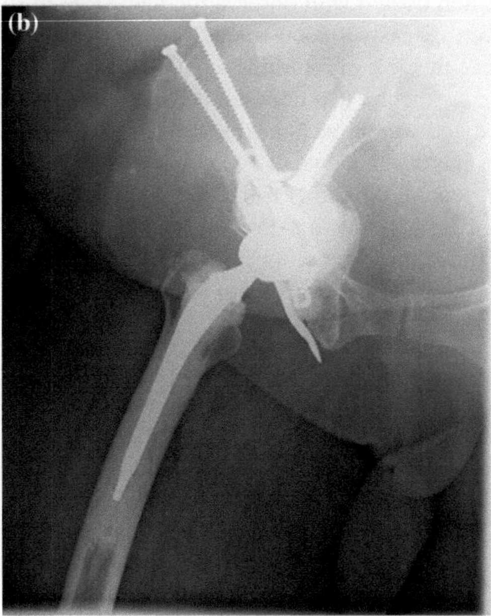

Fig. 6 **a** Preoperative AP pelvis radiograph of a femoral head that has protruded through the acetabulum in a patient with a history of renal cell carcinoma with metastases to bone. **b** Postoperative AP radiograph of the hip demonstrating the large screws that have been used to support the PMMA and the use of the implant to reconstruct this patient's pelvis

7.3.1 Femur

For metastatic disease confined to the femoral head and/or neck, a trial of definitive XRT may be entertained since reconstruction in this region of the femur inevitably involves hemiarthroplasty. A failed period of observation does not necessarily result in additional morbidity but this decision should be made with the assistance of an orthopedic specialist. Once the decision for surgery is made, standard fixation methods for the femoral head and neck have an unacceptably high rate of failure [39]. For this reason, hemiarthroplasty with a conventional length or a long-length stem is indicated. Preoperatively and intraoperatively, particular attention needs to be paid to the ipsilateral acetabulum. If no disease can be identified, acetabulum resurfacing is likely unnecessary.

The peritrochanteric region of the femur is the proximal metaphysis. This area is subjected to tremendous forces and modern implants have been designed with this fact in mind [40]. Current techniques of cephalomedullary fixation utilize mechanics that allow splinting of the entire bone including that of the femoral neck and head. For discrete lesions that are easily accessible, one might entertain curettage prior to intramedullary fixation or PMMA reinforcement of the lesion following fixation. Occasionally, plates and screws are still employed in the treatment of this region of the femur if intramedullary fixation is contraindicated or technically not feasible.

The distal femur is frequently the site of metastatic disease. Due to its very forgiving anatomy, all of the surgical options are routinely used with success. Distal metaphyseal lesions are amenable to intramedullary fixation with or without curettage and cementation. Distal periarticular lesions can be treated with curettage and plate fixation or resection with prosthetic reconstruction. The choice largely depends upon the extent of disease and surgeon preference.

7.3.2 Humerus

Similar principles exist for surgical treatment of the humerus as they do for the femur. A significant difference, however, is that the humerus is largely a non-weight-bearing joint that is much more amenable to nonoperative treatment. Failure of this treatment is not nearly as catastrophic in the majority of patients. Despite this difference, the treatment principles are largely identical to those of the femur with curettage and plate fixation versus prosthetic reconstruction for metaphyseal or periarticular lesions and intramedullary nailing for metastases of the shaft. Special consideration should be paid to the distal humerus if affected. Most authors now agree that dual plate fixation is most likely to allow early, unrestricted, and durable range of motion of the elbow [41].

8   Postsurgical Considerations

The best technically performed surgery may be limited by events that occur in the postoperative period of time. Wound healing, physical therapy restrictions, and adjuvant therapies directed locally to the operative field and systemically to additional sites of disease all impact the quality of life in a patient population that is already facing a diminished quantity of life. A final goal of surgery is the recognition of the confounding factor of time. In addition to restoring function and providing durable fixation that will last the rest of the patient's life, healthcare providers should recommend surgical treatment options that have the reproducibly least complicated postoperative courses. This includes mitigating the risk of postoperative wound healing complications by decreasing operative time, routine use of perioperative antibiotics, and the use of antibiotic-impregnated PMMA when appropriate because the treatments for wound complications negatively impact patients' quality of a life [42–44]. Moreover, the durable fixation methods allow immediate weight bearing and immediate participation in postoperative rehabilitation programs for precisely the same reasons.

Thromboembolic events represent another area of differentiation for this patient population. Due to the pathology of malignancy and some of the treatment protocols, cancer patients may have a hypercoagulable baseline state [45]. The generous use of mechanical prophylaxis and aggressive mobilization will help to lessen the risk of symptomatic and catastrophic thromboembolisms. Additionally, chemical prophylaxis should be judiciously used given the risk of widely metastatic disease including cerebral metastases that will be present in some patients. In high-risk patients that have a contraindication for chemical prophylaxis, consideration should be given to insertion of a vena cava filter in the perioperative period.

One of the most critical postoperative interventions is radiation therapy in the appropriate setting. External beam radiation therapy is recommended for all postoperative treatment regimens that follow an intralesional surgical procedure. This would include prophylactic fixation without curettage, curettage followed by fixation, or an attempted excision of a metastasis with a positive margin suggesting contamination of the surgical field [46]. Radiation should be started once the wound has completely healed and should incorporate the entire surgical field including the complete length of the implant used to stabilize the bone. This is necessary to prevent postoperative disease progression and ultimately failure of the reconstructive effort.

9   Special Considerations

There are some metastatic sites of disease that behave differently enough to warrant a separate but brief note. The location of metastatic sites of disease at times may yield clues to the primary. The discovery of metastases prior to the discovery of a primary (e.g., metastases of unknown origin) is usually related to

Fig. 7 **a** Progression of disease in a patient with a displaced femur fracture in the setting of a metastasis from renal cell carcinoma. Note the failure of the implant despite adjuvant radiation therapy. **b** Salvage procedure utilizing a distal femur endoprosthesis

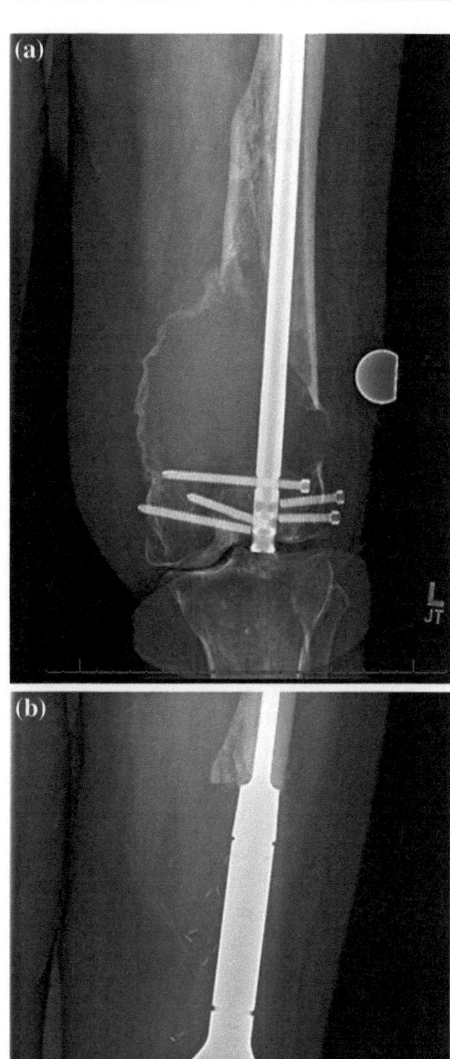

lung carcinoma. Additionally, lung metastases are generally regarded to portend the worst prognosis and have the shortest intervals from diagnosis of skeletal metastasis to death for all metastatic cancers. Their fixation should certainly respect the quantity of time that those patients have left.

Renal carcinomas are one of the most recalcitrant metastases to conventional therapies. They are extremely angiogenic and are generally considered to be largely radioresistant to standard radiation fractionation schedules. Within the treatment algorithm for renal cell carcinoma, metastases lie two important adjuncts to surgery: preoperative embolization and perioperative fractionation schedules that deliver a greater total dose of radiation than is usually given (Fig. 7). Furthermore, a classic teaching of surgically treating an isolated metastasis with wide excision was applied largely to metastases of renal cell carcinoma to bone. Although subsequent studies have not shown a significant increase in survival, there is still some utility in an attempt to resect with clean margins an isolated skeletal metastasis from a renal cell carcinoma primary [47, 48].

10   Conclusions

The treatment of skeletal metastases significantly impacts a patient's quality of life. There are several goals that healthcare providers should keep in mind when treating this unique orthopedic patient population. In the absence of overwhelming confirmatory evidence that a lesion in question is a metastasis, the diagnosis should be confirmed. Metastases should be caught early enough in its natural history to intervene and prevent progression of the local disease and all of the associated morbidities. If the lesion results in an alteration of some type of function, the goal should be to return the patient back to his or her previous level. Impending or displaced pathological fractures warrant some type of intervention. If that intervention is surgical, it should provide fixation that will last the rest of the patient's life and that does not necessarily depend upon the healing of the involved bone to do so. Lastly, healthcare providers should be sensitive to the balance of quality and quantity of life in this patient population. In the absence of an ability to improve upon the quantity, all efforts should focus on quality of life.

References

1. Weber K (2010) Evaluation of the adult patient with a destructive bone lesion. J Am Acad Orthopedic Surgery 18:169–179
2. Coleman R et al (2010) Metastasis and bone loss: advancing treatment and prevention. Cancer Treat Rev 36(8):615–620 (Published online 2010 May 15)
3. Narazaki DK, Alverga Neto CC, Baptista AM, Caiero MT, Camargo OP (2006) Prognostic factors in pathologic fractures secondary to metastatic tumors Clinics 61(4):313–320
4. Coleman R (2006) Clinical features of metastatic bone disease and risk of skeletal morbidity. Clin Cancer Res 12:6243s
5. Jasmin C, Coleman, RE, Coia LR, Capanna R, Saillant G (2005) Textbook of bone metastases. Wiley, London
6. Sivasundaram R, Shah S, Ahmadi S, Wunder JS, Schemitsch EH, Ferguson PC, Zdero R (2013) The biomechanical effect of proximal tumor defect location on femur pathological fractures. J Orthopedic Trauma 27(8):e174–e180

7. Higinbotham NL, Marcove RC (1965) The management of pathological fractures. J Trauma 5:792–798

8. Healey JH, Brown HK (2000) Complications of bone metastases: surgical management. Cancer 88(S12):2940–2951

9. Ahn SG, Lee HM, Cho S-H, Lee SA, Hwang SH, Jeong J, Lee H-D (2013) Prognostic factors for patients with bone-only metastasis in breast cancer. Yonsei Med J 54(5):1168–1177

10. Bloomfield DJ (1998) Should bisphosphonates be part of the standard therapy of patients with multiple myeloma or bone metastases from other cancers? An evidence-based review. J Clin Oncol 16:1218–1225

11. Katzmann JA (2009) Screening panels for monoclonal Gammopathiesltime to change. Clin Biochem Rev 30(3):105–111

12. Jung K et al (2004) Comparison of 10 serum bone turnover markers in prostate carcinoma patients with bone metastatic spread: diagnostic and prognostic implications. Int J Cancer 111(5):783–791

13. Aydiner A (1994) Serum tumor markers for detection of bone metastasis in breast cancer patients. Acta Oncol 33(2):181–186

14. Mundy G (2002) Metastasis to bone: causes, consequences, and therapeutic opportunities. Cancer 2:584–593

15. McNeil BJ (1984) Value of bone scanning in neoplastic disease. Semin Nucl Med 14:277–286

16. Damle NA, Bal C, Bandopadhyaya GP, Kumar L, Kumar P, Malhotra A, Lata S (2013) The role of 18F-fluoride PET-CT in the detection of bone metastases in patients with breast, lung and prostate carcinoma: a comparison with FDG PET/CT and 99mTc-MDP bone scan. Jpn J Radiol 31(4):262–269

17. Rougraff BR, Kneisl JS, Simon MA (1993) Skeletal metastases of unknown origin. A prospective study of a diagnostic strategy. J Bone Joint Surg Am 75:1276–1281

18. Clayer M, Duncan W (2006) Importance of biopsy of new bone lesions in patients with previous carcinoma. Clin Orthop Rel Res 451:208–211

19. Cronin CG, Cashell T, Mhuircheartaigh JN, Swords R, Murray M, O'Sullivan GJ, O'Keeffe D (2009) AJR Am J Roentgenol 193(5):W407–W410

20. Ward WG, Kilpatrick S (2000) Fine-needle aspiration biopsy of primary bone tumors. Clin Orthop Relat Res 373:80–87

21. Yang YJ, Damron TA (2004) Comparison of needle core biopsy and fine-needle aspiration for diagnostic accuracy in musculoskeletal lesions. Arch Pathol Lab Med 128(7):759–764

22. Mankin HJ, Mankin CJ, Simon MA (1996) The hazards of the biopsy, revisited. For the members of the musculoskeletal tumor society. J Bone Joint Surg 78(5):656–663

23. Ward WG, Savage P, Boles C, Kilpatrick SE (2001) Fine-needle aspiration biopsy of sarcomas and related tumors. Cancer Control 8(3):232–238

24. Wong R, Wiffen PJ (2002) Bisphosphonates for the relief of pain secondary to bone metastases. Cochrane Database Syst Rev 2002(2):CD002068

25. Finley RS (2002) Bisphophonates in the treatment of bone meatastases. Sem Onc 29(1)(4):132–138

26. Walkington L, Coleman RE (2011) Advances in management of bone disease in breast cancer. Bone 48(1):80–87

27. Groot MT, Boeken Kruger CGG, Peiger RCM, Uyl-de Groot CA (2003) Costs of prostate cancer, metastatic to the bone in the Netherlands. Eur Urol 43(3):226–232

28. Jeremic B (2001) Single fraction external beam radiation therapy in the treatment of localized metastatic bone pain. a review. J Pain Symptom Manage 22(6):1048–1058

29. Callstrom MR, Dupuy DE, Solomon SB, Beres RA, Littrup PJ, Davis KW, Paz-Fumagalli R, Hoffman C, Atwell TD, Charboneau JW, Schmit GD, Goetz MP, Rubin J, Brown KJ, Novotny PJ, Sloan JA (2013) Percutaneous image-guided cryoablation of painful metastases involving bone: multicenter trial. Cancer 119(5):1033–1041

30. Toyota N, Naito A et al (2005) Radiofrequency ablation therapy combined with cementoplasty for painful bone metastases: initial experience. Cardiovasc Intervent Radiol 28(5):578–583
31. Fidler M (1973) Prophylactic internal fixation of secondary neoplastic deposits in long bones. BMJ 1(5849):341
32. Mirels H (1989) Metastatic disease in long bones a proposed scoring system for diagnosing impending pathologic fractures. Clin Orthop Relat Res 249:256–264
33. Robial N, Charles YP, Bogorin I, Godet J, Beaujeux R, Boujan F, Steib JP (2012) Is preoperative embolization a prerequisite for spinal metastases surgical management? Orthop Traumatol Surg Res 98(5):536–542
34. Fang T, Dong J, Zhou X, McGuire RA Jr, Li X (2012) Comparison of mini-open anterior corpectomy and posterior total en bloc spondylectomy for solitary metastases of the thoracolumbar spine. J Neurosurg Spine 17(4):271–279
35. Nilsson J, Gustafson P, Fornander P, Ornstein E (2000) The Harrington reconstruction for advanced periacetabular metastatic destruction: good outcome in 32 patients. Acta Orthopaedica 71(6):591–596
36. Vena VE, Hsu J, Rosier RN, O'Keefe RJ (1999) Pelvic reconstruction for severe periacetabular metastatic disease. Clin Orthop Relat Res 362:171–180
37. Walker RH (1993) Pelvic reconstruction/total hip arthroplasty for metastatic acetabular insufficiency. Clin Orthop Relat Res 294:170–175
38. Allan DG, Bell RS, Davis A, Langer F (1995) Complex acetabular reconstruction for metastatic tumor. J Arthroplasty 10(3):301–306
39. Wedin R, Bauer HCF (2005) Surgical treatment of skeletal metastatic lesions of the proximal femur Endoproththesis or reconstruction nail? J Bone Joint Surg Br 87(12):1653–1657
40. Ashford RU et al (2012) The modern surgical and non-surgical management of appendicular skeletal metastases. Orthop Trauma 26(3):184–199
41. Frassica FJ, Frassica DA (2003) Evaluation and treatment of metastases to the humerus. Clin Orthop Relat Res 415:S212–S218
42. Hill C et al (1981) Prophylactic cefazolin versus placebo in total hip replacement report of a multicentre double-blind randomised trial. Lancet 1(8224):795–796
43. Donati D, Biscaglia R (1998) The use of antibiotic-impregnated cement in infected reconstructions after resection for bone tumours. J Bone Joint Surg Br 80(6):1045–1050
44. Bickels J, Kollender Y, Wittig JC, Cohen N, Meller I, Malawer MM (2005) Vacuum-assisted wound closure after resection of musculoskeletal tumors. Clin Orthop Relat Res 441:346–350
45. Falanga A, Rickles FR (1999) Pathophysiology of the thrombophilic state in the cancer patient. In: Seminars in thrombosis and hemostasis, vol 25, issue 02. Thieme Medical Publishers Inc, New York, pp 173–182
46. Townsend PW, Rosenthal HG, Smalley SR, Cozad SC, Hassanein RE (1994) Impact of postoperative radiation therapy and other perioperative factors on outcome after orthopedic stabilization of impending or pathologic fractures due to metastatic disease. J Clin Oncol 12(11):2345–2350
47. Fuchs B, Trousdale RT, Rock MG (2005) Solitary bony metastasis from renal cell carcinoma: significance of surgical treatment. Clin Orthop Relat Res 431:187–192
48. Evenski A, Ramasunder S, Fox W, Mounasamy V, Temple HT (2012) Treatment and survival of osseous renal cell carcinoma metastases. J Surg Oncol 106(7):850–855

Clinical Evaluation and Management of Benign Soft Tissue Tumors of the Extremities

Andrew S. Erwteman and Tessa Balach

Abstract

Benign lesions comprise a majority of soft tissue tumors. It has been estimated that their incidence outnumbers that of malignant tumors by a factor of at least 100 [1]. While history and physical examination can start the diagnostic process, imaging including the use of magnetic resonance imaging can be more helpful. Biopsy of these tumors is sometimes necessary and can be performed in a number of ways, often in conjunction with definitive treatment. Specific diagnostic and treatment strategies for a number of the more commonly encountered benign soft tissue tumors including lipomas, pigmented villonodular synovitis and hemangiomas are reviewed. An algorithm for the management of benign soft tissue tumors is discussed.

Keywords

Soft tissue tumor · Benign tumor · Musculoskeletal tumors · Extremity

1 Introduction

Benign lesions make up a majority of soft tissue tumors. They include lesions of cutaneous tissue, subcutaneous adipose tissue, connective tissue, muscle, vascular or lymphatic tissue, and peripheral nerves. It has been estimated that their

A. S. Erwteman · T. Balach (✉)
Department of Orthopaedic Surgery, University of Connecticut Health Center,
263 Farmington Avenue, Farmington, CT, USA
e-mail: balach@uchc.edu

T. D. Peabody and S. Attar (eds.), *Orthopaedic Oncology*,
Cancer Treatment and Research 162, DOI: 10.1007/978-3-319-07323-1_9,
© Springer International Publishing Switzerland 2014

incidence outnumbers that of malignant tumors by a factor of at least 100 [1]. There are many different subtypes of soft tissue tumors with lipomatous tumors being most common. A number of the more prevalent subtypes are discussed in more detail below. This chapter will review a clinical strategy for the diagnosis and treatment of soft tissue tumors, with emphasis on those that are benign.

2 Evaluation

As with any other condition, evaluation of a soft tissue tumor should be thorough and start with a detailed history and physical examination. One should assess when the patient first learned about the lesion, whether it has changed in size, and whether it is symptomatic. There are some clues in a patient's history that may suggest a specific diagnosis. Patients with a soft tissue sarcoma will generally describe a painless enlarging mass. A history of sensitivity to touch or pressure, such as when a patient rolls onto the involved extremity in bed, or radiating pain upon contact with the tumor, may suggest a peripheral nerve sheath tumor. A lesion that first presents after trauma is suspicious for myositis ossificans, though one must keep in mind that the trauma may be circumstantial. Fractures of extremities in patients with a history of severe head injury often results in heterotopic ossification. Fluctuation in the size of the lesion can be seen in vascular lesions, inflammatory lesions, or in cases of lymphadenitis. Eliciting a history of constitutional symptoms such as unintentional weight loss, night sweats, or generalized malaise can be worrisome signs of malignancy or infection. Certain medical conditions are associated with soft tissue masses, making a thorough past medical history important. For example, hyperparathyroidism or renal failure may result in soft tissue calcinosis that can feel like a mass to the patient. Patients with neurofibromatosis often have multiple neurofibromas, which can be palpable or visible soft tissue masses.

On physical examination, in addition to standard inspection, neurovascular examination, and range of motion assessment of the limb, the physician must assess the specific characteristics of the mass. Specifically, it is important to describe the size of the lesion, its consistency, depth, mobility, the presence of tenderness, and the presence of radiating pain with percussion, known as a Tinel's sign. Palpable pulsatile flow suggests a vascular lesion. Proximal lymph nodes in the extremity should be examined for evidence of lymphadenopathy. Large firm lesions that are deep to fascia may represent sarcomas. It should be emphasized that many of the findings on history and physical examination are nonspecific and may not sufficiently narrow down the differential diagnosis. As such, radiologic imaging is a necessary next step in the evaluation process.

3   Imaging Studies

Several imaging modalities exist for the evaluation of soft tissue tumors ranging from radiographs or ultrasounds, that can sometimes be performed in the office, to more advanced imaging modalities such as computed tomography (CT), magnetic resonance imaging (MRI), and positron emission tomography (PET).

MRI is now the imaging modality of choice for the evaluation of most soft tissue lesions. However, radiographs are often obtained first at the time of the initial visit.

Radiographs can be helpful. They can reveal a soft tissue shadow, areas of calcification, and the effects on adjacent bone. In one series of 1,058 individuals with a known soft tissue tumor, 454 had plain radiographs. Of these, 281 (62 %) had positive radiographic findings. Thirty one percent demonstrated a soft tissue mass, and 64 % of radiographs with visible soft tissue masses represented malignant processes. An exception was found in the fingers and toes where lesions were more likely to be benign, most commonly giant cell tumors of tendon sheath, despite the fact that a soft tissue mass was visible [2]. Presence of soft-tissue calcification may be suggestive of specific diagnoses such as myositis ossificans when there is a peripheral distribution, while phleboliths are often found in hemangiomas. In the above-mentioned series, a lesion was more likely to be benign when calcification was present, as only 24 % of malignant tumors demonstrated calcification. Chondroid calcification, however, was more commonly found in sarcomatous lesions such as chondrosarcoma, liposarcoma, epithelioid sarcoma, and synovial sarcoma. Chondroid calcification has a ring and arc pattern due to calcification forming around lobules of cartilage. Sometimes punctate or stippled calcification can also be present in an area of chondroid calcification. Cortical erosion is a nonspecific finding, as this can be seen with both benign lesions, such as PVNS, and with sarcomas. One may also be able to detect intramedullary extension, and periosteal reaction [2].

MRI is essential in the workup of soft tissue lesions. It allows the physician to assess size, shape, depth, relationship to adjacent anatomic structures, and evaluate for the presence of necrosis. Signal characteristics of soft tissue tumors can sometimes point toward specific histologic diagnoses as well. Lesions should be imaged in at least two orthogonal planes. T1-weighted and T2-weighted spin-echo pulse sequences should be obtained. Additional imaging sequences can be obtained as deemed necessary by the radiologist, such as gradient-echo, and Short Tau Inversion Recovery (STIR) imaging. Fat suppression is useful to increase lesion-to-background signal intensity differences for lesions within the marrow or fatty soft tissues. The use of contrast can enhance the signal intensity of many tumors on T1-weighted images, sharpening the demarcation between tumor, surrounding tissues, and edema when present. Contrast also allows for assessment of vascularity within and surrounding the tumor. It is especially useful for visualizing a focus of tumor within an area of hematoma. The tumor, in this case, may not be apparent on T2-weighted imaging, as the entire hematoma will have increased signal intensity. It may also be useful for guiding biopsy by characterizing areas of necrosis within the tumor or revealing cystic regions. While contrast enhancement does provide some additional information, it also increases the cost of the exam and carries the risk of allergic reaction, although that risk is fairly low. Despite the great detail provided by MRI, most lesions have a nonspecific appearance (i.e., low signal intensity on T1, high intensity on T2, and enhancement with the administration of contrast) and the correct histologic diagnosis is reached only 25–35 % of the time based on MR imaging studies alone [3]. In many cases, MRI is limited in its ability to differentiate between benign and malignant lesions. Benign lesions are thought to have smooth well-defined margins, be of a small size, and have a homogenous signal intensity. However, malignant lesions can sometimes take on these characteristics [3]. Based on a multivariate statistical analysis of 10 imaging parameters, De Schepper et al. were able to suggest some loose guidelines. Malignancy was predicted with the highest sensitivity when a lesion had high signal intensity on T2-weighted MR images, was larger than 33 mm in diameter, and had heterogeneous signal intensity on T1-weighted MR images. Signs that had the greatest specificity for malignancy included tumor necrosis, bone or neuro-vascular involvement, and mean diameter of more than 66 mm [4]. Razek et al. looked at diffusion echo-planar MR imaging and assessed its ability to differentiate between benign and malignant lesions. They found that there was a significant difference between the apparent diffusion coefficients (ADC) of malignant compared to benign lesions with a small number of lesions exhibiting crossover. Selection of a threshold ADC value for differentiating malignant soft tissue tumors from benign masses resulted in an accuracy of 91 %, sensitivity of 94 %, and a specificity of 88 %. They acknowledged the small number of subjects within their study and recognized the need for larger studies [5]. A study that evaluated the ability of diffusion-weighted MR imaging to differentiate between benign and malignant breast lesions found a linear inverse correlation between ADC and tumor cellularity that allowed the authors to differentiate between these lesions [6].

Ultrasound is a relatively inexpensive modality with very low risk for morbidity. It can accurately distinguish between cystic and solid tumors, and color Doppler can be used to identify a vascular lesion. Ultrasound can be used for lesion localization, but it is unable to characterize the mass with the same level of detail as MRI. Additionally, some lesions are too deep for reliable examination by ultrasound such as in the pelvis or thigh. Lakkaraju et al. have suggested that ultrasound may have utility as an initial triage modality for primary care physicians before referring to a specialist [7]. In their study of 358 consecutive patients with soft tissue masses, ultrasound was used as the initial imaging modality and divided lesions into 8 groups based on characteristics ranging from normal (group 1) to possible sarcoma (group 8). A group 8 lesion was found to be solid and heterogeneous, with distortion of surrounding anatomy, and disorganized power Doppler flow. Tumors with a high likelihood of being benign (groups 1–5) were sent back to the referring provider for observation. Indeterminate masses or possible sarcomas (groups 6–8) were referred for MRI within 14 days. All of the lesions that were initially diagnosed as benign on US, remained benign at final diagnosis, and a total of 1.68 % of the original cohort, were diagnosed with sarcoma [7].

CT has been replaced by MRI in most institutions due to the superior soft tissue contrast achieved by MRI. It is therefore easier to detect soft tissue masses and delineate their extent [8]. CT, however, can still be useful for imaging soft tissues near the chest wall that are subject to motion artifact with MRI, and in cases where MRI is not an option, such as in those patients with certain pacemaker models, deep brain stimulators, metal or bullet fragments in the brain, or adjacent to other vital organs, cochlear implants, certain types of cerebral aneurysm clips, and some drug infusion devices.

PET is an imaging modality that uses a radioactive substance called a tracer to assess for disease. Unlike other imaging modalities that assess anatomy, PET is used to assess metabolic function and can be used to diagnose, stage, and monitor treatment response for many cancers, and some soft tissue tumors. It may be less desirable in many circumstances due to its great expense, as well as the requirement for an injection of a radioactive substance into the patient. One specific application is in the evaluation of multifocal desmoid tumors, and more specifically, response to treatment. Kasper et al. demonstrated that PET imaging might complement CT and improve the assessment of patients with desmoid tumors. Imatinib, a tyrosine kinase inhibitor, has been shown to successfully stabilize desmoid tumors, and PET imaging has been used to monitor response to imatinib treatment in patients with multifocal desmoids [9].

4   Tissue Diagnosis

Obtaining a tissue diagnosis is the next step in the evaluation of any soft tissue tumor that cannot be reliably diagnosed as a benign lesion by history, physical, and imaging studies. One should always approach tissue biopsy with the assumption that there is a possibility for malignancy, using a well-planned biopsy site. Biopsy can be performed by a surgeon or with imaging guidance by a radiologist for deeper lesions, those adjacent to major neurovascular structures, and for those that are not easily palpable. A biopsy is either performed in an open or closed manner. A closed biopsy can be a fine needle aspiration (FNA), or a core biopsy.

An open biopsy is performed through an incision, often by the surgeon in the operating room, and can be incisional or excisional. Biopsy incisions should be longitudinal and they should be as small as possible to minimize the size of the contaminated biopsy tract. Another important principle of open biopsy is meticulous hemostasis. Careful coagulation of bleeding vessels is important for prevention of a hematoma, which can spread remaining tumor cells throughout the wound bed and surrounding tissues. An incisional biopsy can be used when the tumor is fairly large and there is a possibility of having to do more than local surgical resection. A tissue sample can be sent to pathology for an immediate frozen section. Often times, if the frozen section confirms suspicion for a benign lesion, the remaining tumor can be excised. If the frozen section reveals malignant appearing cells, a wide resection and additional therapy may be necessary. In these cases, the incision should be closed, meticulous hemostasis achieved, and the surgeon should plan to return to the operating room at another time. Depending on the diagnosis, neoadjuvant treatment may be warranted (e.g., chemotherapy or radiation therapy). An excisional biopsy, which removes the entire mass, is appropriate for most small lesions [10, 11].

A closed biopsy is performed percutaneously using a small-bore needle for fine needle aspiration, or a large-bore needle for core biopsy. There is always a tradeoff between obtaining a sufficient amount of tissue for diagnosis and minimizing morbidity. Insufficient samples of tissue can lead to inaccurate pathologic diagnosis. A fine needle aspiration is useful for superficial lesions and provides the pathologist with a limited number of cells, but this is often sufficient to distinguish benign from malignant cells. Sarcomas can also be distinguished from carcinomas, and it is a good option when assessing for local recurrence. The main limitation is the inability to assess the surrounding cellular architecture since it is not maintained with FNA. For an accurate assessment of cellular architecture, one must obtain a core biopsy or an open biopsy specimen. FNA is also less ideal when a large number of stains or cytogenetic analyses must be performed, as there may not be enough tissue [12]. A review of 426 patients with soft tissue tumors who underwent core biopsy yielded 97.6 % accuracy for differentiating soft tissue sarcomas from benign tumors. High grade sarcomas were differentiated from low grade with an accuracy of 86.3 %. Subtype was accurately assigned in 89.5 % of benign tumors and 88 % of sarcomas [13]. Another prospective study of 57 patients with palpable extremity soft tissue masses compared FNA to core needle biopsy. With regard to determining malignancy, FNA and core biopsy had 79.17 and 79.2 % sensitivity, and 72.7 and 81.8 % specificity. Overall accuracy was 75.4 and 80.7 %, respectively [14].

Before deciding to perform a closed biopsy, the physician must ensure that the following criteria are met: (1) the mass should be easily palpable to avoid missing it with the needle, (2) the area of the mass believed to have the most diagnostic tissue is easily identified (i.e., nonfluid portions of a heterogeneous tumor), and (3) the mass should be far enough away from critical neurovascular structures such that risk of injury is minimal. If these criteria are not met, and a closed biopsy is still desired, an image-guided biopsy may be more appropriate. It is important that the treating physician communicate with the radiologist, however, to assist in planning an appropriate biopsy site and needle path. This is determined by the planned surgical approach for excision, if necessary. The path of the needle should avoid contamination of additional compartments, joint-spaces, or neurovascular structures as much as possible, as it is standard to remove the biopsy tract along with the tumor if the final diagnosis is a sarcoma [15–17]. It is important to keep in mind that the consequences of a poorly planned biopsy can alter surgical plans, increase local recurrence rates, and increase morbidity if the mass is found to be malignant [10, 11].

5   Treatment

Once a benign soft tissue lesion is diagnosed, or when there is no suspicion for malignancy, one must discuss treatment options with the patient. Observation is usually an option, but this depends on the natural history of the tumor, its location, presence of symptoms, and risk for malignant transformation. Some soft tissue tumors are aggressive and more likely to show local progression. Asymptomatic, small subcutaneous lesions that are easily palpable can often be observed safely, especially those that are smaller than 5 cm and superficial to fascia, as these lesions are more likely to be benign. Re-evaluation is recommended 6–12 weeks after the initial evaluation, followed by every 3–6 months for approximately 1 year to document lack of growth. Any changes in the mass that are not aligned with its known natural history should prompt additional imaging or possibly biopsy [12].

Surgical excision is always an option as well. For lesions that are smaller than 5 cm, excisional biopsy in the form of marginal excision can be performed with little morbidity. This type of excision is used for benign tumors, as the surgeon tries to avoid damage or excessive resection of the surrounding normal tissues, if possible.

For tumors with concerning features such as those that are larger than 5 cm, deep to fascia, or significantly symptomatic, a tissue diagnosis must be obtained prior to definitive treatment. For malignant tumors, wide excision is the treatment of choice. The goal of wide excision is to remove the tumor en-bloc, ideally, with a cuff of normal tissue surrounding it. This is important for sarcomas where local recurrence rates are high. In some cases, a vital neurovascular structure prevents an adequate cuff of normal tissue [12]. After sarcoma resection, the patient should be followed closely to assess for local and systemic disease. The American College of Radiology recommends repeat MRI of the tumor region at 3–6 month intervals for the first 5 years, followed by annual MRI for at least the next 5 years. Periodic chest CT is recommended as well to evaluate for metastatic disease [18].

Nonsurgical treatment modalities are also available for certain soft tissue lesions and include embolization, sclerotherapy, radiation therapy, and medications. More specific detail about each of these treatment options can be found below in the sections specific to each individual tumor.

---

6   Benign Soft Tissue Lesions

6.1   Lipoma

Lipomas are comprised of fat and are the most common soft tissue lesions, and often occur in the 5th to 7th decades of life without a clear gender predilection [19]. In one large series of 1,331 soft tissue tumors, lipoma was found to account for almost 50 % of the lesions [20]. The prevalence of soft-tissue lipomas has been estimated at 2.1 per 100 people and they are much more frequent than liposarcomas [19]. Only 1 % of superficial lesions are larger than 10 cm in size. Deep lipomas are often larger and more rare and are intramuscular in many cases [1].

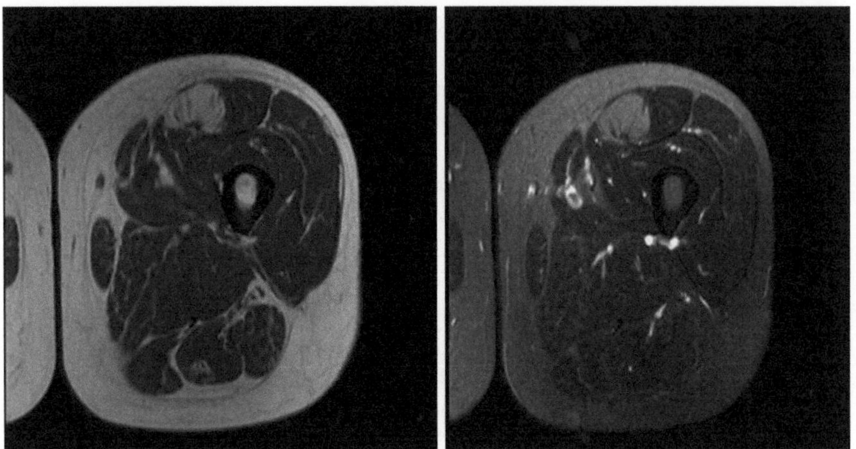

Fig. 1 Intramuscular lipoma of the thigh. Axial MRI images, T1-weighted (*Left*), and T2-Weighted (*Right*)

Superficial, subcutaneous lipomas are the most commonly encountered form. They are frequently found in the upper back, neck, proximal extremities, and abdomen. On physical examination, lipomas are mobile, and have a doughy consistency. They are often solitary, but patients may present with multiple. Lipomas, regardless of their location, are usually asymptomatic, but they can be associated with local pain, limitation of range of motion, and nerve compression in approximately 25 % of patients [19]. Lopez et al. described a case of a lipoma in the region of the greater sciatic notch, which was found to be the cause of severe sciatic nerve compression [21].

The best radiological studies for the diagnosis of a lipoma are CT and MRI. They appear as a homogenous mass with a very similar Hounsfield unit value to subcutaneous fat on CT, and a signal that is isointense to the subcutaneous fat on all MRI pulse sequences. Occasionally, a few thin-walled septae can also be visualized. Well-differentiated liposarcomas are sometimes difficult to distinguish from benign lipomas, but they are generally more heterogeneous lesions and have thicker septae [19] Fig. 1.

A soft tissue lipoma may represent a benign neoplasm, a local hyperplasia of fat cells, or a combination of the above [19]. Grossly, lipomas have a yellow to orange color with a greasy appearance. They are often well circumscribed with a thin capsule separating the mass from the surrounding tissue. Histologically, cells resemble mature adipocytes with uniform eccentric nuclei Fig. 2.

Treatment options for both superficial and deep lipomas include observation or excisional biopsy if they are increasing in size, become symptomatic, or are cosmetically undesirable. If an atypical lipoma or low-grade liposarcoma is a possibility, marginal excision should be performed, as a needle or incisional biopsy alone can yield false negative results [19].

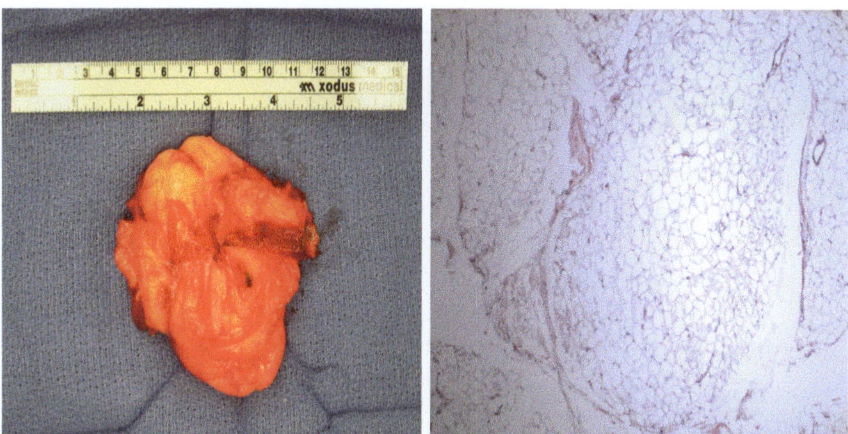

Fig. 2 Intramuscular lipoma, gross specimen (*Left*), and histology (*Right*)

Recurrence rates are estimated at 4–5 % for deep lipomas, as it is sometimes difficult to remove all of the tissue. Fortunately they have no metastatic potential, and malignant transformation is exceedingly rare. In fact, it has only been described in case reports dating back to 1948, and the authors described a focus of liposarcoma within what they believed was a lipoma. It is more likely that these lesions were never really benign lipomas [19, 20, 22].

6.2 Benign Peripheral Nerve Sheath Tumors

Benign peripheral nerve sheath tumors include both schwannomas (neurilemmomas) and neurofibromas. Schwannomas arise from the Schwann cells of the nerve sheath and are encapsulated tumors found within the substance of peripheral nerves. They make up about 5 % of all benign soft tissue tumors [23]. There does not seem to be a gender predilection, and they are most commonly found between the ages of 20 and 50 years. An association has been found with type 2 neurofibromatosis where multiple schwannomas can be present, but in other patients, they are typically solitary lesions that displace the nerve eccentrically within its epineurium.

Neurofibromas are unencapsulated tumors and they often infiltrate the surrounding tissues. They are slightly more common than schwannomas. Ninety percent are solitary and most are not associated with type 1 neurofibromatosis. Neurofibromas are slow growing and most frequently present between the ages of 40–50 years.

On physical examination, these tumors may be palpable, and they are usually firm and somewhat mobile. Schwannomas are often tender to touch and pressure, whereas neurofibromas typically present as a painless mass. Neurologic symptoms are more common when large nerves are involved.

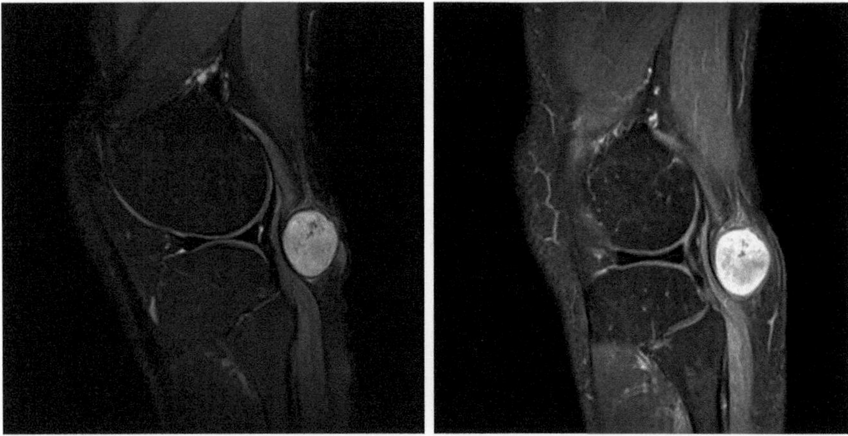

Fig. 3 Peripheral nerve sheath tumor of posterior knee. Sagittal MRI images, T2 without contrast (*Left*), and with contrast (*Right*)

Radiographs may demonstrate a soft tissue shadow, and when large, there may be subtle areas of calcification. Schwannomas and neurofibromas typically appear as a fusiform mass, often displacing the associated neurovascular bundle on MRI. Sometimes the nerve can be visualized as a tubular structure entering, or exiting the mass, giving rise to an image that resembles a tail coming off of the tumor (the tail sign). A large tumor can also displace surrounding intramuscular fat creating the appearance of a thin margin of fat surrounding the tumor known as the split-fat sign. One subtle difference between neurofibromas and schwannomas is that the nerve is eccentric to the tumor in schwannomas, and is centrally located or obliterated by the mass in neurofibromas. Schwannomas typically demonstrate intermediate to moderately high T1-weighted signal and heterogeneously high signal on T2-weighted sequences. Neurofibromas may demonstrate a "target sign," which is an area of low signal intensity centrally and higher signal intensity peripherally on T2-weighted sequences and correlates with the fibrosis and dense collagen found at the center of the neurofibroma, and the more myxoid tissue found peripherally [24]. Jee et al. looked at MRI characteristics of 52 patients with known peripheral nerve sheath tumors. They found that the target sign was more common in neurofibromas, but was still found, on occasion, in schwannomas (58 % of neurofibromas vs. 15 % of schwannomas). Central enhancement with contrast was found in 75 % of neurofibromas and in only 8 % of schwannomas. A combination of these two findings was found in 63 % of neurofibromas compared to only 3 % of schwannomas [25] Fig. 3.

On pathologic analysis, the cut surface of a schwannoma has a yellow-gray color, sometimes with cystic regions. The overlying capsule consists of epineurium, usually with overlying tortuous vessels. Histologically, the schwannoma is

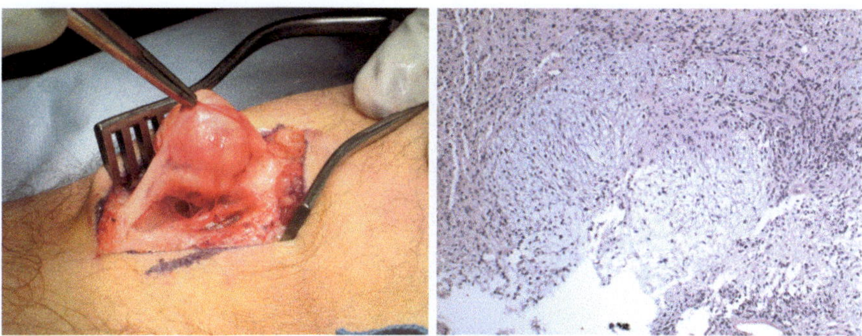

Fig. 4 Peripheral nerve sheath tumor, introperative image of nerve sheath tumor within a peripheral nerve (*Left*), and histology (*Right*)

encapsulated and two tissue types predominate, referred to as Antoni A and Antoni B regions of tissue. Antoni A tissue is cellular and there are areas of nuclear palisading known as as Verocay bodies. Antoni B regions of tissue are myxoid and less cellular [26] Fig. 4.

Neurofibromas are well defined and they are not encapsulated. Histologically, they are made up of spindle-shaped cells in a myxoid stroma, with some collagen fibers. In most cases they can be differentiated from schwannomas by histology, but immunocytochemistry with antibodies to neurofilaments can be helpful if the diagnosis is unclear. Immunostaining for S-100 protein is usually positive in the spindle cells of schwannomas, but negative or only weakly positive in most neurofibromas [26, 27].

Treatment consists of surgical excision or observation with serial MRI scans or ultrasound to provide accurate measurement of the tumor. Schwannomas are thought to be easily enucleated, or "shelled out" of the epineurium, leaving the remaining nerve intact. This is not always the case, however, and neurological deficit may result. This is likely secondary to iatrogenic fascicular injury during the attempted dissection of the tumor, especially in cases where some fascicles are found to be running through the substance of the tumor. Kim et al. evaluated postoperative neurological deficits and potential risk factors associated with this complication. They found an immediate neurological deficit in 76.7 % of their 30 patients, and at final followup, residual deficits persisted in 36.7 % of patients. The risk for deficits was highest in patients with larger tumors. There are other reports that have come to the same conclusions and have hypothesized that there may be a larger number of fascicles running through the substance of the tumor in larger lesions [28, 29]. When neurofibromas are excised, the nerve is sacrificed and neurological deficits may remain especially when larger nerves are involved.

In a series by Lee et al. 78 schwannomas were excised, either via marginal excision, or wide excision. They had no recurrences, and no malignant transformation at 47 months of followup. Seven patients had residual paresthesias [30].

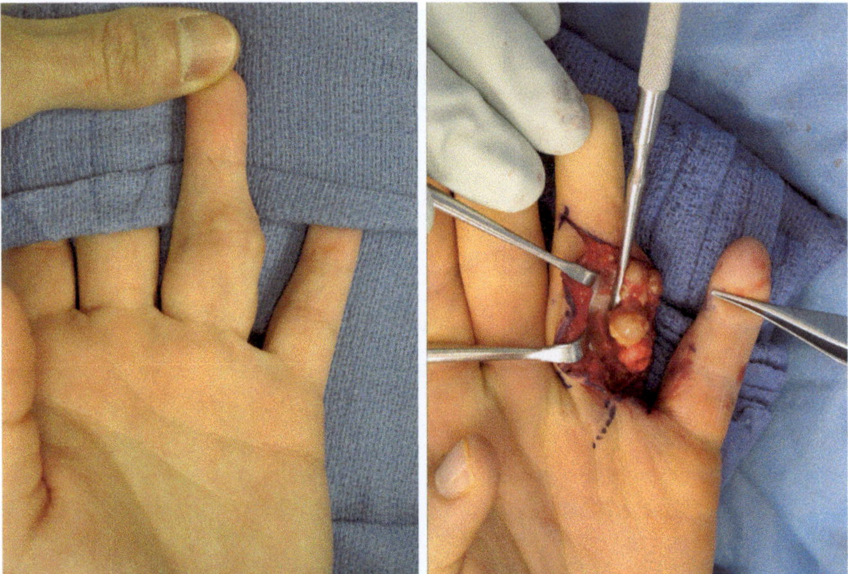

Fig. 5 Giant cell tumor of tendon sheath involving the long finger

6.3　　Giant Cell Tumor of Tendon Sheath

Giant cell tumor of tendon sheath is the most common benign neoplasm of the hand, often found on the fingers [31]. Less commonly, it can be found in the knee, ankle, or foot. It presents more often in women and usually in the fourth to fifth decade of life [31, 32]. On physical examination, this tumor is usually found to be a firm, minimally mobile mass that runs along tendons, and it is usually nontender.

Radiographs are often nonspecific, but cortical erosion of adjacent bone can be seen. Ultrasound can be used to distinguish this solid tumor from a ganglion cyst which will be visualized as a fluid-filled cyst [33]. MRI shows a circumscribed soft tissue mass with occasional degenerative changes. The mass is usually adjacent to a tendon, and is isointense with muscle on T1-weighted images. On T2-weighted images, it can be heterogeneous and either isointense or hypointense to fat. Intense contrast enhancement is commonly seen [24].

On gross examination, the lesion has a dense capsule and, when sectioned, it has a gray-white appearance with variegated pink, brown, or yellow discoloration. Histologically, the predominant cells are mononuclear cells, epithelioid histiocyte-like cells, giant cells, and xanthomatous cells. Another key feature is the presence of hemosiderin-laden macrophages Figs. 5 and 6.

The treatment of choice is excisional biopsy with the goal of excising the entire lesion, though the recurrence rate is as high as 10–20 % [31]. Radiation can be considered in older patients with diffuse or unresectable disease.

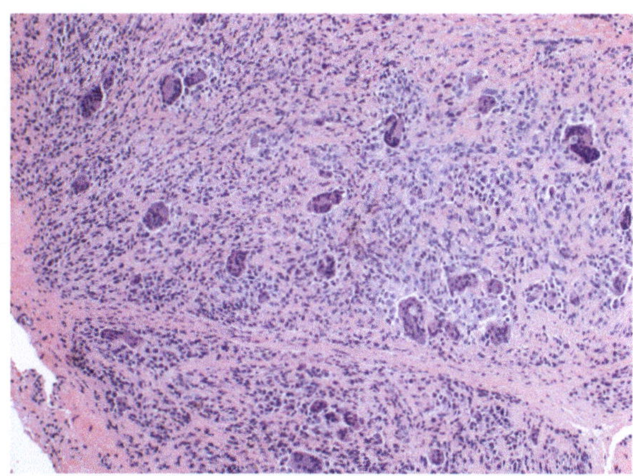

Fig. 6 Giant cell tumor of tendon sheath, histology

6.4 Pigmented Villonodular Synovitis

Pigmented villonodular synovitis (PVNS) is a slowly progressive, benign synovial process that can be either localized to a small area within a joint or diffuse and involve the entire synovium. It is most commonly a monoarticular lesion. Patients usually present in their third or fourth decade, and there is a female predominance. Eighty percent of these lesions occur in the knee, though they can be found in other large joints such as the hip, ankle, shoulder, and elbow [24].

These lesions are often symptomatic and patients present with pain, swelling, and limited range of motion. PVNS can sometimes present with reproducible intra-articular mechanical symptoms.

Radiographs are often normal or can demonstrate a noncalcified soft tissue mass. Radiologic calcification within the mass is extremely unusual and should suggest an alternative diagnosis, such as a calcified loose body or synovial chondromatosis. Well-defined cortical erosions with thin sclerotic borders can be present in up to 50 % of cases. This finding is more common in the hip due to its tight capsule [34]. MRI is the imaging modality of choice for the diagnosis of PVNS where it presents as a disseminated heterogeneous synovial-based process in the diffuse form of the disease and as a well-defined solitary mass in the nodular form. The tumors are typically isointense to hypointense relative to skeletal muscle on both T1- and T2-weighted images. There is frequently enhancement with the administration of contrast. Gradient-echo imaging may display the "blooming" artifact effect because of the paramagnetic effect of hemosiderin in the soft tissues [24] Fig. 7.

PVNS has a very similar pathologic appearance to giant cell tumor of tendon sheath. The synovium often has a nodular texture, and the cut surface has a red-brown or yellow-brown color. The microscopic appearance of the tumor has been described as fingerlike projections of fibrous stroma covered by hyperplastic synovial cells. The yellow color has been attributed to stromal foamy macro-phages. Hemosiderin pigment deposited within this neoplasm is responsible for the

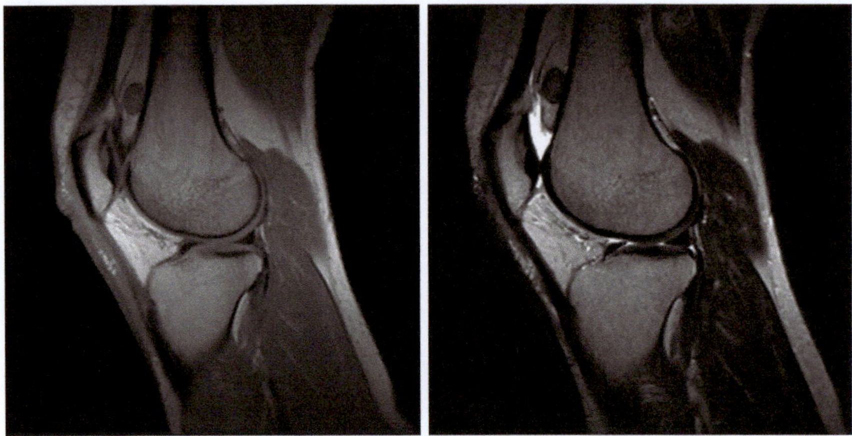

Fig. 7 Pigmented villonodular synovitis. Sagittal MRI images, T1-weighted (*Left*), and T2-weighted (*Right*). Tumor is visualized in the suprapatellar pouch

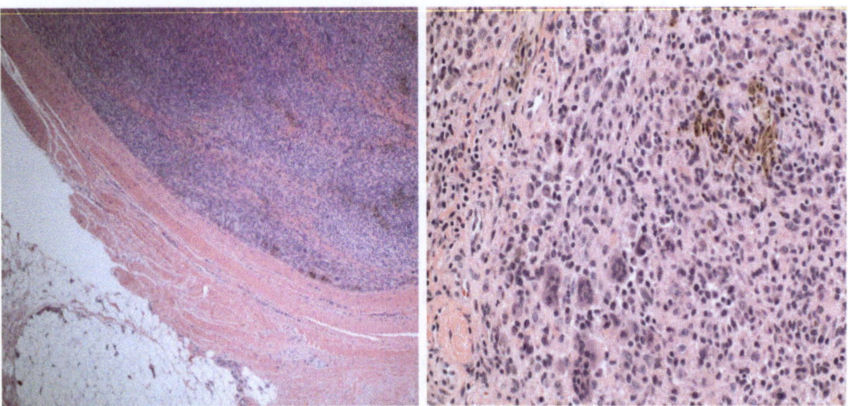

Fig. 8 Pigmented villonodular synovitis, histology. Low power (*Left*), and high power (*Right*) magnification

red-brown color of the lesion. "Rice bodies" can be found in the joint-space and are composed of rounded masses of fibrin that are eventually converted to fibrous tissue with in-growth of capillaries and fibroblasts. The degree of fibrosis increases over time [34] Fig. 8.

Due to its progressive nature and the potential for erosion of the affected joint's articular cartilage, surgical intervention is the standard of care in the form of a synovectomy. This can be done arthroscopically or open, though arthroscopic treatment is contraindicated when the lesion is not accessible such as a lesion that extends beyond the joint, a lesion located within a cyst, or difficult to reach intra-articular regions such as posterior to the PCL [35]. A benefit of arthroscopic synovectomy is reduced postoperative stiffness, which is a good option especially for localized PVNS where a more complete excision can be performed and recurrence rates may be lower. External beam radiation and intra-articular radiation therapy has been used in some cases, but there is no clear benefit over surgical intervention, and there is no benefit of adding radiation as an adjuvant treatment for a primary excision. One must also understand that there are potentially serious complications associated with radiation therapy including skin reactions, joint stiffness, and the risk of sarcomatous transformation. There may be some benefit in using radiation for treating refractory cases and in those with significant extra-articular involvement [36]. The prognosis is good for the localized form, but recurrence rates are high for the diffuse form and have been reported at about 50 % [24, 34].

6.5   Desmoid Tumor (Fibromatosis)

Desmoid tumors are benign fibroblastic neoplasms that can display varying degrees of local aggressiveness. They do not metastasize, but local infiltration of structures can cause significant morbidity or even mortality. They are relatively rare and account for <3 % of all soft tissue tumors that are biopsied. They are often diagnosed in young adults, but can be found between the ages of 15 and 60 years. There is a female predominance and they are especially common in patients with familial adenomatous polyposis (FAP) with an incidence up to 32 % in those with Gardner syndrome, a variant of FAP [37]. Some other proposed risk factors include trauma, surgery, and increased estrogen levels. The most common locations for these tumors are the shoulder, chest wall, back, and thighs.

On physical examination desmoids are firm deep or subcutaneous masses that are minimally mobile and very adherent to surrounding tissues. They are often poorly circumscribed and can be painful. When in close proximity to a joint, range of motion may be limited. Neurological symptoms can be seen if the tumor compresses or invades peripheral motor or sensory nerves.

Radiographs can reveal a soft-tissue shadow to suggest a mass and cortical erosion may be evident. On CT, desmoid tumors have similar attenuation to muscle. MRI is the imaging study of choice where the lesion can be better characterized. Overall, desmoids often have low signal intensity on both T1 and T2 sequences due to the high collagen content of these fibrous lesions, but they frequently enhance after contrast administration Fig. 9.

On gross inspection, desmoid tumors vary in size, they are firm, and they typically infiltrate adjacent tissues. Sectioning of the tumor reveals a glistening, white surface. There may be a capsule, but tumor cells are often found throughout the tissues beyond the macroscopic borders and this is likely the reason for the high incidence of local recurrence. Histologically, they are composed of normal appearing, but relatively sparse fibroblastic cells within a dense fibrous stroma. Macrophages, lymphocytes, and giant cells are often present, as well [37] Fig. 10.

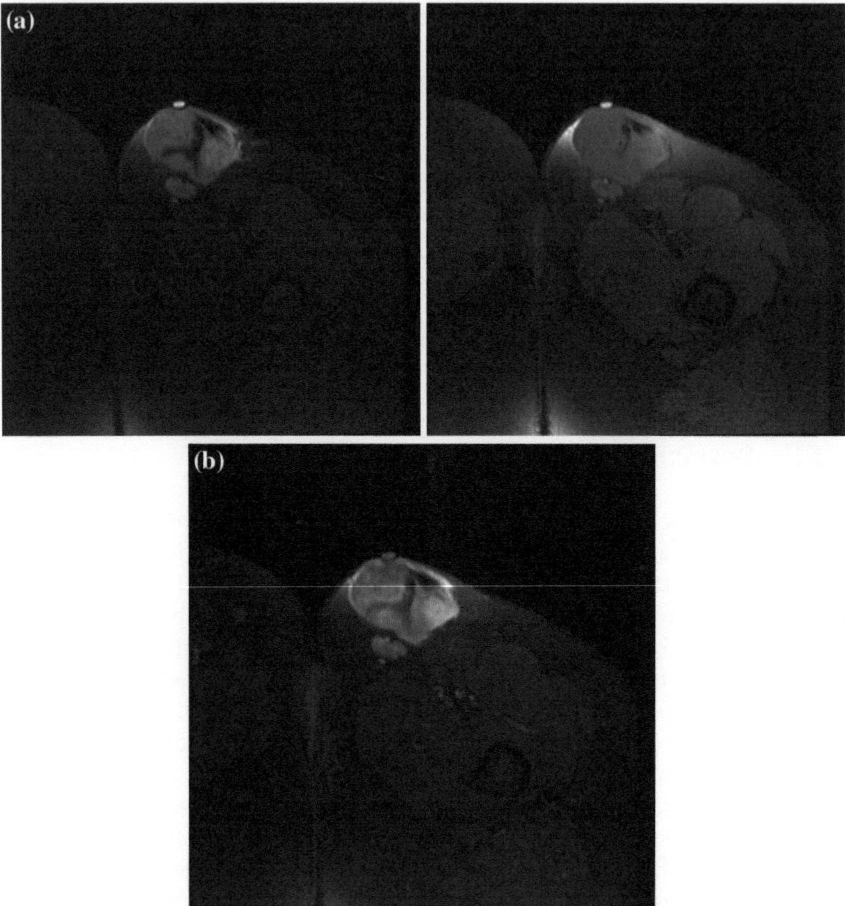

Fig. 9 Desmoid tumor of anterior thigh. Axial MRI images, **a** T1-weighted (*Left*), and T2-weighted (*Right*), **b** contrast-enhanced

Treatment of these tumors should involve a multidisciplinary approach utilizing nonsurgical treatment such as observation, chemotherapy, and radiation therapy, as well as surgical treatment. Observation is reasonable for stable, asymptomatic lesions. More aggressive treatment is warranted for symptomatic or progressive lesions. One must keep in mind the morbidity associated with wide resection of these benign tumors, which has classically been the first line treatment. Due to the high recurrence rate with surgery, adjuvant treatment with radiation has been a commonly used regimen. Five-year disease free survival rates with surgery alone is variable in the literature and has been reported to range from 41 to 75 % in several published series [37]. Recurrence rates were lower when surgery was combined with radiation therapy, and in some series, radiation therapy alone was as successful as surgery with

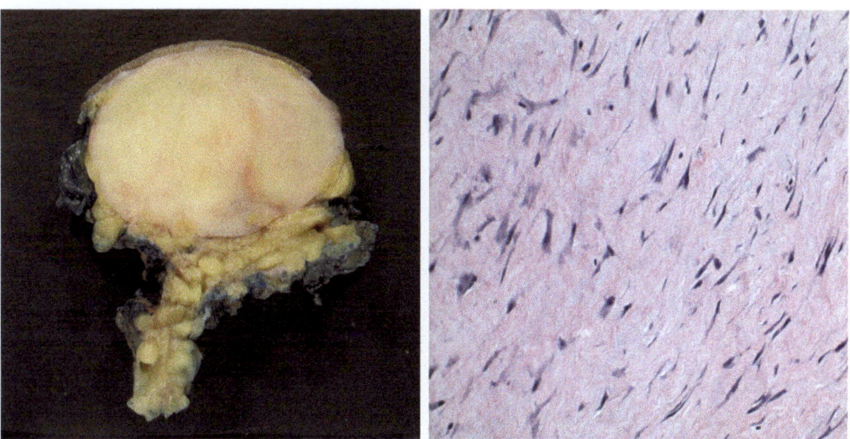

Fig. 10 Desmoid tumor, gross specimen (*Left*), and histology (*Right*)

radiation [38–40]. Optimal radiation dosage is between 50 and 60 Gy based on a study that showed no difference in outcomes when comparing one group who received 50–60 Gy with another group who received >60 Gy. Further, radiation doses >60 Gy were associated with increased morbidity including physeal arrest, soft tissue fibrosis, edema, skin ulceration, cellulitis, neurologic changes, pathologic fracture, and secondary sarcoma [41–43]. Several low-dose chemotherapy regimens have been used for the medical treatment of desmoids with the advantage of having significantly fewer side effects compared to surgery and radiation. One indication is for large lesions where surgical resection will impart significant morbidity. At a mean of 10 years, a noncytotoxic regimen of combination chemotherapy has resulted in an approximately 70 % relapse-free interval [44]. Based on recent studies, Hosalkar et al. have recommended 16 weeks of low-dose chemotherapy [37]. If this fails, another medical regimen can be initiated and can be continued for a period of 3 months beyond maximum regression. These low-dose chemotherapy regimens have consisted of methotrexate, and often, another drug such as vinblastine, or vinorelbine. Doxorubicin-based treatment regimens have been used, but are less common today due to potential side effects which include cardiomyopathy and heart failure [37]. Mace et al. reported on a small series of treatment refractory patients. They demonstrated that desmoids express both PDGF-R and c-kit on their cell surface, both of which are tyrosine kinases receptors. Tyrosine kinases are involved in downstream cell signal transduction that may lead to cell growth. They had some success with imatinib mesylate, a tyrosine kinase inhibitor [45]. A larger series by Chugh et al. consisted of 51 patients in whom surgical treatment was not a good option and they were treated with two different doses of imatinib. Kaplan-Meier estimates of 2- and 4-month progression-free survival rates were 94 and 88 %, respectively, and 1-year progression-free survival was 66 % [46]. Nonsteroidal antiinflammatories have also been used as part of the treatment regimen for desmoid tumors. The proposed mechanism of action is via inhibition of

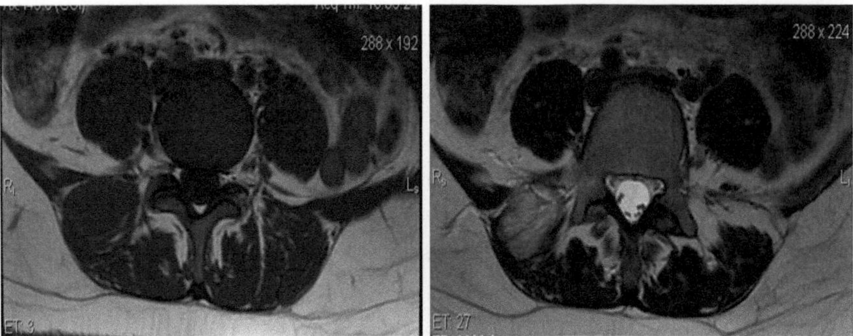

Fig. 11 Hemangioma involving Right paraspinal muscles. Axial MRI images, T1-weighted (*Left*), and T2-weighted (*Right*)

cyclooxygenase-2, an enzyme that has been shown to be expressed by desmoid tumors, and ultimately causes a decrease in cyclic AMP levels with a reduction of proliferative cell signals. It likely alters other cell cycle regulatory proteins such as cyclin D1, as well [47]. Tsukada et al. treated 14 patients with sulindac for intra-abdominal desmoid tumors [48]. One patient experienced a complete response and seven patients experienced a partial response with reduction of tumor size.

6.6   Hemangioma

Hemangiomas are benign vascular lesions that histologically resemble normal blood vessels. They are one of the more common soft tissue tumors, especially in the first few decades of life, accounting for 7 % of benign soft tissue tumors [49]. There seems to be a predilection for females with a ratio of approximately 1.5–1 [50]. The lesion can be classified according to the predominant type of vessel observed. The main subtypes include capillary, cavernous, venous, and arteriovenous.

Patients often present with a mass that can fluctuate in size, and may be painful at rest or with activity. Like other soft tissue tumors, hemangiomas can be superficial, or deep, where they are often intramuscular.

Radiographs may show a soft tissue mass, and up to 90 % of deep hemangiomas contain phleboliths, which are small calcifications visible on imaging. On MRI, hemangiomas appear as masses that are hypointense, or isointense to muscle on T1-weighted sequences, and hyperintense on T2-weighted sequences due to the vascular channels. There is marked enhancement often in a serpentine pattern with the administration of contrast. They are typically well-marginated, heterogeneous masses. Lobulations and septations within these lesions help discriminate them from the round appearance of sarcomas [24]. Ultrasound is useful in characterizing the density of vessels in the lesion. Doppler flow characteristics can differentiate high-flow lesions that contain arterial structures, from low-flow lesions that do not contain arterial structures [51] Fig. 11.

Fig. 12 Hemangioma, histology

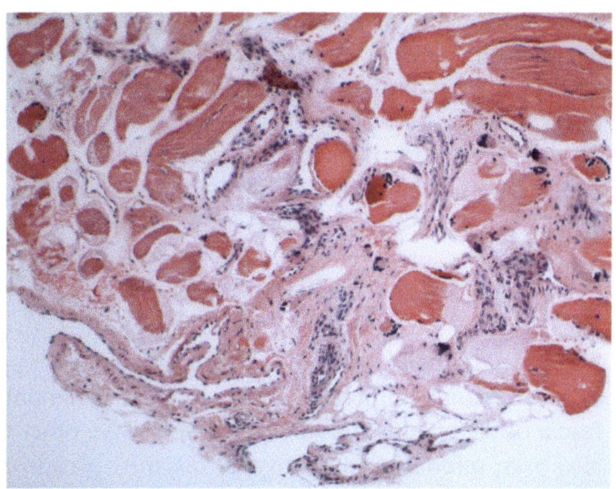

The hemangioma subtype can be specified at the time of histologic examination based on the type of vessels present. Capillary hemangiomas are composed of small mature vessels. These vessels can become massively dilated and are then referred to as cavernous hemangiomas. An arteriovenous hemangioma has the presence of arterial or arteriolar structures, as well as venous structures [50] Fig. 12.

These lesions can be observed, especially the infantile capillary hemangioma subtype, which often regresses by the age of 7. Symptomatic hemangiomas can be treated and there are a number of options including sclerotherapy, embolization, and surgical excision. Complete excision can be challenging due to the vascularity, and the infiltrative nature of these lesions when intramuscular. Failure to completely excise the lesion is the reason for the high recurrence rate of up to 20 % in the literature [52]. Canavese et al. reported no recurrence with wide resection, but higher than 20 % recurrence with marginal resection. Cavernous hemangiomas were the only subtype found to recur, likely because of their deep intramuscular location in most cases. Proximity to neurovascular structures can make wide resection difficult or impossible [49]. Sclerotherapy works by obliterating the lumen leading to fibrosis and growth arrest. This will eventually promote regression of the hemangioma. A variety of agents can be used including ethanol, polidocanol, hypertonic saline, sodium morrhuate, and sodium tetradecyl sulfate (STS). Indications for sclerotherapy include situations where excision is not possible, or when the patient does not wish to undergo surgery. It may also be effectively used to debulk the tumor prior to surgery [53]. Crawford et al. conducted a retrospective review of ethanol sclerotherapy in the treatment of intramuscular hemangiomas. They found that 15 of 19 patients reported some degree of pain relief, and successive treatments provided additional pain relief allowing for long term and in some cases permanent avoidance of surgical treatment. Complications occurred in 28 % of patients, but were minor and resolved with conservative management. Some of the more common complications included extravasation of ethanol leading to tissue necrosis or nerve damage, skin necrosis in superficial lesions, and swelling. Severe systemic complications are possible, but rare, and include arterial thrombosis, hypotension, and death [54]. Embolization has been used as an effective adjunct to surgical treatment for hemangiomas in the spine and liver, but case reports for intramuscular hemangiomas were not found [55]. Due to the reported recurrence rates, it is advisable to follow these patients for a number of years with visits becoming less frequent over time.

6.7 Nodular Fasciitis

Nodular fasciitis is a benign, self-limiting reactive process. It is mainly composed of proliferating fibroblasts and it is most commonly found in the subcutaneous fascia of the upper extremity, but can involve other tissues. In the literature, it has also been referred to as parosteal fasciitis, pseudosarcomatous fasciitis, subcutaneous fibromatosis, nodular fibrositis, and proliferative fasciitis. Most patients are between 20 and 50 years old with male predominance. A small number of cases can be found in the hands, though the distal upper and lower extremities are often spared [56].

The typical history is a rapidly growing, sometimes painful lesion over a period of a few of months. On physical examination, it is mobile, occasionally tender, and there can be multiple.

Radiographs typically do not reveal a shadow from these small soft tissue lesions. T1-weighted MRI sequences show increased signal compared to muscle, and homogenously increased signal on T2-weighted images. The lesion typically enhances diffusely with administration of contrast, but may also enhance in a peripheral pattern [24] Fig. 13a, b.

Macroscopically, nodular fasciitis appears as a fibrous lesion and the cut surface has an irregular, coarse trabecular pattern. Microscopically, spindle cells in a myxomatous stroma are present with occasional normal mitotic figures and giant cells [56] Fig. 14.

Because these are self-limited neoplasms, they often resolve with time. Therefore, close observation is an acceptable treatment. However, because they have a tendency to be painful and grow rapidly, many patients opt for excisional biopsy Recurrence is not thought to occur even if cells are left behind [56].

6.8 Myositis Ossificans Traumatica

Myositis ossificans traumatica (MOT) is a non-neoplastic osseous lesion that typically occurs after blunt trauma to the soft tissues of an extremity. MOT is one subtype of heterotopic ossification, or formation of normal bone at an abnormal anatomical site. The incidence in athletes sustaining a direct blow to an extremity has been reported to be between 9 and 20 % with the most commonly cited location being within the anterior thigh [57].

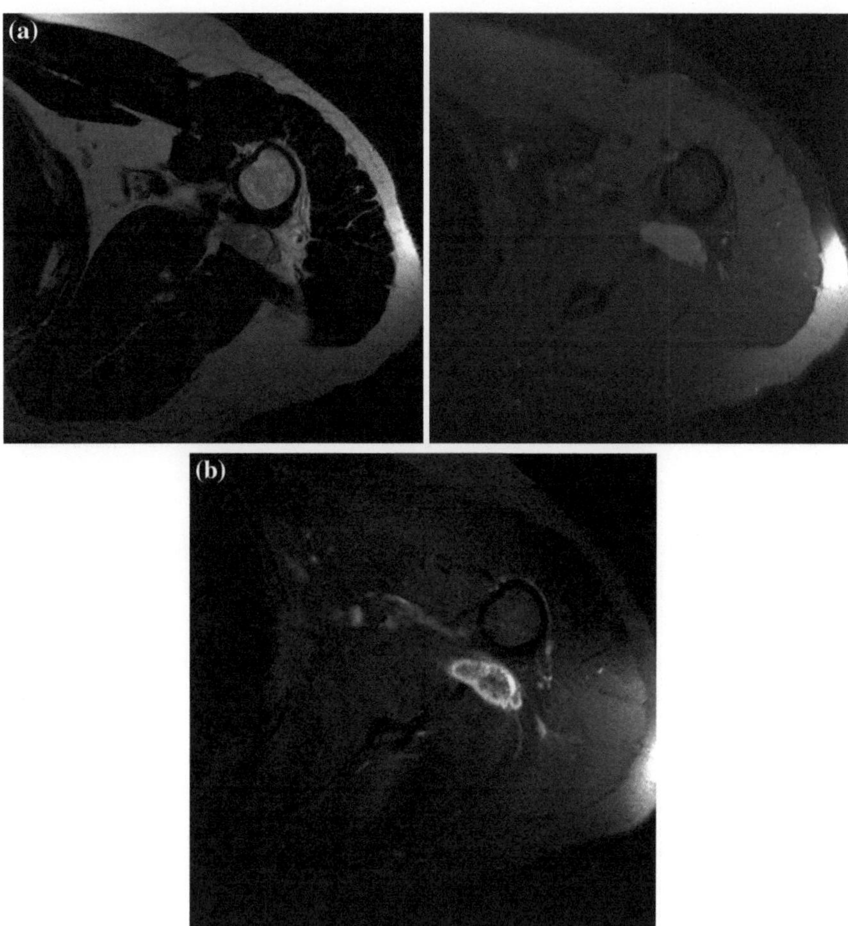

Fig. 13 Nodular fasciitis involving the posterior shoulder. Axial MRI images, **a** T1-weighted (*Left*), and T2-weighted (*Right*), **b** contrast-enhanced

Often, a patient with myositis ossificans has sustained blunt trauma and pain that failed to respond to conservative treatment including rest, ice, compression, elevation, and in some cases initial splinting in a position of muscle tension for 24–48 h (e.g., knee flexed). Patients may report worsening symptoms after 2 weeks including increasing muscle tenderness, swelling, and limited motion of adjacent joints.

Initial imaging should consist of radiographs, which may show some early changes at 2–3 weeks, but should reveal evidence of bone formation at 8 weeks. CT demonstrates bone formation and helps to assess the three dimensional characteristics of the lesion. MRI will reveal increased signal on T2-weighted pulse sequences early on in the region of injury. A triple-phase bone scan may reveal

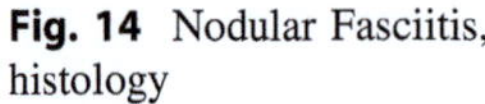

Fig. 14 Nodular Fasciitis, histology

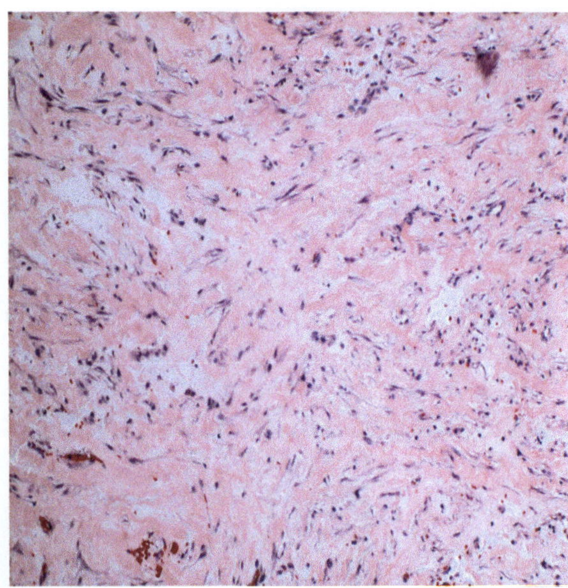

early uptake of radioactive tracer in the soft tissues, even before findings are apparent on plain radiographs [58] Fig. 15a, b.

Macroscopically, MOT has a shell of bone with a soft red-brown center. Microscopically, the typical appearance of MOT has been described as loose connective tissue with a periphery consisting of mature spongy bone, cartilage, and focal aggregations of osteoblasts and osteoclasts [59, 60] Fig. 15c.

The pathophysiology of bone formation is not completely understood, though there are theories. One such theory by Illes et al. is that the presence of rapidly proliferating mesenchymal cells and osteoblasts in the region of injury, leads to heterotopic bone and cartilage formation, possibly as a result of local tissue anoxia [61]. There are three types that have been described in the literature: periosteal, stalk, and intramuscular. The periosteal type consists of flat bone formation adjacent to the diaphysis of bone with disruption of periosteum. The stalk form is an off-shoot of ossification that remains attached to the adjacent bone with damaged periosteum. The intramuscular or disseminated form consists of bone formation without connection to the adjacent bone and without disruption of the periosteum [62].

The patient and their symptoms will guide treatment over time depending on their recovery from injury. Surgical excision is an option, though this should not be done until the bone has fully matured as indicated by the appearance of lamellar bone on radiographs, or minimal to no uptake on bone scan. This often takes 6–12 months, which by default, mandates observation for this period of time. In patients who report a persistent painful mass or significantly limited ROM surgical excision of the mass can be considered. Some have also used Indomethacin, or other nonsteroidal antiinflammatory drugs though there is no good evidence for this approach in treating MOT [63].

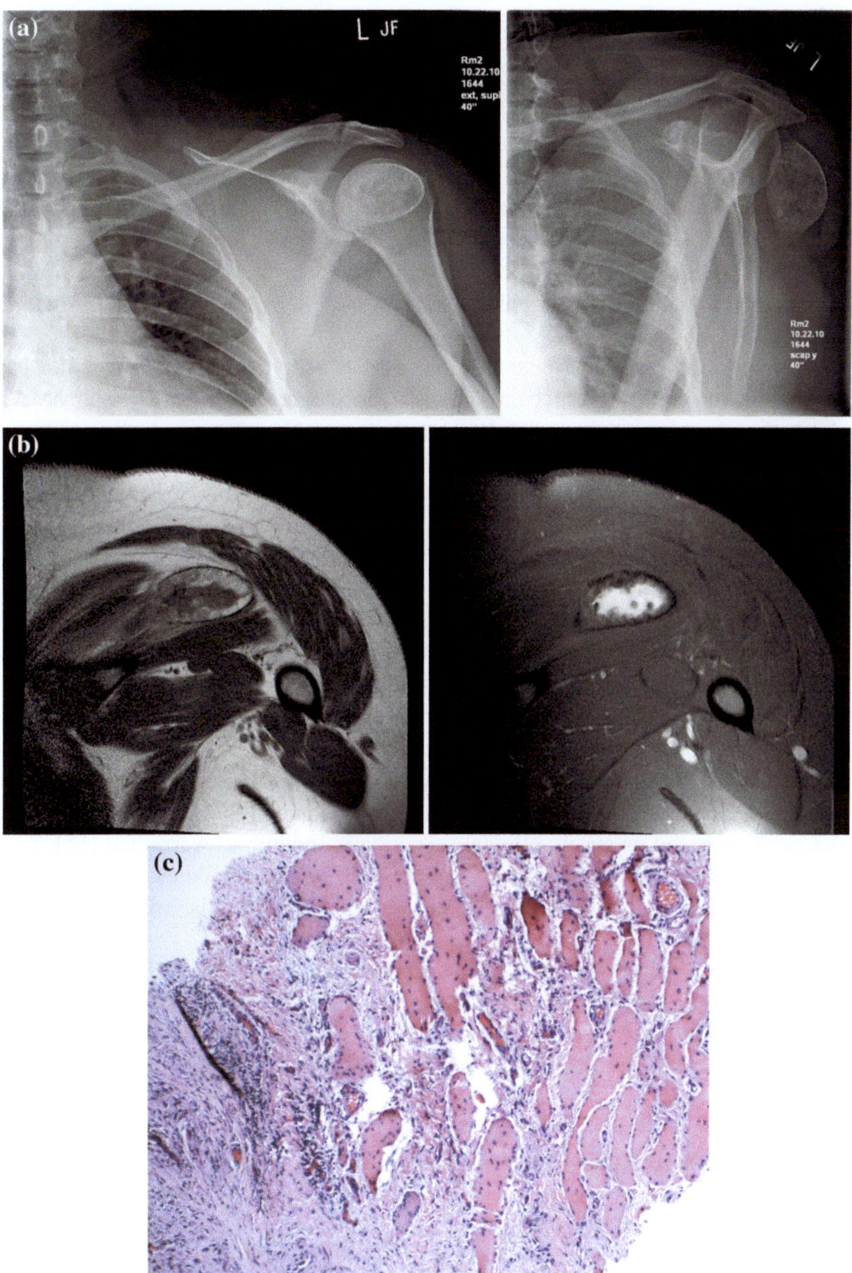

Fig. 15 Myositis ossificans traumatica located in the posterior Left shoulder, **a** AP/Lateral XR of the Left shoulder, **b** coronal MRI T1 (*Left*), and T2 (*Right*) of the Left shoulder, **c** histology

6.9   Glomus Tumor

A glomus tumor is a benign mesenchymal lesion arising from glomus bodies, structures within the dermis that are involved in body temperature regulation via shunting of blood to and from the skin surface. Glomus tumors make up approximately 2 % of soft tissue tumors and are commonly found in the hand, as glomus bodies are concentrated in the digits, especially within the subungual skin. They can also be found in the dermis of the palm, wrist, forearm, or foot, and are most often solitary. A majority of lesions are diagnosed in adults and there is no sex predilection. The subungual form, however, is more commonly found in females [31].

On history and physical examination, a triad of hypersensitivity to cold, paroxysmal pain, and pinpoint pain suggests the diagnosis. Sometimes an area of bluish discoloration at the nail plate can be seen. One described clinical test is Love's pin test, which has been shown to be 100 % sensitive [64]. Love's pin test consists of using the head of a pin, or a paperclip to apply pressure and localize the pain. In a positive test, the patient withdraws the hand complaining of severe pain. Hildreth's test has been shown to be 71.4 % sensitive, and 100 % specific [64]. This test is performed by placing a tourniquet around the base of the involved digit, and repeating Love's pin test. For a positive result, the patient should not experience pain. Another test is the cold sensitivity test that produces an increase in pain when the patient's digit is exposed to cold.

Radiographs are negative, but MRI can be useful as part of the workup for glomus tumors. They often have increased signal intensity on T2-weighted images, and strong contrast enhancement [64]. MRI, however, does not always reveal the glomus tumor as pointed out by Dahlin et al. and they concluded that surgical exploration and excision based on strong clinical suspicion is sometimes warranted [65].

On gross inspection, glomus tumors are small, blue-red nodules. Histologically, they are often composed of glomus cells, smooth muscle cells, and blood vessels Fig. 16.

Treatment consists of excisional biopsy for many patients, as these lesions are symptomatic. There is a risk of local recurrence, which has been estimated to be 10 %. Due to the fact that they are very rarely malignant, observation is an option if the patient wishes to avoid surgery [31, 33].

6.10   Intramuscular Myxoma

Intramuscular myxomas are benign intramuscular neoplasms. Typically patients are older than 40, and it is more common in females. The patient often presents with a painless mass in the extremity, most commonly in the thigh.

Radiographs may show a small soft tissue mass, but are normal in many cases. On ultrasound, a hypoechoic or anechoic mass with multiple cystic areas can be seen. CT is rarely obtained, but the lesion will be visualized as a well-defined,

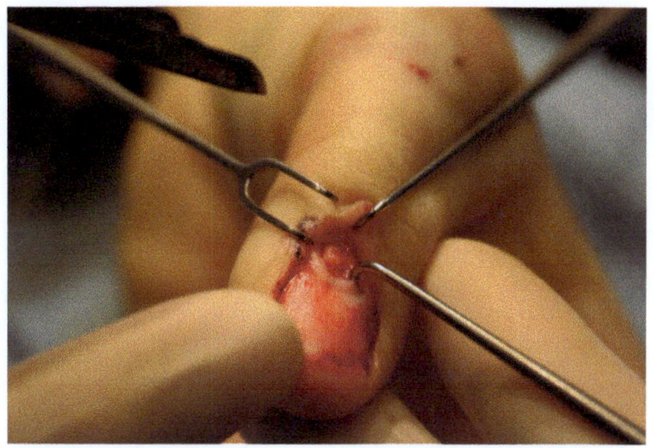

Fig. 16 Glomus tumor located in subungual region of thumb

homogeneous mass with attenuation values between those of water and muscle. On MRI, myxomas are most often homogenous, but can sometimes be heterogeneous with the presence of fat or edema in the surrounding muscles. They are hypointense on T1-weighted images, and hyperintense on T2-weighted images with contrast enhancement internally and peripherally. Cysts may be visualized on occasion. Luna et al. noted that the most distinctive MRI features included a perilesional fat ring and the presence of edema in adjacent muscle [66] Fig. 17.

In that same series by Luna et al. FNA correctly diagnosed intramuscular myxoma in only 1 of 9 cases and, therefore, excisional biopsy was strongly recommended. This finding was likely due to the hypocellularity of the lesion and nonspecific cytologic features [66]. Nielsen et al. described the clinicopathologic features of 51 intramuscular myxomas and noted a few important features. They emphasized that these lesions are mostly hypocellular, but can have regions of hypercellularity and for this reason, can be mistaken for a sarcoma. They had follow-up information for 32 patients at an average of 30 months after excision and noted that no tumor metastasized or recurred. They emphasized that excision is almost always curative, and recurrence is exceedingly rare [67] Fig. 18.

6.11 Synovial Chondromatosis

Synovial chondromatosis, or synovial osteochondromatosis, is a disorder in which cartilaginous nodules are formed within a synovial joint. The nodules then detach from the synovium and may undergo calcification. This is thought to occur most commonly between the third and fifth decades and it affects men approximately twice as often as women. It is a monoarticular process with the knee being the most common joint affected, but it can involve any synovial joint.

Patients typically complain of pain, swelling, stiffness, and sometimes locking of the involved joint. On physical examination, the joint acts much like an arthritic joint with effusion, tenderness, and decreased ROM.

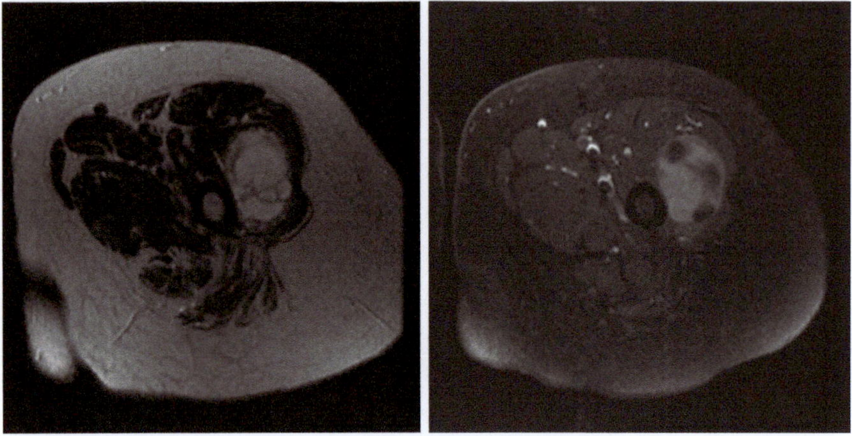

Fig. 17 Intramuscular myxoma of thigh. Axial MRI images, T1-weighted (*Left*), and T2-weighted (*Right*)

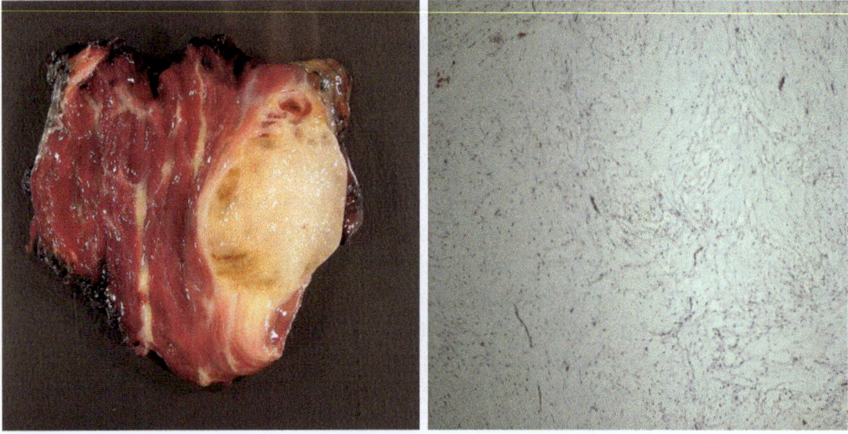

Fig. 18 Intramuscular myxoma, gross specimen (*Left*), and histology (*Right*)

Radiographs demonstrate multiple intra-articular densities when calcified that are usually in a "ring-and-arc" chondroid mineralization pattern. Early on before they become calcified, however, they are not apparent on radiographs. MRI is useful for visualizing radiolucent nodules where they have low signal on T1-weighted images, and increased signal on T2-weighted images. One may see erosive changes of the articular cartilage, and in late stages, there is joint space narrowing, osteophytes, and sclerosis much like an osteoarthritic joint Fig. 19a.

On gross inspection, the synovial nodules, which are composed of hyaline cartilage, typically have a cobblestone appearance. The histologic appearance is that of benign hyaline cartilage, with low to moderate cellularity, and a synovial

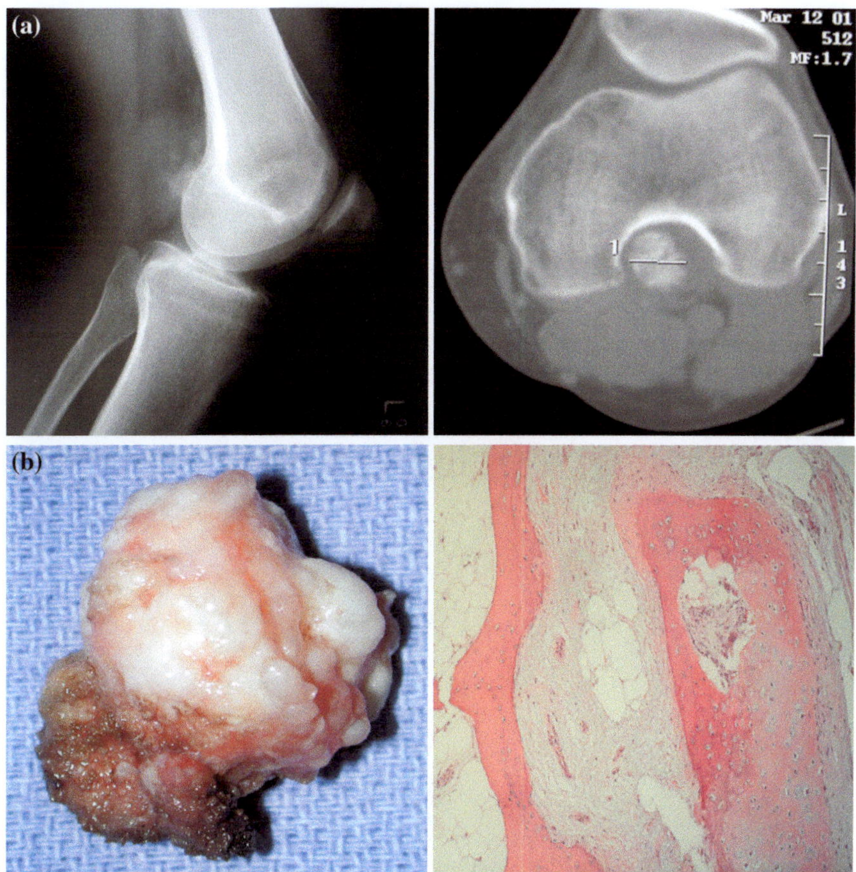

Fig. 19 Synovial chondromatosis visualized in the posterior aspect of the knee joint, **a** Lateral XR (*Left*), and axial CT image (*Right*), **b** gross specimen (*Left*), and histology (*Right*)

tissue lining on the outside. The chondrocytes can demonstrate mild to moderate atypia [68]. This appearance is in contrast to a loose body, or secondary chondromatosis that can result from trauma, or degenerative disease. Loose bodies present with fewer fragments and histologically demonstrate no neoplastic qualities [68]. They are essentially floating pieces of bone or cartilage Fig. 19b.

Treatment should be initiated as soon as possible after diagnosis to prevent disease progression and destruction of articular cartilage. A number of studies have shown unacceptable recurrence rates with simple removal of the nodules, and those authors have recommended synovectomy in addition to nodule removal [69, 70]. Both arthroscopic and open approaches can be used, but significant limitations in ROM have been observed after extensive open approaches. This was not found with arthroscopic methods. Recurrence rates have been reported in the range of 0–31 %

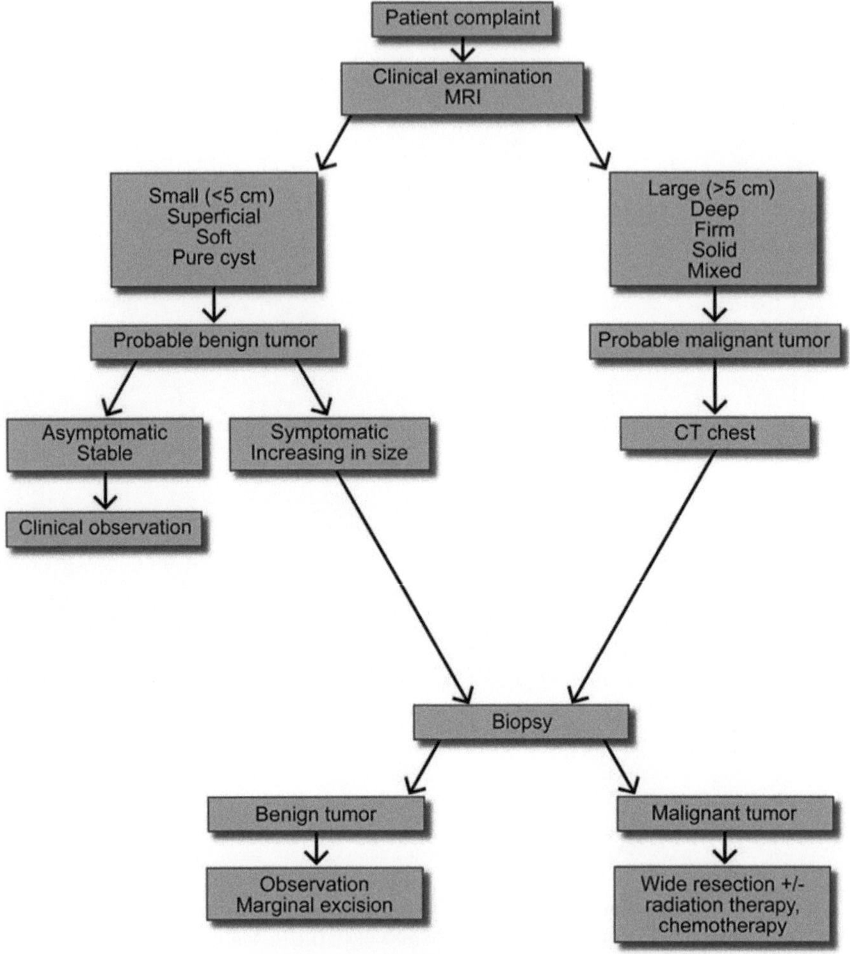

Fig. 20 Algorithm for diagnosis and management of soft tissue tumors of the extremities (Reprinted from [12], with permission from Elsevier)

after both open approaches and arthroscopic approaches. In some cases, repeat arthroscopy can be successful. These patients should be followed long term for both recurrence and development of osteoarthritis in that joint [35]. Synovial chondrosarcoma may be present in the setting of synovial chondromatosis with a reported incidence of 5 %. This should be considered if there are multiple recurrences, a rapid increase in size of the lesion, extra-articular extension, or invasion of the marrow [71].

7   Conclusion

Benign soft tissue tumors are much more common than malignant tumors. A systematic approach including a detailed history and physical examination, radiographs, advanced imaging in some cases, and biopsy when appropriate will often lead to a diagnosis. Multiple treatment options exist and in some cases can be left up to the patient, as is the case for superficial lipomas. Other, more aggressive soft tissue lesions such as desmoids, or intra-articular lesions, may require more aggressive treatment. Some lesions may not have a definitive diagnosis after imaging and will require a biopsy. Others may be painful such as schwannomas, and the patient may choose to have the lesion excised even if it has proven to be stable over time. Patient education, an explanation of advantages and disadvantages of each treatment option, and routine follow-up are all essential parts of appropriate patient care Fig. 20.

References

1. Rydholm A, Berg NO (1983) Size, site and clinical incidence of lipoma. Factors in the differential diagnosis of lipoma and sarcoma. Acta Orthop Scand 54(6):929–934
2. Gartner L, Pearce CJ, Saifuddin A (2009) The role of the plain radiograph in the characterisation of soft tissue tumours. Skeletal Radiol 38(6):549–558
3. Kransdorf MJ, Murphey MD (2000) Radiologic evaluation of soft-tissue masses: a current perspective. AJR Am J Roentgenol 175(3):575–587
4. De Schepper AM, Ramon FA, Degryse HR (1992) Statistical analysis of MRI parameters predicting malignancy in 141 soft tissue masses. Rofo 156(6):587–591
5. Razek A et al (2012) Assessment of soft tissue tumours of the extremities with diffusion echoplanar MR imaging. Radiol Med 117(1):96–101
6. Hatakenaka M et al (2008) Apparent diffusion coefficients of breast tumors: clinical application. Magn Reson Med Sci 7(1):23–29
7. Lakkaraju A et al (2009) Ultrasound for initial evaluation and triage of clinically suspicious soft-tissue masses. Clin Radiol 64(6):615–621
8. Weekes RG et al (1985) Magnetic resonance imaging of soft-tissue tumors: comparison with computed tomography. Magn Reson Imaging 3(4):345–352
9. Kasper B et al (2010) Positron emission tomography in patients with aggressive fibromatosis/ desmoid tumours undergoing therapy with imatinib. Eur J Nucl Med Mol Imaging 37(10):1876–1882
10. Mankin HJ, Lange TA, Spanier SS (1982) The hazards of biopsy in patients with malignant primary bone and soft-tissue tumors. J Bone Joint Surg Am 64(8):1121–1127
11. Mankin HJ, Mankin CJ, Simon MA (1996) The hazards of the biopsy, revisited. Members of the Musculoskeletal Tumor Society. J Bone Joint Surg Am 78(5):656–663
12. Balach T, Stacy GS, Haydon RC (2011) The clinical evaluation of soft tissue tumors. Radiol Clin North Am 49(6):1185–1196, vi
13. Strauss DC et al (2010) The role of core needle biopsy in the diagnosis of suspected soft tissue tumours. J Surg Oncol 102(5):523–529
14. Kasraeian S et al (2010) A comparison of fine-needle aspiration, core biopsy, and surgical biopsy in the diagnosis of extremity soft tissue masses. Clin Orthop Relat Res 468(11):2992–3002
15. Kaffenberger BH, Wakely PE Jr, Mayerson JL (2010) Local recurrence rate of fine-needle aspiration biopsy in primary high-grade sarcomas. J Surg Oncol 101(7):618–621

16. Kilpatrick SE et al (1998) The role of fine-needle aspiration biopsy in the initial diagnosis of pediatric bone and soft tissue tumors: an institutional experience. Mod Pathol 11(10):923–928
17. Schwartz HS, Spengler DM (1997) Needle tract recurrences after closed biopsy for sarcoma: three cases and review of the literature. Ann Surg Oncol 4(3):228–236
18. National Guideline C. ACR Appropriateness Criteria® follow-up of malignant or aggressive musculoskeletal tumors. http://www.guideline.gov/content.aspx?id=32617&search=Malignant+neoplasm+musculoskeletal+. Accessed 14 Dec 2013
19. Murphey MD et al (2004) From the archives of the AFIP: benign musculoskeletal lipomatous lesions. Radiographics 24(5):1433–1466
20. Myhre-Jensen O (1981) A consecutive 7-year series of 1331 benign soft tissue tumours. Clinicopathologic data. Comparison with sarcomas. Acta Orthop Scand 52(3):287–293
21. Lopez-Tomassetti Fernandez EM et al (2012) Intermuscular lipoma of the gluteus muscles compressing the sciatic nerve: an inverted sciatic hernia. J Neurosurg 117(4):795–799
22. Sampson CC et al (1960) Liposarcoma developing in a lipoma. Arch Pathol 69:506–510
23. Murphey MD et al (1999) From the archives of the AFIP. Imaging of musculoskeletal neurogenic tumors: radiologic-pathologic correlation. Radiographics 19(5):1253–1280
24. Bancroft LW et al (2002) Soft tissue tumors of the lower extremities. Radiol Clin North Am 40(5):991–1011
25. Jee WH et al (2004) Extraaxial neurofibromas versus neurilemmomas: discrimination with MRI. AJR Am J Roentgenol 183(3):629–633
26. Kehoe NJ, Reid RP, Semple JC (1995) Solitary benign peripheral-nerve tumours. Review of 32 years' experience. J Bone Joint Surg Br 77(3):497–500
27. Weiss SW, Langloss JM, Enzinger FM (1983) Value of S-100 protein in the diagnosis of soft tissue tumors with particular reference to benign and malignant Schwann cell tumors. Lab Invest 49(3):299–308
28. Kim SM et al (2012) Surgical outcome of schwannomas arising from major peripheral nerves in the lower limb. Int Orthop 36(8):1721–1725
29. Park MJ, Seo KN, Kang HJ (2009) Neurological deficit after surgical enucleation of schwannomas of the upper limb. J Bone Joint Surg Br 91(11):1482–1486
30. Lee SH et al (2001) Results of neurilemoma treatment: a review of 78 cases. Orthopedics 24(10):977–980
31. Mahajan D, Billings SD, Goldblum JR (2011) Acral soft tissue tumors: a review. Adv Anat Pathol 18(2):103–119
32. Monaghan H, Salter DM, Al-Nafussi A (2001) Giant cell tumour of tendon sheath (localised nodular tenosynovitis): clinicopathological features of 71 cases. J Clin Pathol 54(5):404–407
33. Payne WT, Merrell G (2010) Benign bony and soft tissue tumors of the hand. J Hand Surg Am 35(11):1901–1910
34. Dorwart RH et al (1984) Pigmented villonodular synovitis of synovial joints: clinical, pathologic, and radiologic features. AJR Am J Roentgenol 143(4):877–885
35. Adelani MA, Wupperman RM, Holt GE (2008) Benign synovial disorders. J Am Acad Orthop Surg 16(5):268–275
36. Tyler WK et al (2006) Pigmented villonodular synovitis. J Am Acad Orthop Surg 14(6):376–385
37. Hosalkar HS et al (2008) Musculoskeletal desmoid tumors. J Am Acad Orthop Surg 16(4):188–198
38. Gronchi A et al (2003) Quality of surgery and outcome in extra-abdominal aggressive fibromatosis: a series of patients surgically treated at a single institution. J Clin Oncol 21(7):1390–1397
39. Merchant NB et al (1999) Extremity and trunk desmoid tumors: a multifactorial analysis of outcome. Cancer 86(10):2045–2052

40. Spear MA et al (1998) Individualizing management of aggressive fibromatoses. Int J Radiat Oncol Biol Phys 40(3):637–645
41. Acker JC, Bossen EH, Halperin EC (1993) The management of desmoid tumors. Int J Radiat Oncol Biol Phys 26(5):851–858
42. Ballo MT, Zagars GK, Pollack A (1998) Radiation therapy in the management of desmoid tumors. Int J Radiat Oncol Biol Phys 42(5):1007–1014
43. Zlotecki RA et al (2002) External beam radiotherapy for primary and adjuvant management of aggressive fibromatosis. Int J Radiat Oncol Biol Phys 54(1):177–181
44. Azzarelli A et al (2001) Low-dose chemotherapy with methotrexate and vinblastine for patients with advanced aggressive fibromatosis. Cancer 92(5):1259–1264
45. Mace J et al (2002) Response of extraabdominal desmoid tumors to therapy with imatinib mesylate. Cancer 95(11):2373–2379
46. Chugh R et al (2010) Efficacy of imatinib in aggressive fibromatosis: Results of a phase II multicenter Sarcoma Alliance for Research through Collaboration (SARC) trial. Clin Cancer Res 16(19):4884–4891
47. Poon R et al (2001) Cyclooxygenase-two (COX-2) modulates proliferation in aggressive fibromatosis (desmoid tumor). Oncogene 20(4):451–460
48. Tsukada K et al (1992) Noncytotoxic drug therapy for intra-abdominal desmoid tumor in patients with familial adenomatous polyposis. Dis Colon Rectum 35(1):29–33
49. Canavese F et al (2008) Surgical outcome in patients treated for hemangioma during infancy, childhood, and adolescence: a retrospective review of 44 consecutive patients. J Pediatr Orthop 28(3):381–386
50. Tang P et al (2002) Surgical treatment of hemangiomas of soft tissue. Clin Orthop Relat Res 399:205–210
51. Donnelly LF, Adams DM, Bisset GS 3rd (2000) Vascular malformations and hemangiomas: a practical approach in a multidisciplinary clinic. AJR Am J Roentgenol 174(3):597–608
52. Kiran KR et al (2012) Skeletal Muscle Haemangioma: a cause for chronic pain about the knee: a case report. Case Rep Orthop 2012:452651
53. Brown RA, Crichton K, Malouf GM (2004) Intramuscular haemangioma of the thigh in a basketball player. Br J Sports Med 38(3):346–348
54. Crawford EA et al (2009) Ethanol sclerotherapy reduces pain in symptomatic musculoskeletal hemangiomas. Clin Orthop Relat Res 467(11):2955–2961
55. Smith TP et al (1993) Transarterial embolization of vertebral hemangioma. J Vasc Interv Radiol 4(5):681–685
56. Ingari JV, Faillace JJ (2004) Benign tumors of fibrous tissue and adipose tissue in the hand. Hand Clin 20(3):243–248, v
57. King JB (1998) Post-traumatic ectopic calcification in the muscles of athletes: a review. Br J Sports Med 32(4):287–290
58. Drane WE (1984) Myositis ossificans and the three-phase bone scan. AJR Am J Roentgenol 142(1):179–180
59. Takahashi S et al (2008) Adult autopsy case with marked myositis ossificans: association with repetitive physical assault and battery. Leg Med (Tokyo) 10(5):274–276
60. Cushner FD, Morwessel RM (1992) Myositis ossificans traumatica. Orthop Rev 21(11):1319–1326
61. Illes T et al (1992) Characterization of bone forming cells in posttraumatic myositis ossificans by lectins. Pathol Res Pract 188(1–2):172–176
62. Beiner JM, Jokl P (2001) Muscle contusion injuries: current treatment options. J Am Acad Orthop Surg 9(4):227–237
63. Sodl JF et al (2008) Traumatic myositis ossificans as a result of college fraternity hazing. Clin Orthop Relat Res 466(1):225–230
64. McDermott EM, Weiss AP (2006) Glomus tumors. J Hand Surg Am 31(8):1397–1400
65. Dahlin LB, Besjakov J, Veress B (2005) A glomus tumour: classic signs without magnetic resonance imaging findings. Scand J Plast Reconstr Surg Hand Surg 39(2):123–125

66. Luna A, Martinez S, Bossen E (2005) Magnetic resonance imaging of intramuscular myxoma with histological comparison and a review of the literature. Skeletal Radiol 34(1):19–28
67. Nielsen GP, O'Connell JX, Rosenberg AE (1998) Intramuscular myxoma: a clinicopathologic study of 51 cases with emphasis on hypercellular and hypervascular variants. Am J Surg Pathol 22(10):1222–1227
68. Ho YY, Choueka J (2013) Synovial chondromatosis of the upper extremity. J Hand Surg Am 38(4):804–810
69. Ogilvie-Harris DJ, Saleh K (1994) Generalized synovial chondromatosis of the knee: a comparison of removal of the loose bodies alone with arthroscopic synovectomy. Arthroscopy 10(2):166–170
70. Schoeniger R et al (2006) Modified complete synovectomy prevents recurrence in synovial chondromatosis of the hip. Clin Orthop Relat Res 451:195–200
71. Garner HW, Bestic JM (2013) Benign synovial tumors and proliferative processes. Semin Musculoskelet Radiol 17(2):177–178

Soft Tissue Sarcomas

Andre Spiguel

Abstract

Sarcoma is a cancer that arises from cells of mesenchymal origin, such as bone, cartilage, muscle, fat, vascular, or hematopoietic tissue. It is a very rare form of cancer with over 50 histologic subtypes. This chapter discusses selected individual subtypes of sarcomas and characteristics specific to each one. It will broadly go over molecular biology, etiology, risk factors, and the clinical features of this disease. It discusses diagnostic evaluation and the principles of management including imaging, biopsy, staging, treatment, follow-up, and the importance of a multidisciplinary approach.

Keywords

Sarcoma · Clinical features · Diagnosis · Staging · Treatment · Surveillance

1   Introduction

The word sarcoma originates from the Greek word sark or sarx, which means flesh. Soft tissue sarcomas are life-threatening mesenchymal neoplasms that account for less than 1 % of all human cancers. The American Cancer Society predicted that in 2013, there would be 11,410 newly diagnosed soft tissue sarcomas, and 4,390 deaths due to disease. There are more than 50 histological subtypes, and treatment

A. Spiguel (✉)
University of Florida, Department of Orthopaedic Surgery, Division of Oncology,
UF Orthopaedics and Sports Medicine Institute, PO Box 112727, Gainesville,
FL 32611-2727, USA
e-mail: spiguar@ortho.ufl.edu

T. D. Peabody and S. Attar (eds.), *Orthopaedic Oncology*,
Cancer Treatment and Research 162, DOI: 10.1007/978-3-319-07323-1_10,
© Springer International Publishing Switzerland 2014

is often challenging with more than 50 % of newly diagnosed patients dying of disease, a statistic that has changed little in recent decades [1]. They can arise anywhere in the body and have a tendency to become more common with increasing age. Due to the variety of soft tissue sarcomas and the relatively small number of cases, studying this disease and trying to understand it can be quite challenging.

Most soft tissue tumors are benign, with a ratio of 100:1 when compared to malignant sarcomas. Due to the large variety of tumors and the overall prognosis and biologic behavior of each different subtype, it is also very important to obtain a proper diagnosis. The World Health Organization (WHO) divides soft tissue tumors into four main categories: benign, intermediate (locally aggressive), intermediate (rarely metastasizing), and malignant [2]. This chapter will discuss broadly the malignant category of soft tissue sarcomas, describing specific sub-types, and then focus on the management of this disease and the importance of a multidisciplinary approach.

2   Molecular Biology, Etiology, and Risk Factors

Two broad groups have been described: (1) translocation associated sarcomas, which typically occur in young adults due to deregulation induced by fusion genes; (2) and sarcomas with highly aberrant and complex genomes, which have a peak incidence at 50–60 years of age. Most sarcomas are believed to arise sporadically, although there are some predisposing factors that have been identified.

There are certain genetic syndromes that have been associated with the development of soft tissue sarcomas: familial adenomatous polyposis (FAP) and desmoid tumors; neurofibromatosis type 1 (NF1) and malignant peripheral nerve sheath tumors (MPNSTs); Li-Fraumeni syndrome (a rare familial cancer pheno-type associated with a p53 germline mutation) and an elevated risk for the development of a variety of sarcomas; and heritable retinoblastoma (RB1), although in this specific case most of this excess risk can be prevented by limiting their exposure to DNA damaging agents [2–4].

Radiation exposure is another factor that has been identified to cause soft tissue sarcomas. These tumors typically arise in patients treated with radiotherapy whose survival is typically long and can present with a variety of histologic subtypes. The exact mechanism and cause of these lesions is not well understood. They usually arise near the penumbra of the radiation field, possibly due to incomplete damage to normal surrounding tissues. Although these lesions are uncommon, they have a poor prognosis, and studies have shown that they have worse disease-specific survival than sporadic soft tissue sarcomas [2, 3, 5].

Lymphedema is another factor thought to potentially cause specific soft tissue sarcomas—particularly lymphangiosarcoma described by Stewart and Treves in the postmastectomy, postirradiated, lymphedematous arm [6]. Chemical agents such as phenoxy herbicide and dioxin have also been blamed for causing sarco-mas, but studies have failed to show any correlation [2, 3].

3   Selected Histologic Subtypes

3.1   Liposarcoma

Liposarcomas account for at least 20 % of all soft tissue sarcomas in adults. It usually presents in adults ages 50–65, and can occur anywhere in the body, most commonly in the thigh and retroperitoneum:

(1) Well-differentiated liposarcomas (atypical lipomatous tumor)—These tumors represent a locally aggressive malignant neoplasm with mature adipocytic cell proliferation, variation in cell size, and focal nuclear atypia. There is no potential for metastasis unless this tumor undergoes differentiation. Most of these lesions have a supernumerary ring and giant marker chromosomes with gene amplification of chromosome 12. Location is an important predictor of outcome with extremity tumors rarely recurring.

(2) Dedifferentiated liposarcomas—There is a transition within the tumor to a region of nonlipogenic sarcoma with less aggressive features when compared to other high-grade pleomorphic sarcomas.

(3) Myxoid or Round cell liposarcomas—These tumors consist of round, primitive, nonlipogenic mesenchymal cells, and small signet ring lipoblasts in a prominent myxoid stroma. The histologic grade is dependent on the round cell component of the tumor, with greater than 5 % being high grade, and is a predictor of worse outcome. It is important to note that even in the absence of pulmonary metastasis, these tumors can metastasize to unusual locations in the soft tissue (retroperitoneum) and bone, and they are quite sensitive to XRT and certain chemotherapeutic agents.

(4) Pleomorphic liposarcomas—These are highly malignant tumors. 30–50 % will metastasize early, usually to the lungs, with 50 % tumor-associated mortality. Patients with metastasis commonly die within a short period of time [2, 3, 7, 8].

3.2   Fibrosarcoma

Once considered to represent the most common soft tissue sarcoma in adults, the incidence of fibrosarcoma has significantly declined over the past seven decades due to advances in immunohistochemical and molecular genetic techniques. With the evolution of the classification of soft tissue tumors and the recognition of clinically, morphologically, and genetically distinctive subtypes of soft tissue sarcomas, today it is felt to comprise only 1 % of adult sarcomas and 3.6 % of sarcomas arising from the soft tissues. It can be classified according to the WHO as malignant or intermediate (rarely metastasizing). Histologically, it is composed of fibroblasts with variable collagen stroma. Classically, a herring bone pattern to the cellular architecture is appreciated. It usually affects middle-aged adults and can be seen in the extremities, trunk, head, and neck [2, 3, 9].

3.3 Myxofibrosarcoma

Myxofibrosarcoma represents a spectrum of malignant fibroblastic lesions with a variably myxoid stroma and cellular pleomorphism. It is one of the more common sarcomas, typically found in the extremities of elderly adults. Local recurrence is common and is independent of grade or depth. Tumor-associated mortality is obviously higher with metastasis, which occurs in about 35 % of high-grade cases. Low-grade lesions may become higher grade in subsequent recurrences. Common sites of metastasis include the lungs, bone, and lymph nodes (which occur in a small but significant number of patients) with five-year survival rates of 60–70 % [2, 3, 10].

3.4 Dermatofibrosarcoma Protuberans

Dermatofibrosarcoma Protuberans (DFSP) is a low-grade sarcoma that rarely metastasizes, but has a propensity to recur locally (50 % recurrence after simple excision). This lesion can occur anywhere in the body, but more than 50 % occur on the trunk. 10–15 % of these lesions contain areas of fibrosarcoma and these tend to exhibit more aggressive behavior. The lesion starts as a nodular cutaneous mass and growth is usually slow and persistent and eventually becomes protuberant. The central portion of the mass consists of plump fibroblasts and the histology stains positive for CD34. The majority of these tumors (more than 90 %) carry giant chromosomes composed of translocated portions of chromosomes 17 and 22. This tumor is sensitive to imatinib, mainly the tumors with the t(17,22) translocation. Imatinib has been approved by the FDA as a first line of treatment for advanced disease [2, 3, 11, 12].

3.5 High-Grade Pleomorphic Undifferentiated Sarcoma

High-Grade Pleomorphic Undifferentiated Sarcoma (HGPUS) is a group of sarcomas with significant cytological and nuclear pleomorphism and no definable cell line of differentiation. Characteristically, it occurs in late adulthood and presents as a painless, deep-seated mass most commonly found in the lower extremities. The clinical course of HGPUS is typically aggressive with 5 % of people presenting with metastasis, many patients developing metastatic disease within 3 years from diagnosis, and five-year disease-specific survival at 65 % [2, 3].

3.6 Leiomyosarcoma

Leiomyosarcoma is a malignant tumor with smooth muscle features that can arise anywhere and typically affects middle-aged to older adults. It can arise in any blood vessel from deep to subcutaneous and often presents insidiously. It accounts for 10–15 % of sarcomas in the extremity and forms a significant percentage or retroperitoneal sarcomas. The term leiomyosarcoma encompasses a spectrum of disease ranging from low-grade cutaneous lesions with relatively benign behavior to aggressive deep lesions of the abdomen or extremity with significant metastatic potential [2, 3, 13].

3.7 Rhabdomyosarcoma

Rhabdomyosarcoma is the most common soft tissue sarcoma of infants and children, although they can occur in adults. It is a malignant tumor of skeletal muscle differentiation and treatment is usually multimodal, with surgery, radiation, and unlike most other soft tissue sarcomas, the use of chemotherapy.

(1) Embryonal rhabdomyosarcoma—The most common subtype of rhabdomyosarcoma in children. It has phenotypic and biologic features of embryonic skeletal muscle and is usually very responsive to chemotherapy and radiation. Systemic treatment is important because these tumors can disseminate widely. Age is usually a prognostic indicator with worse survival in older patients.

(2) Alveolar rhabdomyosarcoma—Usually found in the extremities of young adults and histologically the tumor is comprised of small blue cells with partial skeletal differentiation. Associated with a specific translocation creating the PAX3-FOX01 fusion gene in the majority of cases. A small subset of patients have the PAX7-FOX01 which is associated with a better prognosis.

(3) Pleomorphic rhabdomyosarcoma—The most common form of rhabdomyosarcoma in adults and it has a very poor prognosis [2, 3].

3.8 Angiosarcoma

Angiosarcoma is a malignant tumor with cells that have morphologic and functional features of normal endothelium. Usually, they are found in the skin or superficial soft tissues. As previously discussed, this disease is sometimes associated with lymphedema and prior radiotherapy and can also develop in chronically lymphadematous extremities (Fig. 1). Most patients present with high-grade histology and multifocal disease. The overall prognosis is generally poor with a propensity for both local recurrence and distant metastasis [3, 14].

3.9 Malignant Peripheral Nerve Sheath Tumor

Malignant peripheral nerve sheath tumor (MPNST) is a highly aggressive sarcoma that rarely occurs sporadically, but has a lifetime incidence in patients with NF1 of 8–13 %. They can occur anywhere but are typically associated with major nerves, typically arising from preexisting plexiform neurofibromas most commonly in the

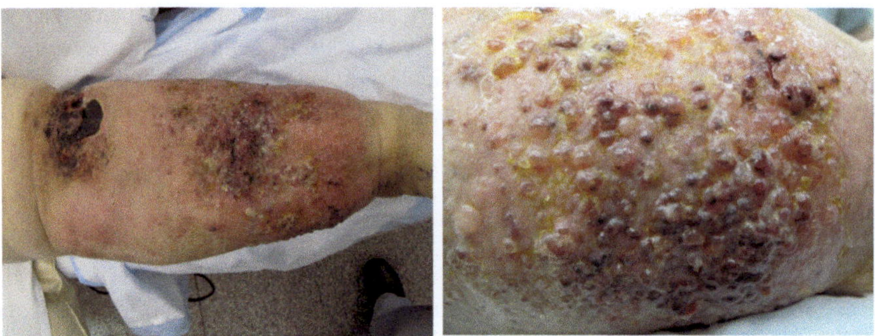

Fig. 1 Angiosarcoma in the setting of chronic lymphedema

lower extremities and retroperitoneum. The majority of these tumors are high grade with pronounced cellular atypia, are difficult to detect, and can metastasize to the lung, liver, brain, soft tissue, bone, regional lymph nodes, skin, and retroperitoneum with poor prognosis. Clinical suspicion should be heightened in patients with NF1 who develop unremitting pain, a rapid increase in size or change in the consistency of a plexiform neurofibroma, or a neurological deficit [3, 15].

3.10 Synovial Sarcoma

Synovial sarcoma is a mesenchymal spindle cell tumor with a specific chromosomal translocation, t(X;18), that can be seen at any age but typically occurs in young to middle-aged adults and accounts for 5–10 % of all soft tissue sarcomas. It generally does not originate from synovial tissue and can be monophasic or biphasic with two morphologically distinct cell types. The genetic translocation that is seen in 100 % of biphasic and 96 % of monophasic tumors involves fusing the SS18 (SYT) gene with either SSX1, SSX2, or SSX4. Chemotherapy does appear to have a more favorable effect on synovial sarcoma when compared to other histologic subtypes of soft tissue sarcomas, and it may be used more often in the treatment of this disease [2, 3].

3.11 Alveolar Soft Part Sarcoma

Alveolar soft part sarcoma (ASPS) is a rare tumor that mainly affects adolescents and young adults. It typically presents as a slow growing asymptomatic mass found in the extremities. The ultimate prognosis is usually quite poor due to early metastasis, most commonly to the lung, brain, and bone. The cure rate is 40–50 % at 10 years with patients sometimes relapsing even after 10 years. Patients will often present with manifestations of metastatic disease prior to diagnosis. ASPS harbors the t(X;17)(p11.2;q25) translocation and, although it is impervious to traditional chemotherapeutic agents, the fusion protein created from the translocation can be targeted. VEGF receptor inhibitors have had some activity giving hope to the use of kinase-targeted agents in progressive disease [2, 3, 16].

3.12   Epithelioid Sarcoma

Epithelioid sarcoma is a rare tumor with a recurrent and protracted course. Patients typically present with a benign-appearing superficial lesion that resembles a subcutaneous nodule. Due to its deceptively harmless appearance, delays in diagnosis are typical. It mainly affects young adults with as many as 50 % of patients presenting with metastatic disease. Histologically, cells have a predominantly epithelioid cytomorphology, although the cell lineage is unknown. Regional lymph node metastasis is also fairly common and it tends to propagate along fascial planes, tendon sheaths, and nerve sheaths making it very difficult to treat. Patients benefit from repeated resections and extended surveillance is indicated with recurrences appearing decades after quiescence [2, 3, 17].

3.13   Clear Cell Sarcoma (Melanoma of Soft Parts)

Clear cell sarcoma shows melanocytic differentiation thought to be derived from neural crest cells and usually involves the tendons and aponeuroses of young adults. Cells contain melanin and regional lymph node metastasis occurs in a significant percentage of cases. It is associated with a poor prognosis, which is why it is important to consider a sentinel node biopsy at the time of surgery. Its distinction from melanoma may be difficult, but it is characterized by a specific chromosomal translocation t(12;22) in up to 90 % of cases, resulting in the fusion of EWSR1 and ATF1 genes. Metastasis is common with five-year survival around 50 % [2, 3, 18].

4   Clinical Features

The clinical symptoms accompanying the diagnosis of soft tissue sarcomas are typically nonspecific. Most sarcomas present as painless, gradually enlarging masses. Even sometimes despite a large tumor volume, they do not typically influence the patient's overall function or general health. Due to their often indolent presentation and relative rarity, they are commonly misinterpreted as benign conditions. The size of the tumor at presentation also typically varies by location for obvious reasons. Sarcomas of the extremities and head or neck are usually smaller and noticed earlier, whereas sarcomas of the thigh or retroperitoneum can be quite large upon presentation. If symptomatic, patients usually present with site-specific complaints, such as increased pressure, paresthesias from nerve compression, distal edema, etc.

As with every new patient, an appropriate workup should begin with a careful history and physical examination. It is important to ask how long ago the mass was noted and what its rate of growth is. Any pain or weakness associated with the mass, numbness, history of trauma, history of any exposure to radiation or toxins, and any personal or family history of cancer should be noted.

The physical examination should explore the size and consistency of the mass, its location, and the involvement of the surrounding structures. It is important to appreciate if the mass is tender to palpation or has a bruit or a thrill. These findings must be considered prior to the biopsy to prevent bleeding or any adverse neurologic issues. A regional lymph node exam and the neurovascular status of the affected extremity is also important.

5   Imaging

Plain radiographs can reveal important details about the mass, and they allow the physician to evaluate if this is a soft tissue mass associated with an underlying primary bone tumor or if there is any bony involvement. A soft tissue shadow can often be seen as well as calcifications or phleboliths, which can occur in certain soft tissue tumors such as synovial sarcomas and hemangiomas. Cortical involvement or remodeling, which is sometimes seen when soft tissue tumors invade or push against the underlying bone, can also be appreciated (Fig. 2).

When evaluating soft tissue tumors, magnetic resonance imaging (MRI) is the modality of choice. It helps to distinguish tumor tissue from surrounding normal tissue. The MRI should be performed with and without gadolinium contrast to evaluate for viable tumor. The MRI helps define the size of the tumor and its relationship to the surrounding muscle compartments and neurovascular structures in multiple planes. It can demonstrate whether there is hemorrhage or necrosis, surrounding peritumoral edema, cystic and myxoid degeneration, and fibrosis. These tumors are typically heterogeneous on MRI, and the T1-weighted images are typically best for evaluating anatomy. With the addition of gadolinium, the delineation between tumor tissue and normal or reactive tissue is even better defined and quite helpful for preoperative planning (Fig. 3). If an MRI is not possible due to patient-specific issues, such as implantable metal devices or a high-risk metallic foreign body, then a computerized tomography (CT) scan with and without IV contrast is recommended. CT scans can also help determine what effect the sarcoma is having on the underlying bone, and if the patient is at risk for fracture (Fig. 4).

The role of positron emission tomography (PET) scanning is still evolving and has shown some promise in the area of soft tissue sarcomas. PET scans allow us to measure biological activity of tissue quantitatively and to relate it to structure, which is unique to this imaging modality (Fig. 5). Fluorine-18 fluorodeoxyglucose (FDG) is a commonly used radionuclide that mimics glucose uptake by tissues and is actively transported into the cell. Once in the cell, it is phosphorylated and trapped and cannot be used for glycolysis. The radionuclide undergoes positron

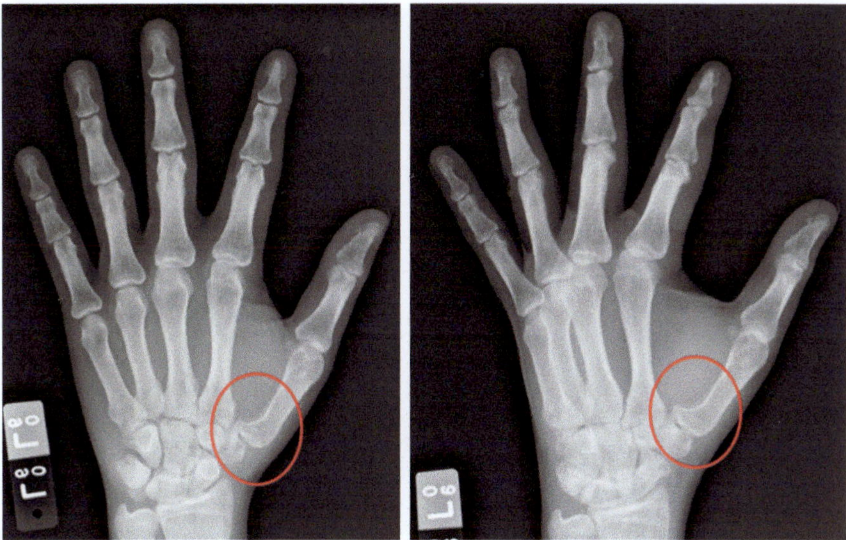

Fig. 2 Patient with a mixed myxoid/round cell liposarcoma of the first intermetacarpal space and scalloping of the base of the first metacarpal

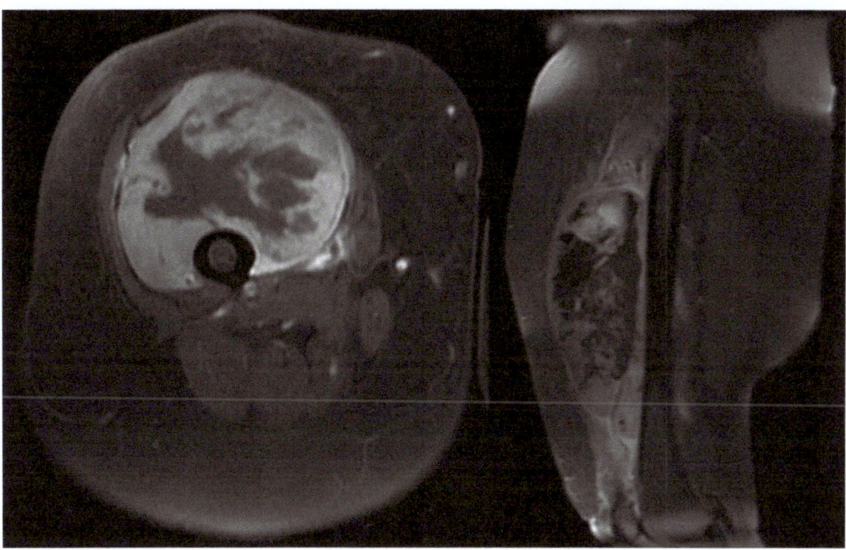

Fig. 3 Post-contrast T1-weighted MRI images of an anterior thigh HGPUS with areas of both viable tumor and necrosis

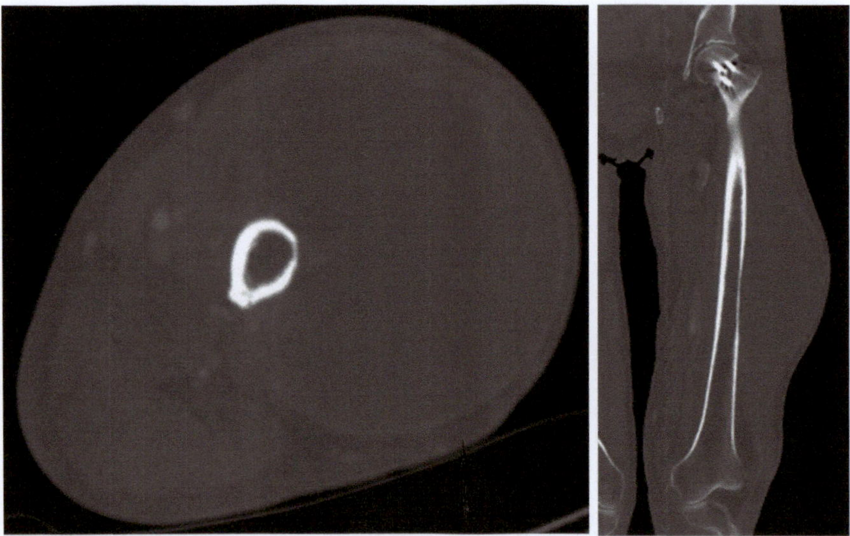

Fig. 4 CT scan of HGPUS of the anterior thigh with bone involvement, cortical thinning, and increased risk of fracture

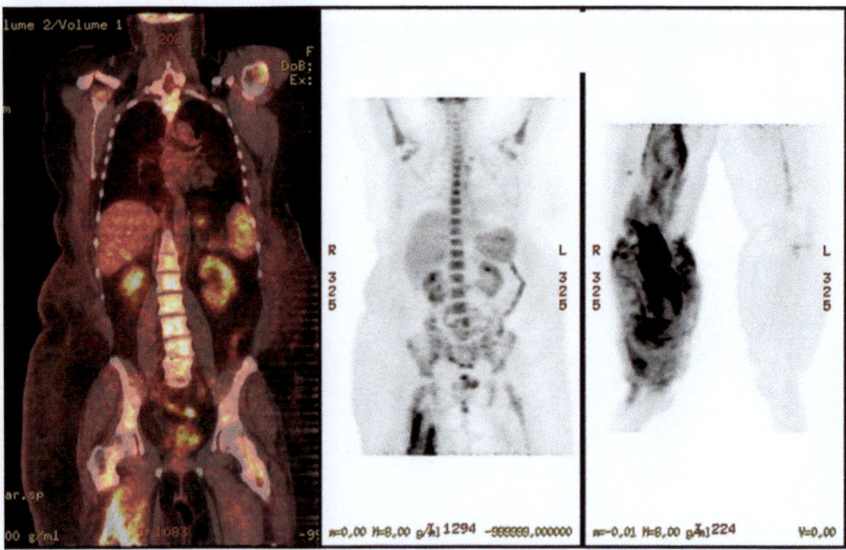

Fig. 5 PET scan from prior clinical photos of angiosarcoma in the setting of chronic lymphedema

decay which collides with electrons to create photons that are registered by the PET scanner. This information is then used to calculate the standardized uptake value (SUV). Studies have shown a significant correlation regarding SUV and both initial sarcoma grade and biological response to preoperative chemotherapy [19, 20]. A recent study has also shown that FDG-PET is useful at accurately detecting local or distant recurrences in patients with a known history of bone or soft tissue sarcoma [21]. The current role of FDG-PET in soft tissue sarcomas is still investigational. It has potential use in identifying unsuspected sites of metastasis in patients with high-grade recurrent tumors at an increased risk for developing metastatic disease.

The evaluation of possible sites of metastasis must be done as well. With soft tissue sarcomas, the majority of metastases go to the lungs and a CT scan of the chest is recommended. A PET scan may also be used to evaluate a pulmonary nodule of questionable significance. Certain histologic subtypes do have a propensity to metastasize to other sites such as the retroperitoneum (myxoid/round cell liposarcomas) and lymph nodes (epithelioid sarcoma, rhabdomyosarcoma, clear cell sarcoma, synovial sarcoma, and angiosarcoma). With these histologic subtypes, a heightened sense of surveillance is needed and further imaging may be warranted.

6   Biopsy

Due to the importance of obtaining an accurate diagnosis, a biopsy is both necessary and appropriate. The biopsy of soft tissue sarcomas, while technically straightforward, is actually a complex procedure requiring significant thought and planning. The biopsy incision or core track should be strategically placed in order to minimize contamination and where it can be completely excised at the time of definitive resection. Poorly executed biopsies and their negative consequences are well documented and have led to diagnostic errors, altered treatment plans, more complex resections, need for adjunctive treatments (chemotherapy and radiation), and unnecessary amputations. It is important for the biopsy to be performed at a sarcoma center where there is multidisciplinary management, and ultimately by the surgeon who will perform the resection [22, 23].

The goal of the biopsy is to obtain an adequate and representative sample in order to establish malignancy, assess histologic grade, and determine the specific histologic type of sarcoma. A treatment plan can then be designed that is tailored to a lesion's predicted pattern of growth, risk of metastasis, and responsiveness to adjuvant and neoadjuvant therapies [2]. When performing a biopsy, the options are a fine-needle aspiration (FNA), a core-needle biopsy, or an incisional biopsy. The open incisional biopsy has long been considered the gold standard. However, most soft tissue masses, especially in the extremities, are usually amenable to a core-needle biopsy. If an open biopsy is performed, longitudinal incisions must be made in line with the planned resection incision. A tourniquet should be used, which should be let down at the conclusion of the biopsy to obtain meticulous hemostasis and prevent a hematoma from contaminating the area.

Core-needle biopsies are minimally invasive, can be done in the outpatient setting under local anesthesia, and unlike FNA it preserves tissue architecture. The diagnostic accuracy of these three modalities has been evaluated over time and as expected the open biopsy has the highest accuracy, with core-needle biopsy being more accurate than FNA. Core-needle biopsies have reported accuracy rates in the literature of 80–91 %, which in all studies is moderately inferior to an open incisional biopsy (94–100 %). However, core-needle biopsy is safe, minimally invasive, and cost effective [24–27].

7   Staging

The staging soft tissue sarcomas compiles all of the gathered information—clinical, radiographic, and histologic—to group patients according to their probability of metastasis, disease-specific survival, or overall survival and prognosis. It also allows for the effective study of treatments and outcomes of patients with similar tumor characteristics and should be practical and reproducible. The major staging system used for soft tissue sarcomas is developed by the American Joint Committee on Cancer (AJCC). The factors thought to carry the most importance are the histologic type, histologic grade, tumor size, depth, regional lymph node involvement, and distant metastasis (Table 1) [28].

Another staging system, which defines prognostically significant progressive stages of risk, is described by Enneking and adopted by the Musculoskeletal Tumor Society. It is a surgical staging system that takes into account the compartmental extent of the tumor and describes three stages: I–low grade; II–high grade; and III–presence of metastases. They are further subdivided by (a) whether the lesion is anatomically confined within well-delineated surgical compartments, or (b) beyond such compartments in ill-defined fascial planes and spaces (Table 2) [30].

The Enneking system goes one step further by defining different types of surgical margins that have predictable local recurrence rates. The surgical margin continues to be the most important prognostic factor for local recurrence. With this system, the goal is to help guide surgical decision making and provide guidelines for the use of adjunctive therapies which could help improve the patient's overall prognosis (Table 3, Fig. 6) [30].

8   Treatment

Surgery remains the mainstay of treatment for soft tissue sarcomas. The extent of surgery required and the use of radiotherapy and chemotherapy as an adjuvant continues to be a topic of controversy and is usually institution dependent. Typically, a treatment plan is designed by a multidisciplinary team with the goal of minimizing local recurrence, maximizing function, and improving patient survival.

Table 1 AJCC soft tissue sarcoma staging criteria [28, 29]

Tumor size				
T1	5 cm or less			
T2	>5 cm			
Location				
a	Superficial			
b	Deep			
Lymph nodes				
N0: no nodal metastases				
N1: nodal metastasis present				
Distant metastases				
M0: no distant metastases				
M1: distant metastases present				
Histologic grade				
G1	Low			
G2	Intermediate			
G3	High			
Group/stage	T	N	M	Histologic grade
IA	T1a	N0	M0	G1
	T1b	N0	M0	G1
IB	T2a	N0	M0	G1
	T2b	N0	M0	G1
IIA	T1a	N0	M0	G2, G3
	T1b	N0	M0	G2, G3
IIB	T2a	N0	M0	G2
	T2b	N0	M0	G2
III	T2a, T2b	N0	M0	G3
IV	Any T	N1	M0	Any G
	Any T	Any N	M1	Any G

A properly executed surgical resection of the tumor is the most important part of the patient's overall treatment. A wide resection, defined above, is clearly desired and results in the highest likelihood of local control. Unfortunately, this is not always possible due to the location and extent of the tumor. It may be in close proximity to critical structures where obtaining an adequate margin would result in a significant functional deficit. In this situation, adjuvant treatments, such as radiotherapy, can be employed to help achieve local control while maintaining functional limb salvage as an option.

Table 2 Enneking/MSTS staging criteria [29, 30]

Tumor grade	
Low grade	1
High grade	2
Location	
Intracompartmental	A
Extracompartmental	B
Stage	Description
IA	Low grade, intracompartmental
IB	Low grade, extracompartmental
IIA	High grade, intracompartmental
IIB	High grade, extracompartmental
III	Metastatic (any grade and location)

Table 3 Surgical margins [30]

Type	Plane of dissection	Result
Intralesional	Piecemeal debulking or curettage	Leaves macroscopic disease
Marginal	Shell out *en bloc* through pseudocapsule or reactive zone	May leave either "satellite" or "skip" lesions
Wide	Intracompartmental *en bloc* with cuff of normal tissue	May leave "skip" lesions
Radical	Extracompartmental *en bloc* entire compartment	No residual

The most extensive resection possible, which is an amputation, is rarely indicated today. Rosenberg et al. published a landmark article in 1982, a prospective randomized trial to evaluate the issue of amputation versus limb-sparing surgery plus radiation therapy in soft tissue sarcomas of the extremity. They found that although local recurrence was greater in the limb-sparing group, disease-free survival was no different [31]. Today, limb-sparing procedures are performed in 90–95 % of cases. However, there are still indications for amputations, and it is usually related to tumor size and involvement of bone and surrounding structures. In the upper extremities, it is best to spare the limb when possible because even a partially functioning hand is better than a prosthesis. In the lower extremities, it has been shown that patients can still function well with resection of the sciatic nerve [32], and patients with peroneal nerve deficits do well with the assistance of an ankle-foot orthotic (AFO). These patients should carefully monitor their feet for minor trauma due the fact that they are insensate and small cuts or sores could ultimately jeopardize the extremity.

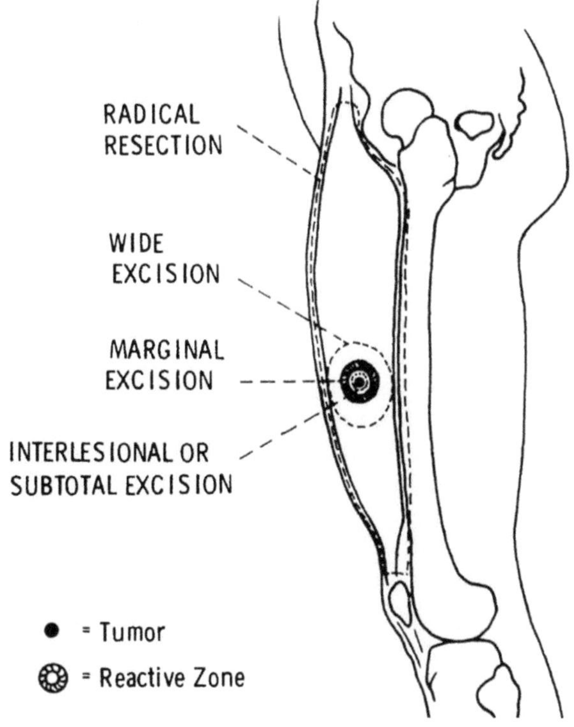

Fig. 6 The various local procedures are shown. The *dotted lines* indicate the plane of dissection and the amount of tissue removed to achieve the various procedures for a theoretical lesion within the anterior compartment of the thigh [30]

The use of surgery alone and withholding radiation therapy to treat soft tissue sarcomas has limited application in carefully selected patients. A study out of the Mayo Clinic that evaluated local control, freedom from distant recurrence, and overall survival in patients treated with limb-conservation surgery alone, found that it is appropriate in the setting of a low-grade tumor resected with negative margins. Of the patients that were analyzed, all local and distant recurrences were found in patients with high-grade tumors [33]. Another study to evaluate this same question found that the only significant risk factor for local recurrence in patients with low-/intermediate-grade tumors less than four centimeters was the size of the closest margin. With this information, surgery alone should be reserved for patients with low-grade tumors which are amenable to complete wide resection who have low risk for local recurrence based on surgical margins, tumor size, and tumor location [34, 35].

The majority of patients require radiation therapy with wide resection for the treatment of their disease. When combined with surgery and negative margins, local control rates have been reported to be 90 % or greater. The goals of radiotherapy in the management of soft tissue sarcomas are to enhance local control, preserve function, and achieve acceptable cosmesis by contributing to tissue preservation [3]. The benefit of radiation is well demonstrated, and whether administered preoperatively or postoperatively, it has been shown to improve the probability of local control and result in cure rates that are comparable to those achieved with more extensive resections [31, 36]. Dagan et al. performed a retrospective review to evaluate the local control and amputation-free survival in patients who received preoperative radiation therapy prior to undergoing a marginal resection for a soft tissue sarcoma of the extremity. The authors concluded that patients can expect excellent rates of local control and limb preservation regardless of whether they have a marginal, wide, or radical resection according to the classic Enneking margin definitions [37].

A standard dose of preoperative radiation therapy involves 50 Gy, delivered over a five-week period. Usually, 3–4 weeks are then required to allow the overlying soft tissues to heal before surgery is attempted. Postoperative radiation doses are higher, usually around 65 Gy and delivered over 6–7 weeks. Usually, 3–6 weeks after surgery is needed to begin treatment to ensure the surgical wound has adequately healed. The effect of radiation is believed to be exerted by sterilizing the tumor capsule and killing microscopic extensions of the tumor. This results in the formation of a fibrous rind or capsule surrounding the tumor which allows the surgeon to spare critical structures in proximity with focally marginal resection planes [29].

The optimal timing of radiotherapy (RT) depends on the clinical situation. Both preoperative and postoperative RT have their advantages and disadvantages. The advantages of preoperative RT are that a lower dose may be used and the irradiated volume is smaller because the treatment volume is well defined. The target is based on anatomic location, and the tumor is contained within undisturbed tissue planes. The likelihood of local control may also be higher. The main disadvantage is that preoperative RT is associated with a higher likelihood of acute wound healing complications. O'Sullivan et al. performed a randomized trial in 2002 to answer this very question and they found that the incidence of wound healing complications was 35 % in the preoperative RT group, compared to 17 % in the postoperative RT group. In this study, they found no significant difference between the two groups regarding rates of local recurrence, metastasis, or progression-free survival. There was a significant difference in overall survival, favoring the preoperative RT group. However, this must be interpreted with caution because the deaths in the postoperative group were not related to progression of the sarcoma alone. Tumor size and anatomic site were also factors that influenced the risk of wound complications [38]. A meta-analysis published in 2010 looking at pre versus postoperative radiation in localized resectable soft tissue sarcomas suggested that the risk of local recurrence may be lower after preoperative radiation, and that a delay in surgical resection to complete preoperative radiation did not increase the risk of metastatic spread [39].

An advantage of postoperative RT is that the entire pathology specimen and final margins are available for analysis. The disadvantage of postoperative RT is that prolonged wound healing from the resection could delay the onset of irradiation. Also, a higher RT dose is sometimes necessary and the irradiated volume is larger because the target is less precisely defined and encompasses all surgically manipulated tissues. This can result in greater late tissue morbidity. These late complications due to the higher doses and higher irradiated volume include joint stiffness, radiation fibrosis, and edema, all of which can lead to decreased function [40]. In addition, increased radiation doses result in higher rates of postradiation fractures [41] and have been correlated with a risk of secondary malignancies. These disadvantages may override the higher frequency of wound complications with preoperative RT.

RT alone can be considered in patients with unresectable disease or medical contraindications to surgery. In this situation, definitive radiation can be used for palliation. The five-year local control rate is 45 %, and overall survival is 35 %. Tumor size had an effect on local control with 51 % five-year local control rates in tumors less than 5 cm, 45 % in tumors 5–10 cm, and 9 % in tumors greater than 10 cm. Patients who received less that 63 Gy had worse outcomes, and those that received greater than 68 Gy had more frequent complications [42].

The ultimate goal of surgery and RT is local control and the use of chemotherapy is to treat systemic disease. Treatment of soft tissue sarcomas with chemotherapy remains controversial and is still investigational. For most patients, chemotherapy is palliative and used to treat unresectable or metastatic disease to try and slow progression. The regimens are highly toxic and have failed to show long-term survival benefits. In 1997, the Sarcoma Meta-Analysis Collaboration published their results of doxorubicin-based chemotherapy regimens combined with surgery for local control. Disease-free survival improved from 45 % for control patients to 55 % for chemotherapy patients, an advantage of only 10 %. The authors were also unable to show a statistically significant benefit to improved survival at 10 years, with survival of patients undergoing chemotherapy at 54 %, compared to the control at 50 % [43].

Another important study that tried to evaluate the benefit of adjuvant chemotherapy for adult soft tissue sarcomas was published in 2001 by the Italian Sarcoma Study Group. They randomized 104 patients with high-grade, deep, extremity tumors greater than 5 cm with no evidence of metastasis to receive no chemotherapy or ifosfamide plus epirubicin. All patients were treated with either pre- or postoperative RT and resection. The trial was stopped early because it had reached its primary end point of improved disease-free survival at both 2 and 4 years. The same cohort was later revisited to update the results at a median follow-up of 89 months and the overall and disease-free survival no longer reached statistical significance [44, 45].

It is important to note that the majority of studies thus far lump all soft tissue sarcomas together, including all of the varying subtypes. This is largely due to the relative rarity of this disease and the difficulty in achieving statistical power to detect small changes in overall survival with small adjuvant chemotherapy trials. There are, however, a few histologic subtypes of soft tissue sarcomas that have a more favorable response to chemotherapy, such as synovial sarcoma, round cell liposarcoma, and pediatric rhabdomyosarcoma. Relative indications include deep high-grade tumors and size greater than 5 cm, especially in younger patients [29]. Although the impact of conventional chemotherapy on soft tissue sarcomas appears to be small, it is important to have a thorough discussion with patients regarding possible options and outcomes.

The treatment of soft tissue sarcomas requires a multidisciplinary approach and the optimal combination of surgery, radiation, and possibly chemotherapy. As previously mentioned, every year approximately 4,000 people die from soft tissue sarcomas in the US and new targeted therapies are needed. The difficulty is identifying the specific alterations that drive sarcomagenesis in such a vast and significantly different group of neoplasms. The use of sequencing technologies to advance our knowledge of mutations, translocations, epigenetic alterations, and aberrant signaling pathways will ultimately help guide treatment with specific sarcoma subtypes. This will enhance the ability to identify and target the critical signaling pathways and proteins driving sarcomagenesis.

9   Surveillance Following Definitive Treatment

After definitive treatment for a primary soft tissue sarcoma, it is important to establish close follow-up for potential development of local recurrence or metastatic disease. 40–60 % of patients will develop local or distant recurrence, and most recurrences occur within 2 years of treatment of the primary tumor [46]. For this reason, early follow-up is more frequent, and eventually spaced out over time. As previously mentioned, pulmonary metastasis is the main concern when treating patients with soft tissue sarcomas. It is the sole site of metastasis 70 % of the time, and the chest should be routinely imaged during the follow-up. Pulmonary metastatic disease carries a poor prognosis with a five-year survival rate of approximately 10 %. This rate can improve significantly with metastectomy, especially in isolated lesions that are amenable to complete resection, and aggressive management of these lesions is usually pursued [47].

Current recommendations for surveillance include a clinical exam and chest radiograph or CT scan every 3 months for the first 2 years, every 4 months for the third year, every 6 months for the following 2 years, and annually thereafter [29, 48, 49]. Local recurrence is monitored with physical exams of the surgical site at routine intervals. If the patient is felt to be at high risk for local recurrence or there is concern on physical exam findings, then an ultrasound or MRI with and without gadolinium should be obtained.

10   Conclusion

Soft tissue sarcomas are a heterogeneous group of rare malignancies that present a unique set of challenges in regard to treatment. It is essential that a treatment plan be devised in a multidisciplinary setting, with input from the surgeon, medical oncologist, radiation oncologist, pathologist, and radiologist. Ideally, the patient should be referred to the sarcoma center prior to any treatment including the biopsy and initial diagnostic evaluation. Today, limb salvage is the standard of care and resection with radiation therapy is most effective at achieving local control. However, the role of chemotherapy in the treatment of sarcomas is not clear and is still evolving. Due to the risk of local recurrence and metastasis, close surveillance following treatment of the primary malignancy is essential.

References

1. Weitz J, Antonescu CR, Brennan MF (2003) Localized extremity soft tissue sarcoma: improved knowledge with unchanged survival over time. J Clin Oncol 21(14):2719–2725
2. Fletcher CDM (2013) World Health Organization., and International Agency for Research on Cancer., WHO classification of tumours of soft tissue and bone, 4th edn. World Health Organization classification of tumours. IARC Press, Lyon, p 468
3. DeVita VT, Hellman S, Rosenberg SA (2005) Cancer, principles and practice of oncology, 7th edn. Philadelphia, Lippincott Williams & Wilkins, lxxv, p 2898
4. Clark MA et al (2005) Soft-tissue sarcomas in adults. N Engl J Med 353(7):701–711
5. Gladdy RA et al (2010) Do radiation-associated soft tissue sarcomas have the same prognosis as sporadic soft tissue sarcomas? J Clin Oncol 28(12):2064–2069
6. Stewart FW, Treves N (1948) Lymphangiosarcoma in postmastectomy lymphedema; a report of six cases in elephantiasis chirurgica. Cancer 1(1):64–81
7. Henze J, Bauer S (2013) Liposarcomas. Hematol Oncol Clin North Am 27(5):939–955
8. Fiore M et al (2007) Myxoid/round cell and pleomorphic liposarcomas: prognostic factors and survival in a series of patients treated at a single institution. Cancer 109(12):2522–2531
9. Folpe AL (2014) Fibrosarcoma: a review and update. Histopathology 64(1):12–25
10. Sanfilippo R et al (2011) Myxofibrosarcoma: prognostic factors and survival in a series of patients treated at a single institution. Ann Surg Oncol 18(3):720–725
11. McArthur GA et al (2005) Molecular and clinical analysis of locally advanced dermatofibrosarcoma protuberans treated with imatinib: Imatinib Target Exploration Consortium Study B2225. J Clin Oncol 23(4):866–873
12. Mendenhall WM, Zlotecki RA, Scarborough MT (2004) Dermatofibrosarcoma protuberans. Cancer 101(11):2503–2508
13. Gladdy RA et al (2013) Predictors of survival and recurrence in primary leiomyosarcoma. Ann Surg Oncol 20(6):1851–1857
14. Mark RJ et al (1996) Angiosarcoma. A report of 67 patients and a review of the literature. Cancer 77(11):2400–2406
15. Ferner RE, Gutmann DH (2002) International consensus statement on malignant peripheral nerve sheath tumors in neurofibromatosis. Cancer Res 62(5):1573–1577
16. Stacchiotti S et al (2011) Sunitinib in advanced alveolar soft part sarcoma: evidence of a direct antitumor effect. Ann Oncol 22(7):1682–1690
17. Guzzetta AA et al (2012) Epithelioid sarcoma: one institution's experience with a rare sarcoma. J Surg Res 177(1):116–122
18. Dim DC, Cooley LD, Miranda RN (2007) Clear cell sarcoma of tendons and aponeuroses: a review. Arch Pathol Lab Med 131(1):152–156
19. Conrad EU 3rd, et al (2004) Fluorodeoxyglucose positron emission tomography scanning: basic principles and imaging of adult soft-tissue sarcomas. J Bone Joint Surg Am 86-A Suppl 2:98–104
20. Evilevitch V et al (2008) Reduction of glucose metabolic activity is more accurate than change in size at predicting histopathologic response to neoadjuvant therapy in high-grade soft-tissue sarcomas. Clin Cancer Res 14(3):715–720
21. Al-Ibraheem A et al (2013) (18) F-fluorodeoxyglucose positron emission tomography/ computed tomography for the detection of recurrent bone and soft tissue sarcoma. Cancer 119(6):1227–1234

22. Simon MA (1982) Biopsy of musculoskeletal tumors. J Bone Joint Surg Am 64(8):1253–1257
23. Mankin HJ, Mankin CJ, Simon MA (1996) The hazards of the biopsy, revisited. Members of the Musculoskeletal Tumor Society. J Bone Joint Surg Am 78(5):656–663
24. Skrzynski MC et al (1996) Diagnostic accuracy and charge-savings of outpatient core needle biopsy compared with open biopsy of musculoskeletal tumors. J Bone Joint Surg Am 78(5):644–649
25. Adams SC et al (2010) Office-based core needle biopsy of bone and soft tissue malignancies: an accurate alternative to open biopsy with infrequent complications. Clin Orthop Relat Res 468(10):2774–2780
26. Pohlig F et al (2012) Percutaneous core needle biopsy versus open biopsy in diagnostics of bone and soft tissue sarcoma: a retrospective study. Eur J Med Res 17:29
27. Kasraeian S et al (2010) A comparison of fine-needle aspiration, core biopsy, and surgical biopsy in the diagnosis of extremity soft tissue masses. Clin Orthop Relat Res 468(11):2992–3002
28. Edge SB (2010) American Joint Committee on Cancer., and American Cancer Society., AJCC cancer staging handbook : from the AJCC cancer staging manual, 7th edn. Springer, New York, xix, p 718
29. Nystrom LM et al (2013) Multidisciplinary management of soft tissue sarcoma. ScientificWorldJournal 2013:852462
30. Enneking WF, Spanier SS, Goodman MA (1980) A system for the surgical staging of musculoskeletal sarcoma. Clin Orthop Relat Res 153:106–120
31. Rosenberg SA et al (1982) The treatment of soft-tissue sarcomas of the extremities: prospective randomized evaluations of (1) limb-sparing surgery plus radiation therapy compared with amputation and (2) the role of adjuvant chemotherapy. Ann Surg 196(3):305–315
32. Bickels J et al (2002) Sciatic nerve resection: is that truly an indication for amputation? Clin Orthop Relat Res 399:201–204
33. Fabrizio PL, Stafford SL, Pritchard DJ (2000) Extremity soft-tissue sarcomas selectively treated with surgery alone. Int J Radiat Oncol Biol Phys 48(1):227–232
34. Baldini EH et al (1999) Long-term outcomes after function-sparing surgery without radiotherapy for soft tissue sarcoma of the extremities and trunk. J Clin Oncol 17(10):3252–3259
35. Yang JC et al (1998) Randomized prospective study of the benefit of adjuvant radiation therapy in the treatment of soft tissue sarcomas of the extremity. J Clin Oncol 16(1):197–203
36. Mendenhall WM et al (2009) The management of adult soft tissue sarcomas. Am J Clin Oncol 32(4):436–442
37. Dagan R et al (2012) The significance of a marginal excision after preoperative radiation therapy for soft tissue sarcoma of the extremity. Cancer 118(12):3199–3207
38. O'Sullivan B et al (2002) Preoperative versus postoperative radiotherapy in soft-tissue sarcoma of the limbs: a randomised trial. Lancet 359(9325):2235–2241
39. Al-Absi E et al (2010) A systematic review and meta-analysis of oncologic outcomes of pre- versus postoperative radiation in localized resectable soft-tissue sarcoma. Ann Surg Oncol 17(5):1367–1374
40. Davis AM et al (2002) Function and health status outcomes in a randomized trial comparing preoperative and postoperative radiotherapy in extremity soft tissue sarcoma. J Clin Oncol 20(22):4472–4477
41. Holt GE et al (2005) Fractures following radiotherapy and limb-salvage surgery for lower extremity soft-tissue sarcomas. A comparison of high-dose and low-dose radiotherapy. J Bone Joint Surg Am 87(2):315–319
42. Tepper JE, Suit HD (1985) Radiation therapy alone for sarcoma of soft tissue. Cancer 56(3):475–479

43. Crowther DA (1997) Adjuvant chemotherapy for localised resectable soft-tissue sarcoma of adults: meta-analysis of individual data. Sarcoma Meta-analysis Collaboration. Lancet 350(9092):1647–1654
44. Frustaci S et al (2001) Adjuvant chemotherapy for adult soft tissue sarcomas of the extremities and girdles: results of the Italian randomized cooperative trial. J Clin Oncol 19(5):1238–1247
45. Frustaci S et al (2003) Ifosfamide in the adjuvant therapy of soft tissue sarcomas. Oncology 65(Suppl 2):80–84
46. Pisters PW et al (1996) Analysis of prognostic factors in 1,041 patients with localized soft tissue sarcomas of the extremities. J Clin Oncol 14(5):1679–1689
47. Kim S et al (2011) Pulmonary resection of metastatic sarcoma: prognostic factors associated with improved outcomes. Ann Thorac Surg 92(5):1780–1786 (discussion 1786–1787)
48. Whooley BP et al (2000) Primary extremity sarcoma: what is the appropriate follow-up? Ann Surg Oncol 7(1):9–14
49. Miller BJ et al (2012) CT scans for pulmonary surveillance may be overused in lower-grade sarcoma. Iowa Orthop J 32:28–34